Boards and Wards

A Review for

USMLE Steps 2 & 3

2nd Edition

Don't miss other books in Blackwell's *Boards and Wards* series!

Boards and Wards
Pathophysiology for the Boards and Wards
Dermatology for the Boards and Wards
Immunology for the Boards and Wards
Microbiology for the Boards and Wards
Behavioral Science for the Boards and Wards
Ophthalmology and Otolaryngology for the Boards and Wards
Pharmacology for the Boards and Wards

Boards and Wards

A Review for

USMLE Steps 2 & 3

2nd Edition

Carlos Ayala, MD
Clinical Fellow in Otology and Laryngology
Harvard Medical School
Resident in Otolaryngology
Harvard Otolaryngology Residency Program
Boston, Massachusetts

Brad Spellberg, MD
Infectious Disease Fellow
Harbor-UCLA Medical Center
Torrance, California

Blackwell
Publishing

© 2003 by Carlos Ayala and Brad Spellberg
Blackwell Publishing

Blackwell Publishing, Inc.,
   350 Main Street, Malden, Massachusetts 02148-5018, USA
Blackwell Publishing Ltd, 9600 Garsington Road, Oxford OX4 2DQ, UK
Blackwell Science Asia Pty Ltd,
   550 Swanston Street, Carlton South, Victoria 3053, Australia
Blackwell Verlag GmbH, Kurfürstendamm 57, 10707 Berlin, Germany

   04 05 06 5 4

ISBN: 1-4051-0341-8

Library of Congress Cataloging-in-Publication Data
Boards and wards : a review for USMLE steps 2&3 / [edited by] Carlos Ayala, Brad Spellberg.—2nd ed.
      p. ; cm.
Includes index.
   ISBN 1-4051-0341-8 (pbk.)
   1. Medicine—Examinations, questions, etc.
   [DNLM: 1. Clinical Medicine—Examination Questions. WB 18.2 B662 2003]   I. Ayala, Carlos, MD.   II. Spellberg, Brad.
R834.5.B63 2003
610'.76—dc21

                                                                                    2002156292

A catalogue record for this title is available from the British Library

Acquisitions: Nancy Anastasi Duffy
Development: Julia Casson
Production: Jennifer Kowalewski
Cover design: Meral Dabcovich
Typesetter: SNP Best-set Typesetter Ltd., Hong Kong
Printed and bound by Edwards Brothers in Michigan

For further information on Blackwell Publishing, visit our website:
www.blackwellmedstudent.com

Notice: The indications and dosages of all drugs in this book have been recommended in the medical literature and conform to the practices of the general community. The medications described do not necessarily have specific approval by the Food and Drug Administration for use in the diseases and dosages for which they are recommended. The package insert for each drug should be consulted for use and dosage as approved by the FDA. Because standards for usage change, it is advisable to keep abreast of revised recommendations, particularly those concerning new drugs.

   Medical knowledge and information is constantly changing. As new research and clinical experience broaden our knowledge, changes in treatment and drug therapy may be required. The authors and editors of the material herein have consulted sources believed to be reliable in their efforts to provide information that is complete and in accord with standards accepted at the time of publication. However, in view of the possibility of human error by the authors, editors or publisher of the work herein, or changes in medical knowledge, neither the authors, editors, publisher, nor any other party who has been involved in the preparation of this work, warrants that the information contained herein is in every respect accurate or complete, and they are not responsible for any errors or omissions or for the results obtained from the use of such information. Readers are encouraged to confirm the information contained herein with other sources.

Figure Credits

Drs. Ayala and Spellberg and Blackwell Science, Inc., wish to thank the following authors for contributing figures to *Boards and Wards*:

- Peter Armstrong, Martin L. Wastie (Figures 1-15, 1-16, 2-15, 2-16, 2-17, 5-1, 7-2, 7-3, 10-1, 10-3 through 10-10, and 10-15 borrowed from *Diagnostic Imaging, 4e,* ©1998 Blackwell Science)
- John Axford (Figures 1-1, 1-8, 1-10 through 1-14, 1-17 through 1-22, 1-24, 1-30, 1-31, 2-3, 2-4, 2-24, 3-5, 3-7, 8-1,10-2, Table 1-42 [adapted], and Plates 1 through 22 borrowed from *Medicine,* ©1996 Blackwell Science)
- Dale Berg (Figures 1-3, 2-16, 9-2, and A-1 borrowed from *Advanced Clinical Skills and Physical Diagnosis,* ©1999 Blackwell Science)
- Geoffrey Chamberlain (Figures 3-10 and 3-11 from *Lecture Notes on Obstetrics, 7e,* ©1996 Blackwell Science)
- Alfred Cuschieri, Thomas P.J. Hennessy, Roger M. Greenhalgh, David I. Rowley, Pierce A. Grace (Figures 2-2, 2-10, 2-19, 2-20 borrowed from *Clinical Surgery,* ©1996 Blackwell Science)
- Harold Ellis, Sir Roy Calne, Christopher Watson (Figures 1-11 and 2-1 borrowed from *Lecture Notes on General Surgery, 9e,* ©1998 Blackwell Science)
- N.C. Hughes-Jones, S.N. Wickramasinghe (Figures 1-29 through 1-32 from *Lecture Notes on Haematology, 6e,* ©1996 Blackwell Science)
- Bruce James, Chris Chew, Anthony Bron (Figures 9-3 through 9-10 and Plates 23 through 30 from *Lecture Notes on Ophthalmology, 8e,* ©1997 Blackwell Science)
- P.R. Patel (Figures 1-6, 1-7, 1-25, 2-6, 2-8, 2-11 through 2-14, 2-21, 2-22, 2-23, 5-2, and 10-11 through 10-14 borrowed from *Lecture Notes on Radiology,* ©1998 Blackwell Science)

Dedication

Dedicated to my wife, Teresa, and to all those who strive to be caring, compassionate physicians.
  Carlos Ayala, MD

I dedicate this book to all those interns manning the front lines of our hospitals, and to all those MS IVs who will soon know their pain.
  Brad Spellberg, MD

Table of Contents

Appendices

Contributors

Carlos Ayala, MD
Clinical Fellow in Otology and Laryngology
Harvard Medical School
Resident in Otolaryngology
Harvard Otolaryngology Residency Program
Boston, Massachusetts

Pedro Cheung, MD
Resident in Family Medicine
Kaiser Permanente
Orange County, California

Eric Daniels, MD
Resident Physician in General Surgery
University of California, Los Angeles School of Medicine
Los Angeles, California

Susan Fisher-Owens, MD, MPH
George Washington University

Michael Gentry, MD
Resident in Radiology
University of California, Los Angeles School of Medicine
Los Angeles, California

Griselda Gutierrez, MD
Resident in Obstetrics and Gynecology
Harbor-UCLA Medical Center
Torrance, California

Charles Lee, MD
Resident in Psychiatry
University of California, San Francisco
San Francisco, California

Danny Liaw, MD, PhD
Clinical Teaching Fellow in Medicine
Harvard Medical School
Resident in Medicine
Beth Israel Deaconess Medical Center
Boston, Massachusetts

Beatriz Mares, MD
Resident in Pediatrics
Oakland Children's Hospital
Oakland, California

Edward C. Miner, MD
Resident in Internal Medicine
Mayo Clinic Foundation
Rochester, Minnesota

Joseph Rosales, MD
Resident in Internal Medicine
Saint Mary's Medical Center
Long Beach, California

Ming-Sing Si, MD
Resident in General Surgery
UC Irvine Medical Center
Irvine, California

Brad Spellberg, MD
Infectious Disease Fellow
Harbor-UCLA Medical Center
Torrance, California

REVIEWERS

Bhushan S. Agharkar, MD
Third year resident, Department of Psychiatry and Behavioral Sciences
Emory School of Medicine
Atlanta, Georgia

Emery Chang, MD
Second year resident, Department of Pediatrics
Tulane School of Medicine
New Orleans, Louisiana

List of Tables

List of Algorithms

Abbreviations Key

↑ (↑↑)	Increases/High (markedly increases/Very high)
↓ (↓↓)	Decreases/Low (markedly decreases/Very low)
→	Causes/Leads to/Analysis shows
1°/2°	Primary/Secondary
BP	Blood pressure
Bx	Biopsy
CA	Carcinoma
CN	Cranial nerve
CNS	Central nervous system
CXR/X-ray	Chest x-ray/X-ray
Dx/DDx	Diagnosis/Differential diagnosis
dz	Disease
HA	Headache
HTN	Hypertension
Hx/FHx	History/Family history
ICP	Intracranial pressure
I&D	Incision and drainage
infxn	Infection
IVIG	Intravenous immunoglobulin
N or Nml	Normal
PE	Physical exam or Pulmonary embolus
pt(s)	Patient(s)
Px	Prognosis
Rx	Prescription/Indicated Drug
Si/Sx/aSx	Sign/Symptom/Asymptomatic
subQ	Subcutaneous
Tx	Treatment/Therapy
Utz	Ultrasound

PREFACE

Scutted-out medical students and exhausted interns have no time to waste studying for the USMLE Steps 2 and 3 exams. That's where we come in. Our book is authored by house staff, like you, training in each of the major fields of medicine tested on the USMLE exams: Internal Medicine, Surgery, Obstetrics-Gynecology, Pediatrics, Family Medicine, Psychiatry, Neurology, Dermatology, and Radiology. However, in contrast to most review texts, we have targeted each chapter toward clinicians *who are not going into that field of medicine*. Thus, Family Medicine is written for surgeons, Obstetrics-Gynecology is written for psychiatrists, Internal Medicine is written for pediatricians, and so on.

None of you surgeons out there wants to spend the five minutes you have before nodding off to sleep "learning" Dermatology for the USMLE Step 2 or 3 exam! Rather, you need a concise review, broad in content but lacking extensive detail, to jar your memory of testable concepts you long ago learned and forgot. Don't waste your precious waking hours poring over voluminous review texts! Remember, sleep when you can sleep. During those few minutes before dozing off in the call room, use a text written by colleagues and designed to help you breeze through subjects you have little interest in and have forgotten most of, but in which you need the most review. Like you, we know and live by the old axiom: study 2 months for the USMLE Step 1 exam, 2 days for the Step 2 exam, and bring a number 2 pencil to the Step 3 exam!

We welcome any feedback you may have about *Boards and Wards*. Please feel free to contact the authors with your comments or suggestions.

> Boards and Wards
> c/o Blackwell Publishing, Inc.
> Commerce Place
> 350 Main Street
> Malden, MA 02148

1. Internal Medicine

Joe Rosales

Carlos Ayala

Brad Spellberg

Cardiology

I. Hypertension (HTN)

Definition = BP ≥ 140/90 measured on 3 separate days

A. Causes

1. 95% of all HTN is idiopathic, called **"essential HTN"**
2. Most of 2° HTN causes can be divided into 3 organ systems & drugs

Table 1-1   Causes of Secondary Hypertension

Cardiovascular	• Aortic regurgitation causes **wide pulse pressure** • Aortic coarctation causes HTN in arms with ↓ **BP in legs**
Renal	• **Glomerular dz commonly presents with proteinuria** • **Renal artery stenosis causes refractory HTN** in older men (atherosclerosis) or young women (fibromuscular dysplasia) • Polycystic kidneys
Endocrine	• Hypersteroidism, typically **Cushing's & Conn's syndromes, which cause HTN with hypokalemia** (↑ aldosterone) • Pheochromocytoma causing episodic autonomic symptoms • Hyperthyroidism causing **isolated systolic HTN**
Drug Induced	• Oral contraceptives, glucocorticoids, phenylephrine, NSAIDs

B. Malignant Hypertension

1. Can be hypertensive urgency or emergency
2. Hypertensive urgency
   a. High BP (e.g., systolic > 200 or diastolic > 110, but numbers vary depending upon source) **without evidence of end-organ damage**
   b. Tx = oral BP medications with goal of slowly reducing BP over several days
3. Hypertensive emergency
   a. Defined as severe HTN with evidence of end-organ compromise (e.g., encephalopathy, renal failure, CHF/ischemia)
   b. Si/Sx = mental status changes, papilledema, focal neurologic findings, anuria, chest pain, or evidence of CHF (e.g., lower extremity edema, elevated JVP, rales on pulmonary exam)
   c. **This is a medical emergency and immediate therapy is needed**
   d. Tx = IV drip with nitroprusside or nitroglycerin (the latter preferred for ischemia), but **do not lower BP by more than ¼ at first or the patient will stroke out**

C. HYPERTENSION TREATMENT

1. Lifestyle modifications first line in pts without comorbid dz
   a. Weight loss, exercise, quitting alcohol & smoking can each significantly lower BP independently—salt restriction may help
   b. ↓ fat intake to ↓ risk of coronary artery dz (CAD); HTN is a cofactor
2. Medications

TABLE 1-2   Medical Treatment of Hypertension

Indications	1) Failure of lifestyle modifications after 6 mo to 1 yr
	2) Immediate use necessary if comorbid organ disease present (e.g., stroke, angina, renal disease)
	3) Immediate use in emergent or urgent hypertensive states (e.g., neurologic impairment, ↑ ICP)
First-line drugs	
No comorbid dz	**Diuretic or β-blocker** (proven to ↓ mortality)
Diabetes	**ACE inhibitors** (proven to ↓ vascular & renal dz)
↓ ejection fraction	**ACE inhibitors** (proven to ↓ mortality)
Myocardial infarction	**β-blocker & ACE inhibitor** (proven to ↓ mortality)
Osteoporosis	**Thiazide diuretics** (↓ Ca^{2+} excretion)
Prostatic hypertrophy	**α-blockers** (treat HTN & BPH concurrently)
Contraindications	
β-blockers	**Chronic obstructive pulmonary dz**, due to bronchospasm
β-blockers (relative)	**Diabetes**, due to alteration in insulin/glucose homeostasis & blockade of autonomic response to hypoglycemia
β-blockers	**Hyperkalemia**, due to risk of ↑ serum K levels
ACE inhibitors	**Pregnancy**, due to teratogenicity
ACE inhibitors	**Renal artery stenosis**, due to precipitation of acute renal failure (GFR dependent on angiotensin-mediated constriction of efferent arteriole)
ACE inhibitors	**Renal failure (creatinine > 1.5)**, due to hyperkalemia morbidity
K⁺ sparing diuretics	**Renal failure (creatinine > 1.5)**, due to hyperkalemia morbidity
Diuretics	**Gout**, due to causation of hyperuricemia
Thiazides	**Diabetes**, due to hyperglycemia

II. Ischemic Heart Disease (Coronary Artery Disease)

A. RISK FACTORS FOR CORONARY ARTERY DISEASE

1. **Major risk factors (memorize these!!!)**
   a. Diabetes (may be the most important)
   b. Smoking
   c. Hypertension
   d. Hypercholesterolemia **(total cholesterol-HDL ratio > 5.0)**
   e. Family history
   f. Age
2. Minor risk factors: obesity, lack of estrogen (males or postmenopausal women not on estrogen replacement), homocystinuria
3. Smoking is the #1 preventable risk factor
4. Diabetes probably imparts the greatest risk of all of them
5. Unlike diabetic microvascular dz (e.g., retinopathy, etc.) **there is no evidence that tight glucose control can diminish onset of CAD**

B. STABLE ANGINA PECTORIS

1. Caused by atherosclerotic CAD, supply of blood to heart < demand
2. Si/Sx = precordial pain radiating to left arm, jaw, back, etc., relieved by rest & nitroglycerin, EKG → **ST depression & T-wave inversion**
3. **Classic Sx often not present in elderly & diabetics (neuropathy)**
4. Dx = clinical, based on Sx, CAD risks, confirm CAD with angiography
5.

TABLE 1-3   Angina Treatment

Acute	Sublingual NTG • Usually acts in 1–2 min • May be taken up to 3 times q3–5 minute intervals • If doesn't relieve pain after 3 doses, pt may be infarcting
Chronic prevention	• Long-acting nitrates effective in prophylaxis • β-blockers ↓ myocardial O_2 consumption in stress/exertion • Aspirin to prevent platelet aggregation in atherosclerotic plaque • Quit smoking! (2 years after quitting, MI risk = nonsmokers) • ↓ LDL levels, ↑ HDL with diet (↓ saturated fat intake more important than actual cholesterol intake), ↑ exercise, ↑ fiber intake, stop smoking, lose weight, HMG-CoA reductase inhibitors • Folate lowers homocysteine levels, but there is controversy over role of ↑ homocysteine in MI, so role of folate Tx is unclear
Endovascular intervention	*Percutaneous Transluminal Coronary Angioplasty (PTCA)* • Indicated with failure of medical management • Morbidity less than surgery but has up to 50% restenosis rate • Stent placement reduces restenosis rate to 20–30% • Platelet gpIIbIIIa antagonists further reduce restenosis rate
Surgery	• Procedure is coronary artery bypass graft (CABG) • Indications = failure of medical Tx, 3 vessel CAD, or 2 vessel dz in diabetes • Comparable mortality rates with PTCA after several years, except in diabetic patients who do better with CABG

C. UNSTABLE ANGINA (USA)

1. Sx similar to stable angina but occur more frequently with less exertion and **may occur at rest**
2. USA is caused by transient clotting of atherosclerotic vessels, clot spontaneously dissolves before infarction occurs
3. EKG during episode usually shows ST depression or flattening of T wave; if ST segment elevation follows, pt is progressing to infarction
4. Labs = cardiac enzymes (CK-MB, troponins) usually negative
5. Tx must be aggressive to prevent infarction, hospitalization is indicated
   a. Immediate IV heparin, with gpIIbIIIa antagonist if labile ST depression on EKG, and aspirin (ASA) to stabilize clotting, pt should continue with ASA after discharge
   b. Nitroglycerin increases O_2 delivery to myocardium
   c. β-blockers decrease myocardial O_2 demand
   d. Once stabilized, pt should undergo evaluation (e.g., exercise stress testing) for risk stratification, usually followed by medical management, PTCA or CABG

D. MYOCARDIAL INFARCT

1. Infarct usually 2° to acute thrombosis in atherosclerotic vessel
2. Si/Sx = crushing substernal pain, as per angina, but not relieved by rest, ⊕ diaphoresis, nausea/vomiting, tachycardia or bradycardia, dyspnea
3. Dx
   a. **EKG → ST elevation & Q waves** (See Figure 1-1)
   b. Enzymes: troponin I or CK-MB—both have similar sensitivities and specificities, but CK-MB normalizes at 72 hrs after infarction, while troponin remains elevated for up to 1 week
   c. Appropriate signs & symptoms with risk factors
4. Tx = reestablish vessel patency
   a. Medical Tx = thrombolysis within 6 hr of the infarct: by using **TPA + heparin** (first line) or streptokinase
   b. PTCA may be more effective, can open vessels mechanically or with local administration of thrombolytics
   c. CABG is longer-term Tx, rarely used for acute process
5. Adjuvant medical therapies
   a. **#1 priority is aspirin! (proven to ↓ mortality)**
   b. **#2 priority is β-blocker (proven to ↓ mortality)**
   c. Statin drugs to lower cholesterol are essential (**LDL must be < 100 postinfarct**, proven to ↓ mortality)
   d. Heparin should be given for 48 hr postinfarct **if tPA was used to lyse the clot** (heparin has no proven benefit if streptokinase was used or if no lysis was performed)
   e. O_2 & morphine for pain control
   f. Nitroglycerin to reduce both pre- & afterloads
   g. ACE inhibitors are excellent late & long-term therapy, ↓ afterload & prevent remodeling
   h. Exercise strengthens heart, develops collateral vessels, ↑ HDL
   i. STOP SMOKING!!!!!!!!!!!!!!!!

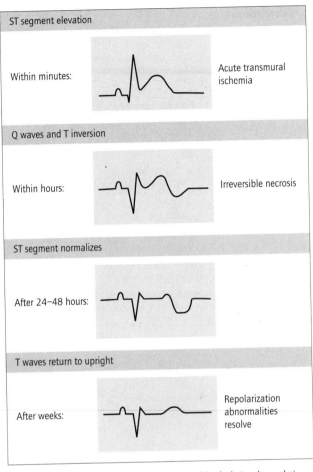

FIGURE 1-1   The changing pattern of the EKG in the affected leads during the evolution of a myocardial infarction.

III. Selected Arrhythmias

A.

TABLE 1-4   Basic Heart Blocks

TYPE	CHARACTERISTICS	PX & TX
1°	• EKG → PR interval > 0.20 seconds • All atrial impulses conducted • May occur in normal individuals due to ↑ vagal tone	Px good, no intervention required
2° Mobitz type I	• Mobitz type I or Wenckebach block • **EKG → PR intervals progressively ↑ from beat to beat** until they become so long the beat is dropped • Following the dropped beat, PR interval resets to baseline & begins to progressively lengthen again • May also occur in normal people or pts taking drugs (e.g., β-blockers, digoxin, Ca-blockers)	Px good, Tx = stop offending drugs if symptomatic
2° Mobitz type II	• Mobitz type II block • **EKG → PR interval fixed at > 0.20 seconds & there is a fixed ratio of dropped beats** • Usually due to block with the His bundle system	Px = poor, ↑ risk progression to 3° Tx = ventricular pacemaker
3°	• Complete heart block • **EKG → absolutely no relationship between P-P intervals & QRS intervals** • Si/Sx = dyspnea, syncope, cannon A waves in jugular veins (See Figure 1-2), wide pulse pressure, may be aSx	Tx = permanent ventricular pacemaker

B. **ATRIAL FIBRILLATION (A-FIB)** (See Table 1-6)
1. Most common chronic arrhythmia
2. Etiologies include ischemia, atrial dilation (often from valve dz), surgery (or any systemic trauma), pulmonary dz, toxicity (e.g., thyrotoxicosis, alcohol intoxication or withdrawal)
3. Pulse is **irregularly irregular, classic descriptor of a-fib**
4. Si/Sx = chest discomfort/palpitations, hypotension/syncope, tachycardia
5. Complications = diffuse embolization, often to brain, of atrial mural thrombi
6. Tx
   a. Rate control with β-blockers, digoxin (not acutely), Ca-blockers (e.g., verapamil & diltiazem)
   b. Convert to normal rhythm (cardioversion) with drugs or electricity
      1) Drug = IV procainamide (first line), sotalol, or amiodarone
      2) Electrical → shocks of 100–200J followed by 360J
      3) All pts with a-fib lasting > 24 hr should be anticoagulated with Coumadin for 3 wk before electrical cardioversion to prevent embolization during cardioversion
   c. If conversion to sinus rhythm does not work, treat with long-term anticoagulation unless pt has a contraindication—Coumadin is 1st line, aspirin second

C. MULTIFOCAL ATRIAL TACHYCARDIA (MFAT)

1. Multiple concurrent pacemakers in the atria, also an irregularly irregular rhythm, usually found in pts with COPD
2. **EKG → tachycardia with ≥ 3 distinct P waves present in 1 rhythm strip** (note: if the pt has ≥ 3 distinct P waves but is not tachycardic, rhythm = wandering pacemaker)
3. Tx = verapamil; also treat underlying condition

D. SUPRAVENTRICULAR TACHYCARDIA (SVT) (See Table 1-6)

1. SVT is a grab-bag of tachyarrhythmias originating "above the ventricle"
2. Pacer can be in atrium or at AV junction, & multiple pacers can be active at any one time (multifocal atrial tachycardia)
3. It can be very difficult to distinguish ventricular tachycardia from SVT if the pt also has a bundle branch block
4. Tx depends on etiology
    a. Correct electrolyte imbalance, ventricular rate control (digoxin, Ca^{2+}-channel blocker, β-blocker, adenosine) & electrical cardioversion in unstable pts
    b. Attempt carotid massage in pts with paroxysmal SVT
    c. Adenosine breaks > 90% of SVT, converting it to sinus rhythm, and failure to break a rhythm with adenosine is a potential diagnostic test to rule out SVT

E. VENTRICULAR TACHYCARDIA (V-TACH) (See Table 1-6)

1. Defined as ≥ 3 consecutive premature ventricular contractions (PVCs)
2. Sustained V-tach lasts minimum of 30 sec, requires immediate intervention due to risk of onset of v-fib (see below)
3. If hypotension or no pulse is coexistent → defibrillate and treat as V-fib
4. Tx depends on symptomatology
    a. If hypotension or no pulse is coexistent → emergency electrical defibrillation, 200–300–360J
    b. If pt is asymptomatic and not hypotensive, first line medical Tx is amiodarone or lidocaine, which can convert rhythm to normal

F. VENTRICULAR FIBRILLATION (V-FIB) (See Table 1-6)

1. Si/Sx = syncope, severe hypotension, sudden death
2. **Emergent electric countershock is the primary therapy** (very rarely precordial chest thump is effective), converts rhythm 95% of the time (200–300–360J) if done quickly enough
3. Second line Tx is amiodarone or lidocaine
4. Without Tx, natural course = total failure of cardiac output → death

TABLE 1-5   Bradyarrhythmias

Complete (Third Degree) AV Block:	
First Degree AV Block:	
Mobitz Type II:	
Mobitz Type I: (Wenckebach Phenomenon)	
Sinus Bradycardia:	
2:1 AV Block:	

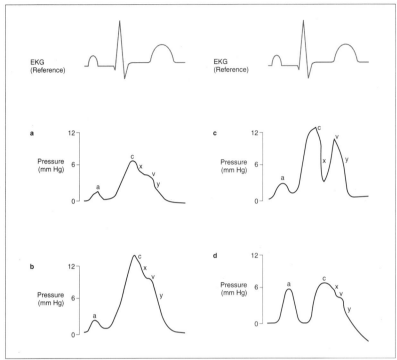

FIGURE 1-2   Jugular venous pressure tracing. (a) Normal: *a* wave, atrial contraction; *c* wave, bulging of tricuspid cusps into the right atrium at the beginning of each systole; *x* descent, relaxation of the right atrium; *v* wave, volume of blood that enters the right atrium during ventricular systole; *y* descent, rapid flow of blood into the right ventricle upon opening of the tricuspid valve. (b) Right ventricular failure: overall increase in jugular venous pulsations and merging of *c* and *v* waves. (c) Tricuspid regurgitation: overall increase in pressure and marked increase in the magnitude of the *x* descent, resulting in separate *c* and *v* waves. (d) Canon *a* waves: marked increase in *a* wave intensity with no increase in jugular venous pulsations (found in AV dissociation).

TABLE 1-6   Tachydysrhythmias

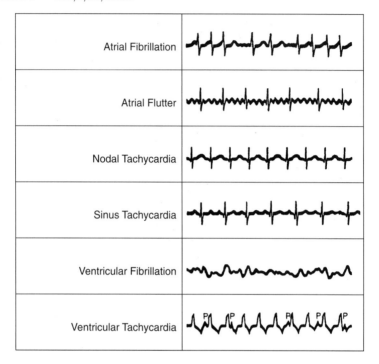

Atrial Fibrillation	
Atrial Flutter	
Nodal Tachycardia	
Sinus Tachycardia	
Ventricular Fibrillation	
Ventricular Tachycardia	

IV. Congestive Heart Failure

A. ETIOLOGIES & DEFINITION
1. Causes = valve dz, MI (acute & chronic), HTN, anemia, pulmonary embolism, cardiomyopathy, thyrotoxicosis, endocarditis
2. Definition = cardiac output insufficient to meet systemic demand, can have right-, left-, or both-sided failure

B. SIGNS & SYMPTOMS & DIAGNOSIS
1. Left-sided failure Si/Sx due to ↓ cardiac output & ↑ cardiac pressures = **exertional dyspnea, orthopnea, paroxysmal nocturnal dyspnea,** cardiomegaly, rales, S3 gallop, renal hypoperfusion → ↑ aldosterone production → Na retention → ↑ total body fluid → worse heart failure
2. Right-sided failure Si/Sx due to blood pooling "upstream" from R-heart = ↑ jugular venous pressure, dependent edema, hepatic congestion with transaminitis, atrial fibrillation, fatigue, weight loss, cyanosis
3. Atrial fibrillation common in CHF, ↑ risk of embolization
4. Dx = echocardiography that reveals ↓ cardiac output

C. TREATMENT
1. 1st line regimen = ACE inhibitor, β-blocker, diuretics (loop and K-sparing), digoxin
2. If pt intolerant of ACE inhibition, use a combination of hydralazine and isosorbide dinitrate

3. **ACE inhibitors proven to ↓ mortality in CHF**
4. β-blockers
   a. **Proven to ↓ mortality**
   b. However, only metoprolol and carvedilol have been reliably shown to do this, and only carvedilol has been shown to do this in class IV (severe) CHF
   c. Furthermore, β-blockers should NEVER be started while the patient is in active failure, as they can definitely worsen failure
   d. Add the β-blockers once the patient is diuresed to dry weight and on stable doses of other medicines
5. **Spironolactone is proven to ↓ mortality in class IV CHF**, and presumed to also ↓ mortality in milder CHF (but not yet proven to)—mechanism not entirely clear for this
6. Loop diuretics (usually furosemide) are almost always used to maintain dry weight in CHF patients
7. Digoxin does not improve mortality in CHF but does improve symptoms and decrease hospitalizations
8. The combination of hydralazine and isosorbide dinitrate is an excellent 2nd-line therapy for patients intolerant of ACE inhibitors because this combination has ALSO been shown to reduce mortality in CHF, but in head to head trials, the mortality benefit is less than ACE inhibitors
9. Beware of giving loop diuretics without spironolactone (a K^+-sparing diuretic), because in the presence of hypokalemia, digoxin can become toxic at formerly therapeutic doses—digoxin toxicity presents as **supraventricular tachycardia with AV block and yellow vision**, and can be acutely treated with anti-digitalis Fab antibodies as well as correction of the underlying potassium deficit

V. Cardiomyopathy

TABLE 1-7   Cardiomyopathy

	DILATED	**HYPERTROPHIC**	**RESTRICTIVE**
Cause	Ischemic, infectious (HIV, Coxsackie virus, Chagas' disease), metabolic, drugs (alcohol, doxorubicin, AZT)	Genetic myosin disorder	Amyloidosis, scleroderma, hemochromatosis, glycogen storage dz, sarcoidosis
Si/Sx	R & L heart failure, a-fib, S3 gallop, mitral regurgitation **Systolic dz**	Exertional syncope, angina, EKG → LVH **Diastolic dz**	Pulmonary HTN, S4 gallop, EKG → ↓ QRS voltage **Diastolic dz**
Px	30% survival at 5 yr	5% annual mortality usually due to sudden death	30% survival at 5 yr
Tx	Stop offending agent, once cardiomyopathy onsets, Tx similar to CHF	• β-blockers & Ca blockers • Surgical excision of myocardium if Sx severe • Dual-chamber pacing with implantable defibrillator	None

VI. Valvular Diseases

A. MITRAL VALVE PROLAPSE (MVP)

1. Seen in 7% of population, in vast majority is a benign finding in young people which is aSx & eventually disappears
2. **Murmur: pathologic prolapse → late systolic murmur with midsystolic click (Barlow's syndrome)**, predisposing to regurgitation
3. Dx = clinical, confirm with echocardiography
4. Tx not required

B. MITRAL VALVE REGURGITATION (MVR)

1. Seen in severe MVP, rheumatic fever, papillary muscle dysfunction (often 2° to MI) & endocarditis
2. Results in dilation of left atrium (LA), ↑ in LA pressure, leading to pulmonary edema/dyspnea
3. See below, Section VIII.A for physical findings
4. Dx = clinical, confirm with echocardiography
5. Tx = ACE inhibitors, vasodilators, diuretics, consider surgery in severe dz

C. MITRAL STENOSIS

1. Almost always due to prior rheumatic fever
2. Decreased flow across the mitral valve leads to left atrial enlargement (LAE) & eventually to right heart failure
3. Si/Sx = dyspnea, orthopnea, hemoptysis, pulmonary edema, a-fib
4. See below, Section VIII.A for physical findings
5. Dx = clinical, confirm with echocardiography
6. Tx
   a. β-blockers to slow HR
   b. Digitalis to slow ventricle in pts with a-fib
   c. Anticoagulants for embolus prophylaxis
   d. Surgical valve replacement for uncontrollable dz
   e. **NEVER give ⊕ inotropic agents for mitral stenosis as are given for other ↓ cardiac output dzs**

D. AORTIC REGURGITATION (AR)

1. Seen in endocarditis, rheumatic fever, VS defect (children), congenital bicuspid aorta, 3° syphilis, aortic dissection, Marfan's syndrome, trauma
2. **There are 3 murmurs in AR** (see below, Section VIII.A)
3. AR has numerous classic signs
   a. **Water-Hammer pulse** = wide pulse pressure presenting with forceful arterial pulse upswing with rapid fall-off
   b. **Traube's sign** = pistol-shot bruit over femoral pulse
   c. **Corrigan's pulse** = unusually large carotid pulsations
   d. **Quincke's sign** = pulsatile blanching & reddening of fingernails upon light pressure
   e. **de Musset's sign** = head bobbing caused by carotid pulsations
   f. **Muller's sign** = pulsatile bobbing of the uvula
   g. **Duroziez's sign** = to-&-fro murmur over femoral artery heard best with mild pressure applied to the artery

4. Dx = clinical, confirm by echocardiography
5. Tx
   a. ↓ afterload with ACE inhibitors or vasodilators (e.g., hydralazine)
   b. Antibiotic prophylaxis prior to procedures (e.g., dental work)
   c. Consider valve replacement if dz is fulminant or refractory to drugs

E. AORTIC STENOSIS (AS)

1. Frequently congenital, also seen in rheumatic fever, mild degenerative calcification = aortic sclerosis that is a normal part of aging
2. Obstructive hypertrophic subaortic stenosis (OHSS)
   a. Also called "hypertrophic obstructive cardiomyopathy"
   b. Ventricular septum hypertrophies inferior to the valve
   c. Stenosis due to septal wall impinging upon anterior leaflet (rarely posterior leaflet) of mitral valve during systole
3. **Si/Sx = classic triad of syncope, angina, exertional dyspnea**
4. Dx = clinical, confirm by echocardiography
5. Tx is surgery for all symptomatic pts who can tolerate it
   a. Either mechanical or bioprosthesis required, pt anticoagulated chronically after surgery
   b. Use balloon valvuloplasty of aortic valve for poor surgical candidates
   c. Tx with digitalis effective only in mild dz
   d. Patients need endocarditis prophylaxis prior to procedures
   e. **NEVER give AS patients β-blockers or afterload reducers (vasodilators & ACE inhibitors)—peripheral vasculature is maximally constricted to maintain BP, so administration of such agents will cause pt to go into shock**

F. TRICUSPID & PULMONARY VALVES

1. Both undergo fibrosis in carcinoid syndrome
2. Endocarditis prophylaxis required prior to procedures (e.g., dental work)
3. Tricuspid stenosis → **diastolic rumble easily confused with mitral stenosis, differentiate from MS by ↑ loud with inspiration** (see below, Section VIII.A)
4. Tricuspid regurgitation → holosystolic murmur (see below, Section VIII.A), look for jugular & hepatic systolic pulsations
5. Pulmonary stenosis → dz of children, or in adults with carcinoid syndrome, with midsystolic ejection murmur
6. Pulmonary regurgitation → develops 2° to pulmonary HTN, endocarditis, or carcinoid syndrome, due to valve ring widening, **Graham Steell murmur** = diastolic murmur at left sternal border, mimicking AR murmur
7. Tx for stenosis = balloon valvuloplasty, valve replacement rarely done

G. ENDOCARDITIS

1. Acute endocarditis is usually caused by *Staphylococcus aureus*
2. Subacute dz (insidious onset, Sx less severe) usually caused by viridans group *Streptococcus* (oral flora), *Streptococcus* spp. and *Enterococcus*
3. Marantic endocarditis is due to cancer seeding of heart valves during metastasis, very poor Px, malignant emboli → cerebral infarcts
4. Culture negative endocarditis is caused by hard-to-culture organisms known as the HACEK group: **H**aemophilus parainfluenzae, **A**ctinobacillus, **C**ardiobacterium, **E**ikenella, **K**ingela kingai

5. SLE causes **Libman-Sacks endocarditis,** may be due to autoantibody damage of valves—usually endocarditis is aSx, but murmur can be heard
6. Si/Sx = splenomegaly, **splinter hemorrhages** in fingernails, **Osler's nodes** (painful red nodules on digits), **Roth spots** (retinal hemorrhages with clear central areas), **Janeway lesions** (dark macules on palms/soles), conjunctival petechiae, brain/kidney/splenic abscesses → focal neuro findings/hematuria/abdominal or shoulder pain
7. Dx based upon the Duke criteria

TABLE 1-8   Duke Criteria for Endocarditis Diagnosis*

Major criteria	1) ⊕ blood cultures (×2) of common organisms
	2) ⊕ echocardiogram or onset of new murmur (transesophageal should be used, as transthoracic only 50–60% sensitive)
Minor criteria	1) Presence of predisposing condition (i.e., valve abnormality)
	2) Fever > 38°C
	3) Embolic disease (e.g., splenic, renal, hepatic, cerebral)
	4) Immunologic phenomena (i.e., Roth spots, Osler's nodes)
	5) ⊕ blood culture ×1 or rare organisms cultured

*80% specific if 2 major or 1 major + 3 minor, or 5 minor criteria are met.

8. Tx = prolonged antibiotics, 4–6 wk typically required (new research indicates sometimes 2 wk can be used for certain organisms)
9. Empiric Tx is often a combination of a β-lactam + aminoglycoside, and therapy is then tailored based upon sensitivities of the organism cultured from blood
10. Surgery required for severe heart disease or large, expanding abscesses

H. RHEUMATIC FEVER/HEART DISEASE

1. Presents usually in 5–15-year-olds after group A Strep infection
2. Dx = Jones criteria (2 major & 1 minor)
3. Major criteria (**mnemonic: J♥NES**)
   a. **J**oints (migratory polyarthritis), responds to NSAIDs
   b. **♥**carditis (pancarditis, Carey-Coombs murmur = middiastolic)
   c. **N**odules (subcutaneous)
   d. **E**rythema marginatum (serpiginous skin rash)
   e. **S**ydenham's chorea (face, tongue, upper-limb chorea)
4. Minor criteria = fever, ↑ ESR, arthralgia, long EKG PR interval
5. In addition to Jones criteria, need evidence of prior strep infection by either culture or ⊕ antistreptolysin O (ASO) antibody titers
6. Tx = penicillin

VII. Pericardial Disease

A. PERICARDIAL FLUID

1. Pericardial effusion can result from any disease causing systemic edema
2. Hemopericardium is blood in the pericardial sac, often 2° to trauma, metastatic cancer, viral/bacterial infections
3. Both can lead to cardiac tamponade
   a. **Classic Beck's triad: distant heart sounds, distended jugular veins, hypotension**
   b. **Look for pulsus paradoxus, which is ≥ 10 mm Hg fall in BP during inspiration**

    c. EKG shows **electrical alternans**, which is beat-to-beat alternating height of QRS complex

  4. Dx = clinical, confirm with echocardiography

  5. Tx = immediate pericardiocentesis in tamponade, otherwise treat the underlying condition & allow the fluid to resorb

B. PERICARDITIS

  1. Caused by bacterial, viral, or fungal infections, also in generalized serositis 2° to rheumatoid arthritis (RA), SLE, scleroderma, uremia

  2. Si/Sx = retrosternal pain relieved when sitting up, often following URI, not affected by activity or food, listen for pleural friction rub

  3. **EKG → ST elevation in all leads**, also see PR depression

  4. Dx = clinical, confirm with echocardiography

  5. Tx = NSAIDs for viral, antimicrobial agents for more severe dz, pericardiectomy reserved for recurrent dz

VIII. Murmurs

A.

TABLE 1-9   Summary of Major Murmurs*

DISEASE	MURMUR	PHYSICAL EXAM
Mitral stenosis	**Diastolic apical rumble** & opening snap	Feel for RV lift 2° to RVH
Mitral valve prolapse	**Late systolic murmur with midsystolic click (Barlow's syndrome)**	Valsalva → click earlier in systole, murmur prolonged
Mitral regurgitation	High-pitched **apical blowing holosystolic murmur radiate to axilla**	Laterally displaced PMI, systolic thrill
Tricuspid stenosis	**Diastolic rumble** often confused with MS	**Murmur louder with inspiration**
Tricuspid regurgitation	High-pitched **blowing holosystolic** murmur at left sternal border	**Jugular & hepatic pulsations, murmur louder with inspiration**
Aortic stenosis (AS)	**Midsystolic crescendo-decrescendo murmur at second right interspace, radiates to carotids & apex, with S_4 due to atrial kick,** systolic ejection click	**Pulsus parvus et tardus =** peripheral pulses are weak & late compared to heart sounds, systolic thrill second interspace
Aortic sclerosis	Peaks earlier in systole than AS	None
Aortic regurgitation	3 murmurs: • **Blowing early diastolic** at aorta & LSB • **Austin Flint = apical diastolic rumble** like mitral stenosis but no opening snap • Midsystolic flow murmur at base	Laterally displaced PMI, **wide pulse pressure, pulsus bisferiens** (double-peaked arterial pulse): see text for classic eponym physical findings
Hypertrophic subaortic stenosis	Systolic murmur at apex & left sternal border that is poorly transmitted to carotids	**Murmur increases with standing & Valsalva**

*The authors thank Dr. J. Michael Criley & Dr. Richard D. Spellberg for assistance with creation of this table.

B.

TABLE 1-10   Physical Exam Differential Diagnosis for Murmurs*

TIMING	POSSIBLE DISEASE: DIFFERENTIATING CHARACTERISTICS		
Midsystolic ("Ejection")	**Aortic stenosis/ sclerosis**: crescendo-decrescendo, second right interspace	**Pulmonic stenosis**: second left interspace, EKG → RVH	Any high flow state → "flow murmur": **aortic regurgitation** (listen for other AR murmurs), **A-S defect** (fixed split S₂), **anemia, pregnancy, adolescence**
Late Systolic	**Aortic stenosis**: worse dz → later peak	**Mitral valve prolapse**: apical murmur	**Hypertrophic subaortic stenosis**: murmur louder with Valsalva
Holosystolic	**Mitral regurgitation**: radiates to axilla	**V-S defect**: diffuse across precordium	**Tricuspid regurgitation**: louder with inspiration
Early Diastolic	**Aortic regurgitation**: blowing aortic murmur		**Pulmonic regurgitation**: Graham Steell murmur
Middiastolic	**Mitral stenosis**: opening snap, no change with inspiration	**Aortic regurgitation** (Austin Flint murmur): apical, resembles MS	**A-S defect**: listen for fixed split S₂, diastolic rumble	**Tricuspid stenosis**: louder with inspiration
Continuous	**Patent ductus**: machinery murmur loudest in back	**Mammary souffle**: harmless, heard in pregnancy due to ↑ flow in mammary artery	**Coarctation of aorta**: upper/lower extremity pulse discrepancy	**A-V fistula**

*The authors thank Dr. J. Michael Criley & Dr. Richard D. Spellberg for assistance with creation of this table.

Pulmonary

I. Hypoxemia

A. DIFFERENTIAL DIAGNOSIS

TABLE 1-11   Five Mechanisms of Hypoxemia

CAUSE	PCO₂	PA-aO₂*	EFFECT OF O₂	DLCO	TX
↓ FIO₂	Nml	Nml	⊕	Nml	O₂
Hypoventilation	↑	Nml	⊕	Nml	O₂
Diffusion impairment	Nml	↑	⊕	↓	O₂
V/Q Mismatch	↑/Nml	↑	⊕	Nml	O₂
Shunt	↑/Nml	↑	—	Nml	Reverse cause

*PAO_2 - PaO_2 gradient (PA-aO_2) ≡ PO_2 in **alveoli** minus PO_2 in **arteries**.
Normal gradient = 10, ↑ by 5–6 per decade above age 50.

$$PAO_2 = FIO_2(P_{breath} - P_{H_2O}) - (PaCO_2/R)$$
At sea level: FIO_2 = .21, P_{H_2O} = 47, P_{breath} = 760: $\mathbf{PAO_2 = 150 - (PaCO_2/R)}$
$PaCO_2$ is measured by lab analysis of arterial blood, R = .8

B. CAUSES

1. Low inspired FIO_2 most often caused by high altitude
2. Hypoventilation
   a. Can be due to hypopnea ($\downarrow$ respiratory rate) or $\downarrow$ vital capacity
   b. Hypopnea causes = CNS dz (e.g., narcotics, trauma, infection, etc.)
   c. $\downarrow$ vital capacity causes = chest wall neuromuscular dz (e.g., amyotrophic lateral sclerosis, kyphoscoliosis, etc.), airflow obstruction (e.g., sleep apnea), or any parenchymal lung dz
3. Diffusion impairment causes = $\uparrow$ diffusion path (fibrosis) or $\downarrow$ blood transit time through lung ($\uparrow$ cardiac output, anemia)
4. V/Q inequality causes = pulmonary embolism, parenchymal lung disease
5. R-L shunt causes = pulmonary edema, pneumonia, atelectasis, atrial & ventricular septal defects, & chronic liver disease

C. PRESENTATION

1. Symptoms = tachycardia (very sensitive; primary compensation for hypoxia is to increase tissue blood flow), dyspnea/tachypnea, feeling of "inability to breathe enough" (dyspnea) usually precedes increase in breaths per minute
2. Si = crackles & rales present in some pulmonary parenchymal disorders, clubbing/cyanosis (not just in lung dz, but can be correlated to long-term hypoxemic states)

D. TREATMENT

1. Requires Tx for hypoxemia along with correction of underlying disorder
2. $\uparrow$ FIO_2 $\rightarrow$ $\uparrow$ PaO_2 & $\uparrow$ hemoglobin O_2 saturation
3. Give O_2 by nasal cannula (NC), face mask, CPAP, intubation, tracheostomy
   a. General rule, 1 L/min O_2 $\uparrow$ FIO_2 by 3% (e.g., giving pt 1 L/min O_2 $\rightarrow$ FIO_2 = 24%)
   b. Nasal cannula cannot administer > 40% FIO_2 even if flow rate is > 7 L/min
   c. Face mask $\uparrow$ maximum FIO_2 to 50–60%, nonrebreather face mask $\uparrow$ maximum FIO_2 to > 60%
   d. CPAP = tightly-fitting face mask connected to generator that creates continuous positive pressure, can $\uparrow$ maximum FIO_2 to 80%
   e. Intubation/tracheostomy $\uparrow$ maximum FIO_2 to 100%
4. **Note that $\uparrow$ FIO_2 will not improve hypoxemia caused by R-L shunt!** (because alveoli are not ventilated & blood will not come in close contact with O_2)
5. Oxygen toxicity seen with FIO_2 > 50–60% for longer than 48 hr, presents with neurologic dz & ARDS-like findings
6. Cannot just rely on O_2 supplementation, must also Tx underlying cause
7. High-altitude hypoxemia is self-limiting & stabilizes in weeks to months

HYPOXEMIA[a]

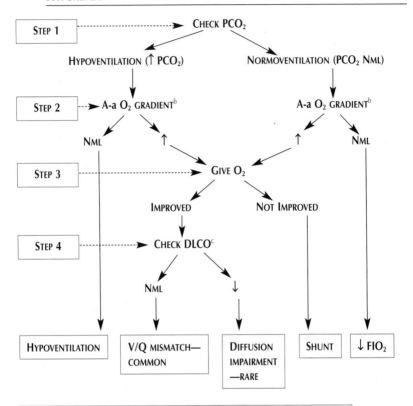

[a] The authors thank Dr. Arian Torbati for his assistance with this algorithm.
[b] A-a O_2 gradient = difference in alveolar and arterial O_2 concentrations.
[c] DLCO = diffusion limited carbon monoxide, a measurement of diffusion capacity.

II. Chronic Obstructive Pulmonary Disease (COPD)

↓ **FEV/FVC** & Nml/↑ TLC
(Forced expiratory volume at 1 min/Forced vital capacity & total lung capacity)

TABLE 1-12 Diagnosis and Treatment of Obstructive Lung Disease

DISEASE	CHARACTERISTICS	TX
Emphysema (Pink puffer)	• **Dilation of air spaces with alveolar wall destruction** • **Smoking is by far the most common cause**, α-1-antitrypsin deficiency causes **panacinar** disease • Si/Sx = hypoxia, hyperventilation, barrel chest, **classic pursed lips breathing**, ↓ breath sounds • CXR → loss of lung markings & **lung hyperinflation** • Dx = clinical	• Ambulatory O_2 including home O_2 • Stop smoking!!! • Bronchodilators • Steroid pulses for acute desaturations
Chronic bronchitis (Blue bloater)	• Defined as **expectoration on most days during ≥3 consecutive months for ≥2 consecutive years** • Si/Sx = as per emphysema but **hypoxia is more severe**, plus pulmonary hypertension with right ventricular hypertrophy, distended neck veins, hepatomegaly • Dx clinical, confirmed by lung biopsy → ↑ Reid index (gland layer is >50% of total bronchial wall thickness)	As per emphysema, use of antibiotics very controversial
Asthma	• Bronchial hyperresponsiveness → **reversible bronchoconstriction** due to smooth muscle contraction • Usually starts in childhood, in which case it often resolves by age 12, can start in adulthood • Acute asthma attacks are the most common cause of pediatric ER visits • Si/Sx = episodic dyspnea & **expiratory wheezing, reversible with bronchodilation** • Dx = ≥ 10% ↑ in FEV with bronchodilator therapy • Status asthmaticus (refractory attack lasting for days, can cause death) is a major complication	• Albuterol/atrovent inhalers are mainstay • Add inhaled steroids for improved long-term control • Pulse with steroids for acute attacks • Intubate as needed to protect airway
Bronchiectasis	• Permanent abnormal dilation of bronchioles commonly due to cystic fibrosis, chronic infxn (often tuberculosis, fungal infxn, or lung abscess), or obstruction (e.g., tumor) • Si/Sx = foul breath, purulent sputum, hemoptysis, CXR → **tram-track lung markings**, CT → thickened bronchial walls with dilated airways • Dx = clinical with radiologic support	• Ambulatory O_2 • Aggressive antibiotic use for frequent infections • Consider lung transplant for long-term cure

III. Restrictive Lung Disease

Nml/↑ FEV/FVC & ↓ TLC

TABLE 1-13   Diagnosis and Treatment of Restrictive Lung Disease

DISEASE	CHARACTERISTICS	TX
↓ Lung tissue	• Causes = atelectasis, airway obstruction (tumor, foreign body), surgical excision	• Ambulate pt • Incentive spirometer to encourage lung expansion • Remove foreign body/tumor
Parenchymal disease	• Causes = inflammatory (e.g., vasculitis & sarcoidosis), idiopathic pulmonary fibrosis, chemotherapy (the **B's**, **b**usulfan & **b**leomycin), amiodarone, radiation, chronic infections (TB, fungal), & toxic inhalation (e.g., asbestos & silica) • Dx = clinical, biopsy to rule out infection	• Antibiotics for chronic infection • Steroids for vasculitis, sarcoidosis, & toxic inhalations
Interstitial fibrosis	• Chronic injury caused by asbestos, oxygen toxicity, organic dusts, chronic infection (e.g., TB, fungi, CMV, idiopathic pulmonary fibrosis & collagen-vascular dz) • **CXR → "honeycomb" lung**	• Ambulatory O_2 • Steroids for collagen-vascular dz • Add PEEP to reduce FIO_2 for O_2 toxicity
Extrapulmonary disease	• Neuromuscular dz (e.g., multiple sclerosis, kyphoscoliosis, amyotrophic lateral sclerosis, Guillain-Barré, spinal cord trauma) • ↑ diaphragm pressure (e.g., pregnancy, obesity, ascites)	Supportive

Pleural effusion	• ↑ fluid in the pleural space, transudative or exudative
	• Transudate
	  ◊ **Low protein content** due to ↓ oncotic pressure
	  ◊ causes = CHF, nephrotic syndrome, hepatic cirrhosis
	• Exudate
	  ◊ High protein content due to ↑ hydrostatic pressure
	  ◊ Causes = malignancy, pneumonia ("parapneumonic effusion"), collagen-vascular dz, pulmonary embolism
		Thoracentesis (see below)

TABLE 1-14   Lab Analysis of Pleural Effusions

STUDY	TRANSUDATE	EXUDATE
Effusion protein	≤3.0 g/dL (≤0.5 of serum)	>3.0 g/dL* (>0.5 of serum)
Effusion LDH	≤200 IU/L (≤0.6 of serum)	>200 IU/L* (>0.6 of serum)
Specific gravity	≤1.015	>1.015
pH	≥7.2	<7.2 → parapneumonic effusion
Gram's stain	No organisms	ANY organism → parapneumonic
Cell count	WBC ≤1000	WBC >1000 (lymphocytes → TB)
Glucose	≥50 mg/dL	<50 mg/dL → infxn, neoplasm, collagen-vascular dz (≤10 → RA)
Amylase	↑ in pancreatitis, esophageal rupture, malignancy	
RF	Titer > 1:320 → virtually pathognomonic for RA (pH often <7.2)	
ANA	Titer > 1:160 → highly indicative for SLE (pH often >7.4)	

*Either of these findings rules out transudative effusion, rules in exudative effusion.

IV. Pulmonary Vascular Disease

A. PULMONARY EDEMA & ACUTE RESPIRATORY DISTRESS SYNDROME (ARDS) (See Figure 1-3)
   1. Si/Sx = dyspnea, tachypnea, resistant hypoxia, diffuse alveolar infiltrate
   2. Differential for pulmonary edema
      a. **If pulmonary capillary wedge pressure < 12 = ARDS**
      b. **If pulmonary capillary wedge pressure > 15 = cardiogenic**
   3. Tx = O_2, diuretics, positive end-expiratory pressure (PEEP) ventilation
   4. Purpose of PEEP
      a. Helps prevent airway collapse in a failing lung
      b. ↑ functional residual capacity (maintain lung volume) & ↓ shunting
      c. Expands alveoli for better diffusion

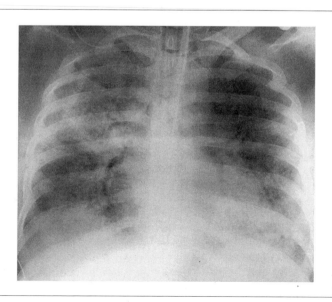

FIGURE 1-3   Adult respiratory distress syndrome (ARDS). There is widespread consolidation of the lungs. This patient had suffered extensive trauma to the limbs.

B. PULMONARY EMBOLISM (PE)

    1. 95% of emboli are from leg deep venous thrombi (DVT)

    2. Si/Sx = swollen, painful leg, sudden dyspnea/tachypnea, tachycardia, hemoptysis—
are often no Sx at all, most emboli are clinically silent

    3. Risk factors = **Virchow's triad = endothelial cell trauma, stasis, hypercoagulable
states** (nephrosis, DIC, tumor, postpartum amniotic fluid exposure, antithrombin III
deficiency, protein C or S deficiency, factor V Leiden deficiency, oral contraceptives,
smoking)

    4. PE can cause lung infarctions

        a. 75% occur in lower lobes

        b. **Classic CXR finding is "Hampton's hump,"** a wedge-shaped opacification at
distal edges of lung fields

    5. EKG findings

        a. Classically (but rarely) → S wave in I, Q in III, inverted T III ($S_I Q_{III} T_{III}$)

        b. **Most common finding is simply sinus tachycardia**

    6. Dx = leg Utz to check for DVT, **spiral CT of chest & V/Q scan best to rule out PE,** &
pulmonary angiography (gold standard)

    7. Tx = prevention with heparin, IVC filter, or Coumadin, use tPA thrombolysis in
massive PE or hemodynamic compromise

C. PULMONARY HYPERTENSION

    1. Defined as pulmonary pressure ≥ $\frac{1}{4}$ systemic (should be 1/8)

    2. Can be active (1° pulmonary dz) or passive (2° to heart dz)

        a. 1° dz includes idiopathic pulmonary HTN (rare, occurs in young women), COPD
& interstitial restrictive diseases

        b. 2° dz seen in any heart disease, **commonly seen in HIV**

    3. Si/Sx: loud S_2, tricuspid regurgitation, audible crackles, ↓ breath sounds, pulsatile
liver, EKG → right atrial enlargement, CXR → large hilar shadow

    4. Dx = clinical, confirm with heart catheterization

    5. Tx = home O_2 and try prostaglandins

V. Respiratory Tract Cancers

A. EPIDEMIOLOGY

    1. **#1 cause of cancer deaths & second most frequent cancers**

    2. Can only be seen on x-rays if > 1 cm in size, by that time they have usually already
metastasized, **so x-rays not a good screening tool**

    3. Si/Sx = cough, hemoptysis, hoarseness (recurrent laryngeal nerve paralysis), weight
loss, fatigue, recurrent pneumonia

B. PARENCHYMAL LUNG CANCERS

    1. Diseases & characteristics

TABLE 1-15   Parenchymal Lung Cancers

CANCER	CHARACTERISTICS
Adenocarcinoma	• Most frequent lung CA in nonsmokers • Presents in subpleura & lung periphery • Presents in preexisting scars, "scar cancer" • Carcinoembryonic antigen (CEA) ⊕, used to follow Tx, not for screening due to ↓ specificity
Bronchoalveolar carcinoma	• Subtype of adenocarcinoma **not related to smoking** • **Presents in lung periphery**
Large cell carcinoma	• **Presents in lung periphery** • Highly anaplastic, undifferentiated cancer • Poor prognosis
Squamous cell carcinoma	• **Central hilar masses arising from bronchus** • **Strong link to smoking**
Bronchogenic carcinoma	• **Causes hypercalcemia due to secretion of PTHrp** (parathyroid hormone related peptide)
Small cell (Oat cell) carcinoma	• **Usually has central hilar location** • **Often already metastatic at Dx, very poor Px** • **Strong link to smoking (99% are smokers)** • Causes numerous endocrine syndromes ◊ ACTH secretion (cushingoid) ◊ Secretes ADH, causing SIADH
Bronchial carcinoid tumors	• Carcinoid syndrome = serotonin (5-HT) secretion • **Si/Sx = recurrent diarrhea, skin flushing, asthmatic wheezing & carcinoid heart dz** • Dx by ↑ 5-HIAA metabolite in urine • Tx = methysergide, a 5-HT antagonist
Lymphangio-leiomyomatosis	• Neoplasm of lung smooth muscle → cystic obstructions of bronchioles, vessels & lymph • **Almost always seen in menstruating women** • Classic presentation = **pneumothorax** • Tx = progesterone or lung transplant

2. Tx differs from small cell vs. non-small cell lung CA
   a. Small cell → radiation & chemotherapy
   b. Non-small cell CA
      1) Local disease → lung resection +/– radiation
      2) Metastatic disease → radiation + chemotherapy

C. OTHER CANCER SYNDROMES
   1. **Superior sulcus tumor (Pancoast tumor)** (See Figure 1-4)
      a. **Horner's syndrome** (ptosis, miosis, anhydrosis) by damaging the sympathetic cervical ganglion in the lower neck
      b. **Superior vena cava syndrome** = obstructed SVC → facial swelling, cyanosis, & dilation of veins of head & neck
   2. Small cell carcinoma can cause a **myasthenia gravis-like condition known as the Lambert-Eaton syndrome** due to induction of Abs to tumor that cross-reacts with presynaptic Ca channel
   3. Renal cell CA metastatic to lung can cause 2° polycythemia by ectopic production of erythropoietin

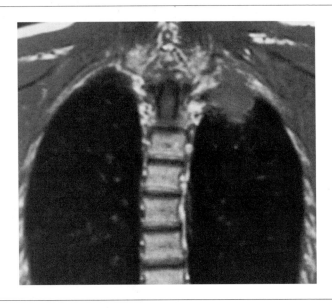

FIGURE 1-4   Pancoast tumor. This carcinoma of the lung can be seen invading the root of the neck on this coronal MRI scan (T1-weighted).

VI. Mediastinal Tumors

TABLE 1-16   Mediastinal Tumors (See Figure 1-5)

ANTERIOR[a]	MIDDLE	POSTERIOR[b]
Thymoma	Lymphoma	Neuroblastoma
Thyroid tumor	Pericardial cyst	Schwannoma
Teratoma	Bronchial cyst	Neurofibroma
Terrible lymphoma		
Tx = excision for all, add radiation/chemotherapy as needed		

[a] The four T's.
[b] Neural tumors.

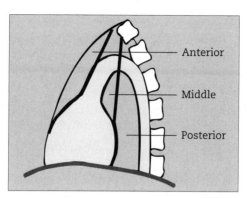

FIGURE 1-5   Mediastinal compartments.

VII. Tuberculosis (See Figure 1-6)

A. PRIMARY TB
1. Classically affects lower lobes (bacilli deposited in dependent portion of lung during inspiration)
2. Usually asymptomatic
3. **Classic radiologic finding is "Ghon complex"** = calcified nodule at primary focus ⊕ calcified hilar lymph nodes

B. SECONDARY (REACTIVATION) TB
1. Reactivates in **apical lung** due to ↑ oxygen tension in upper lobes
2. Si/Sx = insidious fevers, night sweats, weight loss, cough, hemoptysis, upper lobe infiltration or scarring on CXR
3. Risk factors = HIV, imprisonment, homelessness, malnourishment

C. MILIARY (DISSEMINATED) TB
1. Hematogenous **dissemination involving any organ**, often the liver, spleen, bone, kidneys, pericardium, spine, meninges
2. Presents in any patient with immune deficiency
3. Classic syndromes
   a. Pott's dz = TB of spine, presents with multiple compression fractures
   b. Scrofula = TB causing massive cervical lymphadenopathy
   c. Gastroenteritis with profuse diarrhea & colitis

D. DIAGNOSIS & TREATMENT
1. Latent infection (new terminology and guidelines as of 2000)
   a. Latent infection is defined by positive PPD status with no Si/Sx of active disease and no active disease on CXR
   b. PPD test is a **screening test for latent infection**, it is **NOT** a diagnostic test for active tuberculosis
   c. Guidelines for interpretation of PPD
      1) ≥ 5 mm induration is a positive test for latent infection if the patient:
         a) has HIV
         b) has been in close contact with someone with active TB
         c) has fibrotic changes on CXR consistent with old TB

        d) is taking immunosuppressive medicines (e.g., > 15 mg/d of prednisone for > 1 mo, cyclosporin, etc.)

     2) ≥ 10 mm induration is a positive test for a latent infection if the patient:

        a) is a recent immigrant from a high-risk country (most developing countries)

        b) is an injection drug user

        c) works or resides in a prison/jail, nursing home, health care facility (that's you and us!), or a homeless shelter

        d) has a chronic debilitating illness such as renal failure, cancer, or diabetes mellitus

     3) ≥ 15 mm induration is a positive test for latent infection if the patient does not meet any of the above categories

    d. Treatment of latent infection (formerly known as "prophylaxis") is isoniazid × 9 mos (alternate regimens should only be given by specialists)

2. Active infection

    a. To reiterate a point made above: **PPD is not intended as a diagnostic test for active TB**—it is commonly falsely negative in pts with active dz, and a positive test only indicates latent infection, not active disease, thus it is neither sensitive nor specific for active disease

    b. Active infection is diagnosed based on 3 components: clinical assessment, CXR, and sputum (or other body fluid if miliary disease is considered)

     1) Clinical indicators of active dz include subacute/chronic cough, night sweats, weight loss, hemoptysis, etc.

     2) CXR indicators of active dz include upper lobe infiltrates or scarring, and cavitary lesions in a patient with symptoms

     3) Sputum for acid fast staining is the diagnostic study of choice

    c. Treatment

     1) Start regimen with 4 drugs: isoniazid, rifampin, ethambutol, pyrizinamide

     2) Narrow regimen based on sensitivities of culture organism

     3) If culture negative, narrow to 2 drugs at 2 months (isoniazid & rifampin)

     4) Treat for a minimum of 6 months

     5) Treatment should be given by specialists in TB care

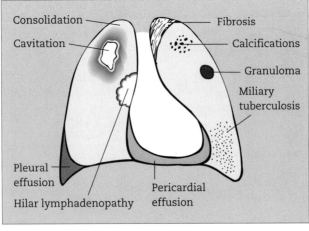

FIGURE 1-6   Manifestations of pulmonary tuberculosis.

VIII. Pneumonia

TABLE 1-17   Pneumonia

ORGANISM	CHARACTERISTICS	TX
Typical Bacterial Pneumonia		
Streptococcus pneumoniae	Children, elderly, immunosuppressed pts, ↑ frequency in asplenic and AIDS, presents with acute onset cough with shaking rigors, can rapidly progress, #1 cause of CAP[a] (70%)	Ceftriaxone, macrolide, or fluoroquinolone (resistance to all increasing)
Haemophilus	*H. influenzae* causes 10% CAP[a], same patients as *S. pneumoniae*	Ceftriaxone, macrolide, or fluoroquinolone (resistance to all increasing)
Moraxella catarrhalis	Causes 5% CAP[a], common in COPD & immunosuppressed	Ceftriaxone, macrolide, or fluoroquinolone (resistance to all increasing)
Staphylococcus aureus	2° infects after influenza virus, commonly → pleural effusion	Oxacillin[b]
Gram-negative rods	Often nosocomial infections	3rd generation cephalosporin or fluoroquinolone
Pseudomonas	Often in cystic fibrosis, commonly nosocomial, cavitates, rapid antibiotic resistance (use 2 antibiotics!)	3rd generation cephalosporin or fluoroquinolone
Klebsiella	Seen in alcoholics, diabetics, nosocomial, classically sputum is "currant jelly" bloody red, antibiotic resistant	3rd generation cephalosporin or fluoroquinolone
Anaerobes	Aspiration pneumonia seen in loss of consciousness, dementia, alcoholic → abscess, foul sputum, dz in dependent lung lobes	Metronidazole/clindamycin
Atypical Pneumonia		
Mycoplasma pneumoniae	Classically young adults (college), causes 10% of CAP*, after 2–4 wk incubation → tracheobronchitis & nocturnal cough	Doxycycline, macrolide, or quinolone
Legionella pneumophila	Seen in alcoholic, transplant pts, COPD, malignancy, diabetes, water exposure (e.g., air conditioner): 25% lethal with Tx, classic Si/Sx = hyponatremia, CNS changes, LDH > 700, diarrhea	Doxycycline, macrolide, or quinolone
Chlamydia pneumoniae	Seen in elderly pts, Sx = sore throat, hoarse voice, sinusitis	Doxycycline, macrolide, or quinolone
Chlamydia psittaci	Contracted from birds (often parrots), bird may show signs of illness also (e.g., ruffled feathers)	Doxycycline, macrolide, or quinolone
Coxiella burnetii	Called "Q-fever," contracted from farm animals (e.g., cattle, goats), inhalation or ingestion of milk, etc.	Doxycycline, macrolide, or quinolone
Francisella tularensis	Found in hunters, butchers, etc., classically contracted from rabbits, but other animals & ticks as well	Streptomycin
Actinomyces israelii	50% → empyema, crosses tissue planes (e.g., pericardium, spine), look for sinus tract drainage through anterior chest wall	Penicillin (6–12 mo)
Nocardia asteroides	Gram-positive acid fast aerobe, mimics TB, Si/Sx = fever, night sweats, **eosinophilia**, seen in AIDS as opportunistic infection	Bactrim
Fungal Pneumonia		
Pneumocystis carinii	Insidious onset of dry cough/dyspnea, bilateral infiltrates, not pleural effusions (very rare), Dx → sputum silver stain, ↑ LDH: AIDS pts with CD4 <200 get prophylaxis with Bactrim (See Figure 1-7)	Bactrim
Coccidioides immitis	"San Joaquin Valley Fever," major risks = travel to SW desert (e.g., California, Arizona, New Mexico, Texas), imprisonment, ↑ incidence after earthquakes, Filipinos & blacks have ↑ rate disseminated dz, Dx best by sputum cytology → budding yeast	Amphotericin (ampB) or fluconazole (flucon)

TABLE 1-17 *Continued*

ORGANISM	CHARACTERISTICS	Tx
Histoplasma	Exposure to Ohio/Mississippi River valleys, bat or bird dung	AmpB/flucon
Aspergillus	Seen in neutropenic pts, CXR → "fungus-ball" with cavitation	AmpB/itracon[c]
Cryptococcus	Seen in AIDS patients or any immunosuppressed	AmpB/flucon
	Viral Pneumonia	
Influenza	Presents in patients >65 yr, can be deadly in them	Amantadine/oseltamivir/ zanamivir
Hantavirus	Children/young adults exposed to SW desert rodents, 50% fatal with Tx, 3–6 day prodromal fever & myalgias → acute ARDS	Supportive (intubation)
Other	RSV, adenovirus, parainfluenza, less severe than influenza	Supportive

[a] CAP = community-acquired pneumonia.
[b] Vancomycin if resistant to oxacillin.
[c] Itracon = itraconazole.

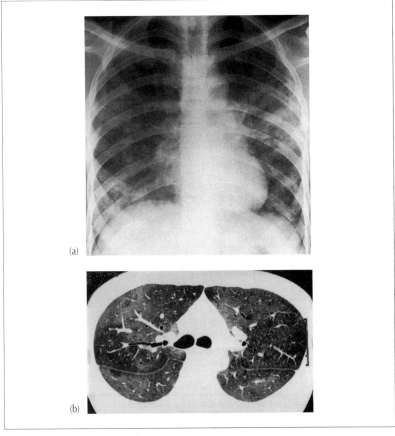

(a)

(b)

FIGURE 1-7 *Pneumocystis carinii* pneumonia in a patient with AIDS showing (a) typical widespread low-density air space shadowing on chest x-ray; (b) high-resolution CT in another patient with similar but less advanced changes.

Gastroenterology and Hepatology

I. Gastroesophageal Disease

A. CHRONIC (NONEROSIVE) GASTRITIS (ATROPHIC GASTRITIS)

1. Type A (fundal) = autoimmune (pernicious anemia, thyroiditis, etc.)
2. Type B (antral) due to *Helicobacter pylori* (*H.p.*), NSAIDs, herpes, CMV
3. NSAIDs are #1 cause of chronic gastritis (in antrum, not fundus)
4. Si/Sx = usually aSx, may cause pain, nausea/vomiting, anorexia, upper GI bleeding manifested as coffee grounds emesis or hematemesis
5. Dx = upper endoscopy
6. *H.p.* infxn Dx by urease breath test, can screen with serum IgG test (less expensive but less sensitive & does not indicate **active** infection), can confirm with endoscopic Bx
7. Tx depends on etiology
   a. Tx *H.p.* gastritis with proton pump inhibitor +2 antibiotics (tetracycline + clarithromycin or metronidazole) + bismuth compound
   b. If drug induced, stop offending agent (usually NSAIDs), add sucralfate, H2 blocker, or proton pump inhibitor
   c. Pernicious anemia Tx = vitamin B_{12} replenishment
   d. Stress ulcer (especially in ICU setting), Tx with sucralfate or H2 blocker IV infusion

B. GASTRIC ULCERS (GU)

1. *H.p.* found in 70% of GU, 10% caused by ulcerating malignancy
2. **As opposed to duodenal ulcers, GUs are NOT caused by acid hypersecretion—** patients with GU have low-to-normal acid secretion, may have ↓ mucosal protection from acid
3. Si/Sx = gnawing/burning pain in midepigastrium, **worse with food intake**, if ulcer erodes into artery can cause hemorrhage & peritonitis, may be guaiac positive
4. Dx = endoscopy with Bx to confirm not malignant, *H.p.* testing as above
5. Tx = mucosal protectors (e.g., bismuth, sucralfate, misoprostol), H2 blockers or proton pump inhibitors & antibiotics for *H.p.*

II. Small Intestine

A. DUODENAL ULCER (DU)

1. Almost all DU pts have ↑ acid production, 80% have ↑ nocturnal secretion
2. *H.p.* found in 90% of duodenal ulcers
3. Smoking & excessive alcohol intake ↑ risk for peptic ulcer
4. Sx/Si = burning or gnawing epigastric pain 1–3 hr postprandial, **relieved by food/antacids**, pain typically awakens patient at night, melena
5. Dx = endoscopy, barium swallow if endoscopy unavailable
6. Tx = as for GU above, quit smoking
7. Sequelae
   a. Upper GI bleed
      1) Usually see hematemesis, melena, or (rarely) hematochezia if briskly bleeding ulcer

    2) Dx with endoscopy

    3) Tx = endoscopic coagulation or sclerosant, surgery rarely necessary

  b. Perforation

    1) Change in pain pattern is suspicious for perforation

    2) Plain abd films may show free air, can perform UGI series with water-soluble contrast (barium contraindicated)

    3) Tx is emergency surgery

B. CROHN'S DISEASE (INFLAMMATORY BOWEL DISEASE)

1. A GI inflammatory disease that may be <u>infectious</u> in nature
2. Affects any part of GI from mouth to <u>rectum</u>, but usually the intestines
3. Si/Sx = abdominal pain, diarrhea, malabsorption, fever, stricture causing obstruction, fistulae, see below for extraintestinal manifestations
4. Dx = colonoscopy with biopsy of affected areas → transmural, **noncaseating granulomas, cobblestone mucosal morphology, skip lesions, creeping fat on gross dissection is pathognomonic**
5. Tx
  a. Sulfasalazine (5-ASA), better for colonic dz but also helps in small bowel
  b. Steroids for acute exacerbation, but no effect on underlying dz
  c. Immunotherapy (azathioprine & mercaptopurine) – useful in pts with unresponsive dz
  d. Newest Tx is anti-tumor necrosis factor (TNF) antibody, infliximab

C. CARCINOID SYNDROME

1. APUDoma (**a**mine **p**recursor **u**ptake & **d**ecarboxylate)
2. Occurs most frequently in the appendix
3. Carcinoid results from liver mets that secrete serotonin (5-HT)
4. Si/Sx = flushing, watery diarrhea & abdominal cramps, bronchospasm, right-sided heart valve lesions
5. Dx = ↑ levels of urine 5-HIAA (false ⊕ seen if eat lots of bananas)
6. Tx = somatostatin & methysergide

III. Large Intestine

A. ULCERATIVE COLITIS (UC) (INFLAMMATORY BOWEL DISEASE)

1. An idiopathic <u>autoinflamm</u>atory disorder of the colon
2. Always starts in rectum & spreads proximal
3. If confined to rectum = ulcerative proctitis, a benign subtype
4. Si/Sx = bloody diarrhea, colicky abdominal pain, can progress to generalized peritonitis, watch for toxic megacolon!
5. Dx = colonoscopy with biopsy → crypt abscess with numerous PMNs, friable mucosal patches that bleed easily
6. Tx depends on site & severity of dz
  a. Distal colitis → topical mesalamine & corticosteroids
  b. Moderate colitis (above sigmoid) → oral steroids, mesalamine & sulfasalazine
  c. Severe colitis → IV steroids, cyclosporine & surgical resection if unresponsive
  d. Fulminant colitis (rapidly progressive) → broad-spectrum abx
7. Comparison of inflammatory bowel disease (IBD)

TABLE 1-18   Comparison of Inflammatory Bowel Disease

	ULCERATIVE COLITIS	CROHN'S DISEASE
Location	Isolated to colon	Anywhere in GI tract
Lesions	Contiguously proximal from colon	Skip lesions, disseminated
Inflammation	Limited to mucosa/submucosa	Transmural
Neoplasms	Very high risk for development	Lower risk for development
Fissures	None	Extend through submucosa
Fistula	None	Frequent: can be enterocutaneous
Granulomas	None	Noncaseating are characteristic
Extraintestinal manifestations	Seen in both: • Arthritis, iritis, erythema nodosum, pyoderma gangrenosum • Sclerosing cholangitis = chronic, fibrosing, inflammation of biliary system leading to cholestasis & portal hypertension	

IV. Liver

A. JAUNDICE—VISIBLE WHEN SERUM BILIRUBIN EXCEEDS 2 MG/DL
1.

TABLE 1-19   Congenital Hyperbilirubinemia

SYNDROME	CHARACTERISTICS	TX
Gilbert's	• Mild defect of glucuronyl transferase in 5% of population • Si/Sx = ↑ serum **unconjugated bilirubin** → jaundice in stressful situations, completely benign	None required
Crigler-Najjar	• Genetic deficiency of glucuronyl transferase → ↑ serum **unconjugated bilirubin** • Type 1 = severe, presents in neonates with markedly ↑ bilirubin levels → death from kernicterus by age 1 • Type 2 = mild, pts suffer no severe clinical deficits	Phenobarbitol
Dubin-Johnson	• ↑ **conjugated bilirubin** due to defective bilirubin excretion • Si/Sx = jaundice, liver turns black, no serious clinical deficits	None required
Rotor	• ↑ **conjugated bilirubin** similar to Dubin-Johnson • Defect is in bilirubin storage, not excretion	None required

2. Hemolytic Anemias
   a. Excess production → ↑ unconjugated bilirubin
   b. Si/Sx = as per any anemia (weakness, fatigue, etc.), others depend on etiology of hemolytic anemia [see Hematology section]
   c. Dx = ⊕ Coombs' test, ↓ haptoglobin, ⊕ urine hemosiderin
   d. Tx depends on etiology [see Hematology section]
3. Intrahepatic cholestasis (hepatocellular)
   a. May be due to viral hepatitis or cirrhosis
   b. May be due to drug-induced hepatitis (acetaminophen, methotrexate, oral contraceptives, phenothiazines, INH, fluconazole)

c. Dx = ↑ transaminases, liver biopsy to confirm hepatitis

d. Tx = cessation of drugs, or supportive for viral infection

4. Extrahepatic

    a. Myriad causes include choledocholithiasis (but not cholelithiasis), CA of biliary system or pancreas, cholangitis, biliary cirrhosis

    b. Primary biliary cirrhosis

        1) An autoimmune disorder usually seen in women

        2) Si/Sx = jaundice, pruritus, hypercholesterolemia, **antimitochondrial antibody test is 90% sensitive**

        3) Dx = clinical ⊕ serology, confirm with biopsy

        4) Tx = liver transplant, otherwise supportive

    c. Secondary biliary cirrhosis results from long-standing biliary obstruction due to any cause (e.g., cholangitis)

    d. Si/Sx of acquired jaundice = acholic stools (pale), urinary bilirubin, fat malabsorption, pruritus, ↑ serum cholesterol, xanthomas

    e. Dx may require abdominal CT or endoscopic retrograde cholangiopancreaticoduodenoscopy (ERCP) to rule out malignancy or obstruction of bile pathway

    f. Tx depends on etiology

B. Hepatitis

1. General Si/Sx = jaundice, abdominal pain, diarrhea, malaise, fever, ↑ AST & ALT

2.

Table 1-20   Hepatitis Diagnosis and Treatment

Type	Characteristics	Tx
Fulminant	• Complication of acute hepatitis, progresses over less than 4 wk • Can be 2° to viral hepatitis, drugs (INH), toxins & some metabolic disorders like Wilson's dz • Elevated PT & hepatic encephalopathy	Urgent liver transplant

Viral	• Hepatitis A → fecal-oral transmission, transient influenza-like illness
	• Hepatitis B & C → blood transmission, B also sex & vertical → chronic hepatitis
	• 5–10% of HBV & >50% of HCV infxn → chronic
	• Dx = serologies & ↑ ALT & AST—ratio ≅ 1:1 (See Figure 1-10)
	  ◊ HBV surface antigen = active infection
	  ◊ anti-HBV surface antibody = immunity
	  ◊ anti-HBV core antibody = immunity
	  ◊ HBV e antigen = highly infectious
	  ◊ HCV antibody = exposure, not immune
		Interferon-α +/− lamivudine for HBV (*New Engl J Med* 1997, 339:61–8), Interferon-α +/− ribavirin for HCV (*New Engl J Med* 1998, 339:1485–1492 & 1493–1499)—both ↓ risk of chronic infxn

Granulomatous	• Causes = TB, fungal (e.g., *Coccidioides*, *Candida*, *Aspergillus*), sarcoidosis, brucella, rickettsia, syphilis, leptospirosis • Dx = liver biopsy	Antibiotics, prednisone for sarcoidosis

TABLE 1-20   *Continued*

TYPE	CHARACTERISTICS	TX
Alcoholic	• Most common form of liver disease in US • Si/Sx = as per other hepatitis with specific alcohol signs = palmar erythema, Dupuytren's contractures, spider angiomas, gynecomastia • Dx = clinical, ↑ AST & ALT, with AST : ALT = 2 : 1 is highly suggestive	Cessation of alcohol can reverse dz if early in course, otherwise → cirrhosis & only Tx is transplant
Autoimmune	• Type I occurs in young women, ⊕ ANA, ⊕ anti–smooth muscle Ab • Type II occurs mostly in children, linked to Mediterranean ancestry, ⊕ anti–liver-kidney-muscle (anti-LKM) antibody • Si/Sx as for any other hepatitis	Tx = prednisone +/– azathioprine

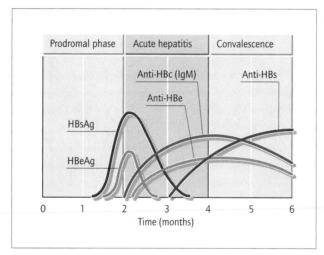

FIGURE 1-8   Time course of events leading to acute hepatitis B infection.

C. CIRRHOSIS

1. Most commonly due to alcoholism, also to chronic viral hepatitis
2. Si/Sx = purpura & bleeding & ↑ PT/PTT, jaundice, ascites 2° to ↓ albumin & portal hypertension, spontaneous bacterial peritonitis, encephalopathy, asterixis
   a.

TABLE 1-21   Ascites Differential Diagnosis

	PORTAL HYPERTENSION	NO PORTAL HYPERTENSION
Serum/ascites albumin gradient	> 1.1 g/dL	< 1.1 g/dL
Causes	Cirrhosis, alcoholic hepatitis, Budd-Chiari, CHF	Pancreatic dz, nephrosis, TB, peritoneal mets, idiopathic
Other labs	Ascites total protein > 2.5 → heart dz Ascites total protein ≤ 2.5 → liver dz	Amylase ↑ in pancreatic dz

    b. Spontaneous bacterial peritonitis
       1) Usually low protein ascites with no Sx of infxn
       2) Dx = ascitic fluid with absolute neutrophil count of >250 or ⊕ Gram's stain/culture of ascitic fluid
       3) Common organisms include *E. coli, Klebsiella, Enterococcus* & *S. pneumoniae*
       4) Tx = ceftriaxone or cefotaxime, plus IV albumin to maintain renal perfusion pressure
    c. Encephalopathy
       1) Due to ↑ levels of toxins, likely related to ammonia, but ammonia levels do not correlate well with encephalopathy
       2) Characterized by asterixis (flapping tremor of the wrist upon flexion) & altered mental status
       3) Tx of encephalopathy is to lower ammonia levels
         a) Lactulose metabolized by bacteria, acidifies the bowel, $NH_3 \rightarrow NH_4^+$, which cannot be absorbed
         b) Neomycin kills bacteria making NH_3 in gut
    d. Alcohol withdrawal has 4 phases—any given pt can go through any of these phases but does not have to go through all of them, and the phases occurring during a prior withdrawal episode are predictive for what will happen the next time withdrawal occurs
       1) Tremor—occurs within hours of last drink, so it's the 1st sign of withdrawal
       2) Seizure—occurs at several hours to about 48 hours after the last drink, these can be fatal and are best treated with benzodiazepines, not standard anti-seizure medicines
       3) Hallucinosis—occurs at 48–72 hours after the last drink, this is NOT delirium tremens (DTs), but rather is simply auditory or tactile hallucinations, also best treated with benzodiazepines
       4) Delirium tremens—at about 72 hours after the last drink the autonomic insta-bility that defines DTs begins with dangerous tachycardia and hypertension, and can be accompanied by each of the other 3 phases (tremor, seizure, hal-lucinosis)—the autonomic instability is also best treated with benzodiazepines
    e. Treatment of inpatient alcoholics
       1) IV thiamine & B_{12} supplements to correct deficiency (very common), also **must give thiamine before IV glucose or will precipitate Wernicke's encephalopathy**
       2) Give IV glucose, fluids & electrolytes
       3) Correct any underlying coagulopathy
       4) Benzodiazepine for prevention & Tx of delirium tremens

D. HEPATIC ABSCESS

  1. Caused by (in order of frequency in the US) bacteria, parasites (usually amebic) or fungal
  2. Bacterial abscesses usually result from direct extension of infection from gallbladder, hematogenous spread via the portal vein from appendicitis of diverticulitis, or via the hepatic artery from distant sources such as from a pneumonia or bacterial endocarditis
  3. Organisms in pyogenic hepatic abscesses are usually of enteric origin (e.g., *E. coli, K. pneumoniae, Bacteroides* & *Enterococcus*)
  4. Si/Sx = high fever, malaise, rigors, jaundice, epigastric or RUQ pain & referred pain to the right shoulder

5. Labs → leukocytosis, anemia, ↑ alkaline phosphatase
6. Dx = Utz or CT scan
7. Tx
    a. IV ampicillin/gentamicin/metronidazole
    b. Percutaneous or surgical drainage
    c. For amebic abscesses (caused by *Entamoeba histolytica*) use metronidazole
8. Complications = intrahepatic spread of infxn, sepsis & abscess rupture
9. Mortality of hepatic abscesses is 15%, higher with coexistent malignancy

E. PORTAL HYPERTENSION

1. Defined as portal vein pressure >12 mm Hg (normal = 6–8 mm Hg)
2. Si/Sx = ascites, hepatosplenomegaly, variceal bleeding, encephalopathy
3. Can be presinusoidal, intrahepatic, or postsinusoidal in nature

TABLE 1-22   Causes of Portal Hypertension

PREHEPATIC	INTRAHEPATIC		POSTHEPATIC
• Portal vein thrombosis	• Cirrhosis	• Idiopathic portal hypertension	• Severe right-sided heart failure
• Splenomegaly	• Schistosomiasis	• Granulomatous dz (e.g., tuberculosis, sarcoidosis)	• Hepatic vein thrombosis (Budd-Chiari syndrome)
• Arteriovenous fistula	• Massive fatty change		• Constrictive pericarditis
	• Nodular regenerative hyperplasia		• Hepatic veno-occlusive disease

4. Dx = endoscopy & angiography (variceal bleeding), & Utz (dilated vessels) (See Figure 1-9)
5. Tx
    a. Acute variceal bleeding controlled by sclerotherapy
    b. If continued bleeding, use Sengstaken-Blakemore tube to tamponade bleeding
    c. Pharmacotherapy = IV infusion of vasopressin or Octeotide
    d. Long term → propranolol once varices are identified (↓ bleeding risk but effect on long-term survival is variable)
    e. Decompressive shunts—most efficacious way of stopping bleeding
    f. **Indication for liver transplant is end-stage liver disease, not variceal bleeding**
6. **Budd-Chiari syndrome**
    a. Rarely congenital, usually acquired thrombosis occluding hepatic vein or hepatic stretch of inferior vena cava
    b. Associated with hypercoagulability (e.g., polycythemia vera, hepatocellular or other CA, pregnancy, etc.)
    c. Sx = acute onset of abdominal pain, jaundice, ascites
    d. Hepatitis quickly develops, leading to cirrhosis & portal hypertension
    e. Dx = right upper quadrant ultrasound
    f. Tx = clot lysis or hepatic transplant
    g. Px poor, less than 1/3 pts survive at 1 yr

SYSTEMIC SHUNTS IN PORTAL HYPERTENSION

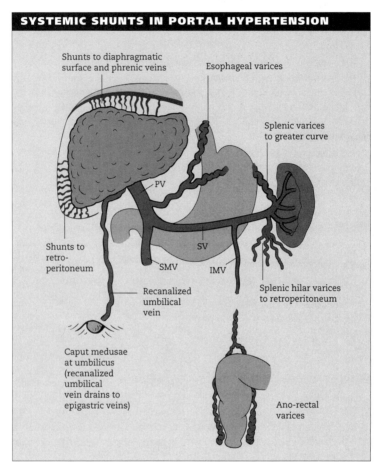

FIGURE 1-9   The sites of occurrence of portal-systemic communications in patients with portal hypertension. PV = portal vein; SMV = superior mesenteric vein; IMV = inferior mesenteric vein; SV = splenic vein.

7. Veno-occlusive disease (VOD)
   a. Occlusion of hepatic venules (not large veins)
   b. Associated with graft vs. host disease, chemotherapy & radiation therapy
   c. Px = 50% mortality at 1 yr
   d. Tx = hepatic transplant, sometimes is self-limiting

Nephrology

I. Renal Tubular and Interstitial Disorders

A. DRUG-INDUCED INTERSTITIAL NEPHRITIS
1. Penicillin, sulfonamides, diuretics & NSAIDs cause hypersensitivity
2. Si/Sx = pyuria, maculopapular rash, eosinophilia, proteinuria, hematuria, oliguria, flank pain, fever, eosinophiluria—**eosinophiluria is rare, but is pathognomonic for hypersensitivity TIN or atheroembolic dz**
3. Dx = clinical, improvement following withdrawal of offending drug can help confirm Dx, but sometimes the dz can be irreversible
4. Tx = removal of underlying cause, consider corticosteroids for allergic dz

B. ACUTE RENAL FAILURE (ARF)
1. Rapid $\uparrow$ azotemia ($\uparrow$ creatinine & BUN), +/– oliguria ($\equiv$ <500 mL/day urine)
2. Causes = 1) prerenal (hypoperfusion), 2) postrenal (obstruction), 3) renal
3. Prerenal failure caused by volume depletion, heart failure, liver failure, sepsis, heat-stroke (myoglobinuria), burns & bilateral renal artery stenosis
4. Postrenal ARF due to obstruction 2° to BPH, bladder/pelvic tumors, calculi
5. Intrinsic renal causes = acute tubular necrosis (most common, see below), others include nephrotoxin exposure & renal ischemia
6. Si/Sx = hyperkalemia → arrhythmias, oliguria, metabolic acidosis
7. Dx

TABLE 1-23   Laboratory Characteristics of Acute Renal Failure

TEST/INDEX	PRERENAL	POSTRENAL	RENAL
Urine osmolality	**>500**	<350	<350
Urine Na	**<20**	>40	>20
FE_{Na}*	<1%	>4%	>2%
BUN/Creatinine	>20	>15	**<15**

*FE_{Na} = (U/P sodium) / (U/P creatinine).

    a. Urinary eosinophils suggest allergic nephriti or atheroembolic dz
    b. **RBC casts virtually pathognomonic for glomerulonephritis**
8. Tx
    a. IV fluids to maintain urine output, diurese to prevent volume overload
    b. Closely monitor electrolyte abnormalities
    c. Indications for dialysis: recalcitrant volume overload status, critical electrolyte abnormalities, unresponsive metabolic acidosis, toxic ingestion, uremia

C. ACUTE TUBULAR NECROSIS (ATN)
1. Most common cause of ARF, falls into the intrinsic renal category
2. ATN causes = renal ischemia 2° to sepsis, trauma, hemorrhage, crush injury or rhab-domyolysis → myoglobinuria, direct toxins (e.g., amphotericin, aminoglycosides, radiocontrast dyes)

3. 3 phases of injury: 1) prodromal, 2) oliguric, 3) postoliguric
4. Tx = resolution of precipitating cause, IV fluids to maintain urinary output, monitor electrolytes, diurese as needed to prevent fluid overload

D. RENAL TUBULE FUNCTIONAL DISORDERS

1. Renal tubular acidosis (RTA)

TABLE 1-24   Renal Tubular Acidosis*

TYPE	CHARACTERISTIC	URINARY PH
Type I	• **Distal tubular defect** of urinary H^+ gradient	**Urine pH > 5.5**
Type II	• **Proximal tubule failure** to resorb HCO_3	Urine pH > 5.5 early, then → < 5.5 as acidosis worsens
Type IV	• ↓ **Aldosterone** → hyperkalemia & hyperchloremia • Usually due to ↓ secretion (**hyporeninemic hypoaldosteronism**), seen in diabetes, interstitial nephritis, NSAID use, ACE inhibitors & heparin • Also due to aldosterone resistance, seen in urinary obstruction & sickle cell dz	**Urine pH < 5.5**

*There is no RTA III for historical reasons.

2. Diabetes insipidus (DI)
   a. ↓ ADH secretion (central) or ADH resistance (nephrogenic)
   b. Si/Sx = polyuria, polydipsia, nocturia, urine specific gravity <1.010, urine osmolality (U_{osm}) ≤ 200, serum osmolality (S_{osm}) ≥ 300
   c. Central DI
      1) 1° (idiopathic) or 2° (acquired via trauma, infarction, granulomatous infiltration, fungal or TB infection of pituitary)
      2) Tx = DDAVP (ADH analogue) nasal spray
   d. Nephrogenic DI
      1) 1° dz is X-linked, seen in infants, may regress with time
      2) 2° dz in sickle cell, pyelonephritis, nephrosis, amyloid, multiple myeloma, drugs (aminoglycoside, lithium, demeclocycline)
      3) Tx = ↑ water intake, sodium restriction
   e. **Dx = water deprivation test**
      1) Hold all water, administer vasopressin
      2) Central DI: U_{osm} after deprivation no greater than S_{osm}, but ↑ ≥ 10% after vasopressin given
      3) Nephrogenic DI: U_{osm} after deprivation no greater than S_{osm}, & vasopressin does not ↑ U_{osm}
3. Syndrome of inappropriate antidiuretic hormone (SIADH)
   a. Etiologies
      1) CNS dz: trauma, tumor, Guillain-Barré, hydrocephalus
      2) Pulmonary dz: pneumonia, tumor, abscess, COPD
      3) Endocrine dz: hypothyroidism, Conn's syndrome

4) Drugs: NSAIDs, antidepressants, chemotherapy, diuretics, phenothiazine, oral hypoglycemics

b. Dx = hyponatremia with U_{osm} >300 mmol/kg

c. Tx = usually self-limiting, otherwise give normal saline, demeclocycline for resistant cases—**beware of central pontine myelinolysis with rapid correction of hyponatremia**

E. CHRONIC RENAL FAILURE

1. Always associated with azotemia of renal origin
2. Uremia = biochemical & clinical syndrome of the following characteristics
   a. Azotemia
   b. Acidosis due to accumulation of sulfates, phosphates, organic acids
   c. Hyperkalemia due to inability to excrete K^+ in urine
   d. Fluid volume disorder (early can't concentrate urine, late can't dilute)
   e. Hypocalcemia due to lack of vitamin D production
   f. Anemia due to lack of EPO production
   g. Hypertension $2°$ to activated renin-angiotensin axis
3. Si/Sx = anorexia, nausea/vomit, dementia, convulsions, eventually coma, bleeding due to platelet dysfunction, fibrinous pericarditis
4. Dx = renal Utz → small kidneys in chronic dz, anemia from chronic lack of EPO, diffuse osteopenia
5. Tx = salt & water restriction, diuresis to prevent fluid overload, dialysis to correct acid-base or severe electrolyte disorders

II. Glomerular Diseases

A. NEPHROTIC SYNDROME

1. Si/Sx = proteinuria >3.5 g/day, generalized edema (anasarca), lipiduria with hyperlipidemia, marked ↓ albumin, hypercoagulation
2. Dx of type made by renal biopsy
3. General Tx = protein restriction, salt restriction & diuretic therapy for edema, HMG-CoA reductase inhibitor for hyperlipidemia
4.

TABLE 1-25   Nephrotic Glomerulopathies

DISEASE	CHARACTERISTICS
Minimal change disease (MCD)	• Classically seen in young children • Tx = prednisone, disease is very responsive, Px is excellent
Focal segmental glomerulosclerosis	• Clinically similar to MCD, but occurs in adults with refractory HTN • Usually idiopathic, but heroin, HIV, diabetes, sickle cell are associated • Idiopathic typically presents in young, hypertensive black males • Tx = prednisone + cyclophosphamide, dz is refractory, Px poor

TABLE 1-25 *Continued*

DISEASE	CHARACTERISTICS
Membranous glomerulonephritis	• Most common primary cause of nephrotic syndrome in adults • Slowly progressive disorder with ↓ response to steroid treatment seen • Causes of this disease are numerous ◊ Infections include HBV, HCV, syphilis, malaria ◊ Drugs include gold salts, penicillamine (note, both used in RA) ◊ Occult malignancy ◊ SLE (10% of patients develop) • Tx = prednisone +/– cyclophosphamide, 50% → end-stage renal failure
Membranoproliferative glomerulonephritis	• Disease as 2 forms ◊ Type I often slowly progressive ◊ Type II more aggressive, often have an autoantibody against C3 convertase "C3 nephritic factor" → ↓ serum levels of C3 • Tx = prednisone +/– plasmapheresis or interferon-α, Px very poor
Systemic diseases	See Table 1-26

5.

TABLE 1-26 Systemic Glomerulonephropathies

DISEASE	CHARACTERISTIC NEPHROPATHY
Diabetes	• Most common cause of end-stage renal disease in US • Early manifestation is microalbuminuria ◊ ACE inhibitors ↓ progression to renal failure if started early ◊ Strict glycemic & hypertensive control also ↓ progression • Biopsy shows pathognomonic Kimmelstiel-Wilson nodules • As dz progresses only Tx is renal transplant
HIV	• Usually seen in HIV acquired by intravenous drug abuse • Presents with focal segmental glomerulonephritis • Early Tx with antiretrovirals may help kidney disease
Renal amyloidosis	• Dx → birefringence with Congo Red stain • Tx = transplant, dz is refractory & often recurrent
Lupus	
Type I	No renal involvement
Type II	• **Mesangial disease** with focal segmental glomerular pattern • Tx not typically required for kidney involvement
Type III	• **Focal proliferative disease** • Tx = aggressive prednisone +/– cyclophosphamide
Type IV	• **Diffuse proliferative disease**, the most severe form of lupus nephropathy • Presents with a combination of nephrotic/nephritic disease • Classic LM → wire-loop abnormality • Tx = prednisone + cyclophosphamide, transplant may be required
Type V	• **Membranous disease**, indistinguishable from other 1° membranous GNs • Tx = consider prednisone, may not be required

B. NEPHRITIC SYNDROME

1. Results from diffuse glomerular inflammation
2. Si/Sx = acute onset hematuria (smoky-brown urine), ↓ GFR resulting in azotemia (↑ BUN & creatinine), oliguria, hypertension & edema

3.

TABLE 1-27   Nephritic Glomerulonephropathies

DISEASE	CHARACTERISTICS
Poststreptococcal (Postinfectious) Glomerulonephritis (PSGN/PIGN)	• Prototype of nephritic syndrome (acute glomerulonephritis) • Classically follows infection with group A β-hemolytic streptococci (*S. pyogenes*), but can follow infxn by virtually any organism, viral or bacterial • Lab → urine red cells & casts, azotemia, ↓ serum C3, ↑ ASO titer • Immunofluorescence → coarse granular IgG or C3 deposits • Tx typically not needed, dz usually self-limiting
Crescentic (rapidly progressive) glomerulonephritis	• Nephritis progresses to renal failure within weeks or months • May be part of PIGN or other systemic diseases • Goodpasture's disease ◊ **Disease causes glomerulonephritis with pneumonitis** ◊ **90% pts present with hemoptysis**, only later get glomerulonephritis ◊ Peak incidence in men in mid-20s ◊ **Classic immunofluorescence → smooth, linear deposition of IgG** • Tx = prednisone & plasmapheresis, minority → end-stage renal dz
Berger's disease (IgA nephropathy)	• **Most common worldwide nephropathy** • Due to IgA deposition in the mesangium • Si/Sx = recurrent hematuria with low-grade proteinuria • Whereas PIGN presents weeks after infection, **Berger's presents concurrently or within several days of infection** • 25% of pts slowly progress to renal failure, otherwise harmless • Tx = prednisone for acute flares, will not halt dz progression
Henoch-Schönlein purpura (HSP)	• Also an IgA nephropathy, but almost always presents in children • Presents with abdominal pain, vomiting, hematuria & GI bleeding • **Classic physical finding = "palpable purpura" on buttocks & legs in kids** • Often follows respiratory infection • Tx not required, dz is self-limiting
Multiple myeloma	↑ production of light chains → tubular plugging by Bence-Jones proteins • 2° hypercalcemia also contributes to development of "myeloma kidney" • Myeloma cells can directly invade kidney parenchyma • Defect in normal antibody production leaves pt susceptible to chronic infections by encapsulated bacteria (e.g., *E. coli*) → chronic renal failure • Tx is directed at underlying myeloma

C.

TABLE 1-28   Urinalysis in Primary Glomerular Diseases

	NEPHROTIC SYNDROME	NEPHRITIC SYNDROME	CHRONIC DISEASE
Proteinuria	↑↑↑↑	+/–	+/–
Hematuria	+/–	↑↑↑↑	+/–
Cells	—	⊕ RBCs ⊕ WBCs	+/–
Casts	Fatty casts	RBC & granular casts	Waxy & pigmented granular casts
Lipids	Free fat droplets, oval fat bodies	—	—

III. Renal Artery Stenosis (RAS)

A. PRESENTATION
1. **Classic dyad = sudden hypertension with low K⁺** (pt not on diuretic)
2. Causes are atherosclerotic plaques & fibromuscular dysplasia
3. Screening Dx = oral captopril induces ↑ renin
4. Dx confirmed with angiography
5. Tx = surgery vs. angioplasty

IV. Urinary Tract Obstruction

A. GENERAL CHARACTERISTICS
1. Most common causes in children are congenital
2. Most common causes in adults are BPH & stones
3. Obstruction → urinary stasis → ↑ risk of UTI

B. NEPHROLITHIASIS
1. Calcium pyrophosphate stones
   a. 80–85% stones, are **radiopaque**, associated with hypercalciuria
   b. Hypercalciuria can be idiopathic or due to ↑ intestinal calcium absorption, ↑ 1° renal calcium excretion, or hypercalcemia
   c. **50% associated with idiopathic hypercalciuria**
   d. Tx = vigorous hydration, loop diuretics if necessary
2. Ammonium magnesium phosphate stones ("struvite stones")
   a. Second most common form of stones, are **radiopaque**
   b. Most often due to urease ⊕ *Proteus* or *Staph. saprophyticus*
   c. Can form large staghorn or struvite calculi
   d. Tx = directed at underlying infection
3. Uric acid stones
   a. 50% of pts with stones have hyperuricemia
   b. 2° to gout or ↑ cell turnover (leukemia, myeloproliferative dz)
   c. Stones are **radiolucent**
   d. Tx = alkalinize urine, treat underlying disorder
4. Si/Sx of stones = urinary colic = sharp, 10/10 pain, often described as the worst pain in the pt's life, radiates from back → anterior pelvis/groin
5. Tx = vigorous hydration, loop diuretics as needed

V. Tumors of the Kidney

A. RENAL CELL CARCINOMA
1. Most common renal malignancy, occurs in male smokers aged 50–70
2. **Hematogenously disseminates by invading renal veins or the vena cava**
3. Si/Sx = hematuria, palpable mass, flank pain, fever, 2° polycythemia
4. Tx = resection, systemic interleukin-2 immunotherapy, poor Px

B. WILMS' TUMOR
1. Most common renal malignancy of childhood, incidence peaks at 2–4 yr
2. Si/Sx = palpable flank mass (often huge)

3. Can be part of **WAGR** complex = **W**ilms' tumor, **A**niridia, **G**enitourinary malformations, mental motor **R**etardation
4. **Also associated with hemihypertrophy of the body**
5. Tx = nephrectomy plus chemotherapy &/or radiation

Endocrinology

I. The Hypothalamic Pituitary Axis

A. PROLACTINOMA
1. Si/Sx = headache, diplopia, CN III palsy, impotence, amenorrhea, gynecomastia, galactorrhea, ↑ androgens in females → virilization
2. **50% cause hypopituitarism, caused by mass effect of the tumor**
3. Dx = MRI/CT confirmation of tumor
4. Tx
   a. First line = dopamine agonist (e.g., bromocriptine)
   b. Large tumors or refractory → transsphenoidal surgical resection
   c. Radiation therapy for nonresectable macroadenomas

B. ACROMEGALY
1. Almost always due to pituitary adenoma secreting growth hormone
2. Childhood secretion prior to skeletal epiphyseal closure → gigantism
3. If secretion begins after epiphyseal closure → acromegaly
4. Si/Sx = adult whose glove, ring, or shoe size acutely ↑, coarsening of skin/facial features, prognathism, voice deepening, joint erosions, peripheral neuropathies due to nerve compression
5. Dx = ↑ insulin-like growth factor 1 &/or MRI/CT confirmation of neoplasm
6. Tx = surgery or radiation to ablate the enlarged pituitary, octreotide (somatostatin analogue) second line for refractory tumors

II. Diabetes

A. TYPE I DIABETES
1. Autoinflammatory destruction of pancreas → insulin deficiency
2. Si/Sx = polyphagia, polydipsia, polyuria, weight loss in child or adolescent, can lead to diabetic ketoacidosis (DKA) when pt is stressed (e.g., infection)
3. Dx = see type II below for criteria
4. **Tx = insulin replacement required—oral hypoglycemics will not work!**
5. Complication of type I diabetes = diabetic ketoacidosis (DKA)
6. Sx/Si of DKA = **Kussmaul hyperpnea** (slow & deep breaths), **abdominal pain, dehydration, ⊕ anion gap**, urine/blood ketones, hyperkalemia, hyperglycemia, *Mucor* sinusitis = rapidly fatal fungal infxn seen in DKA
7. DKA Tx
   a. **1° Tx = FLUIDS!!!**
   b. **2° = K⁺ & insulin**
   c. **3° = add glucose to insulin drip if pt becomes normoglycemic**—insulin is given to shut down ketogenesis, NOT to ↓ glucose, so insulin must be given until ketones are gone despite normal glucose!

B. TYPE II DIABETES

1. Peripheral insulin resistance—a metabolic dz, not autoinflammatory!
2. Usually adult onset, not ketosis prone, often strong FHx
3. Si/Sx
    a. Acute = dehydration, polydipsia/-phagia/-uria, fatigue, weight loss
    b. Subacute = infections (yeast vaginitis, *Mucor, S. aureus* boils)
    c. Chronic (See Figure 1-10)
        1) Macrovascular = stroke, coronary artery disease
        2) Microvascular = retinitis, nephritis
        3) Neuropathy = ↓ sensation, paresthesias, glove-in-hand burning pain, auto-nomic insufficiency
4. Dx of any diabetes (type I or II)
    a. Random plasma glucose over 200 with symptoms or
    b. Fasting glucose over 125 twice or
    c. 2-hr oral glucose tolerance test glucose >200 with or without Sx
5. Tx
    a. Oral hypoglycemics first line for mild to moderate hyperglycemia
        1) Metformin is first line, unknown mechanism, watch for GI upset and lactic acidosis
        2) Sulfonylureas (e.g., glyburide, glipizide), ↑ β-cell insulin secretion
        3) Thiazolidinediones (e.g., pioglitazone & rosiglitazone) increases tissue sensitivity to insulin
    b. Dz refractory to oral hypoglycemics requires insulin
    c. Diet & nutrition education
    d. ACE inhibitors slow progression of nephropathy
6. Monitoring: glycosylated hemoglobin A1c (HgA1c)
    a. Because of serum half-life of hemoglobin, HgA1c is a marker of the prior 3 mo of therapeutic regimen
    b. **Tight glucose control has been shown to reduce complications & mortality in IDDM & NIDDM**, thus HgA1c is a crucial key tool to follow efficacy & compli-ance of diabetic Tx regimens
    c. HgAlC of <8 is recommended
7. Complication = hyperosmolar hyperglycemic nonketotic coma (HHNK)
    a. 2° to hypovolemia, precipitated by acute stress (e.g., infxn, trauma)
    b. Glucose often >1000 mg/dL, no acidosis, ⊕ renal failure & confusion
    c. Tx = rehydrate (may require 10 L), mortality approaches 50%

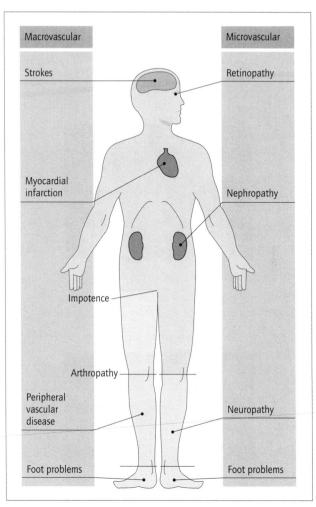

FIGURE 1-10   Macro- and microvascular complications of DM.

III. Adrenal Disorders

A. CUSHING'S SYNDROME

1. Usually iatrogenic (cortisol Tx) or due to pituitary adenoma = Cushing's disease, rarely due to adrenal hyperplasia, ectopic ACTH/CRH production
2. Si/Sx = **buffalo hump** (See Figure 1-11), **truncal obesity** (See Figure 1-12), **moon facies**, **striae** (See Figure 1-13), hirsutism, hyperglycemia, hypertension, purpura, amenorrhea, impotence, acne
3. Dx = 24 hr urine cortisol & high dose dexamethasone suppression test

4. Tx
   a. Excision of tumor with postop glucocorticoid replacement
   b. Mitotane (adrenolytic), ketoconazole (inhibits P450), metyrapone (blocks adrenal enzyme synthesis), or aminoglutethimide (inhibits P450) for nonexcisable tumors

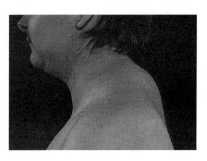

FIGURE 1-11   Buffalo hump.

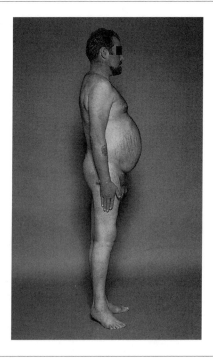

FIGURE 1-12   Truncal obesity with abdominal striae.

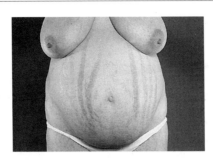

Figure 1-13   Abdominal striae.

B. Adrenal Insufficiency

1. Can be 1° (Addison's disease) or 2° (↓ ACTH production by pituitary)
2. Addison's disease
   a. Causes = autoimmune (most common), granulomatous disease, infarction, HIV, DIC (Waterhouse-Friderichsen syndrome)
   b. **Waterhouse-Friderichsen** = hemorrhagic necrosis of adrenal medulla during the course of meningococcemia
   c. Si/Sx = fatigue, anorexia, nausea/vomit, constipation, diarrhea, salt craving (pica), hypotension, **hyponatremia, hyperkalemia**
   d. **Dx = hyperpigmentation, ↑ACTH, ↓cortisol response to ACTH**
3. 2° Dz → **NO hyperpigmentation**, ↓ **ACTH**, ↑ cortisol response to ACTH
4. Acute adrenal crisis
   a. Due to stress (e.g., surgery or trauma), usually in setting of treated chronic insufficiency or withdrawal of Tx
   b. Can occur in pituitary apoplexy (infarction)
5. Tx = cortisol replacement, ↑ replacement for times of illness or stress—**must taper replacement off slowly to allow HPA axis to restore itself**

C. Adrenal Cortical Hyperfunction

1. 1° hyperaldosteronism = Conn's syndrome
   a. Adenoma or hyperplasia of zona glomerulosa
   b. Si/Sx = **HTN**, ↑**Na**, ↑**Cl**, ↓ **K**, **alkalosis**, ↓ renin (feedback inhibition)
   c. Dx = ↑ aldosterone, ↓ renin, CT → adrenal neoplasm
   d. Tx = excision of adenoma—bilateral hyperplasia → spironolactone; bilateral adrenalectomy should NOT be performed
2. 2° hyperaldosteronism
   a. Due to increased renin production 2° to renal ischemia (e.g., CHF, shock, renal artery stenosis), cirrhosis, or tumor
   b. Dx = ↑ renin (renin levels differentiate 1° vs. 2° hyperaldosteronism)
   c. Tx = underlying cause, β-blocker or diuretic for hypertension

D. Adrenal Medulla

1. Pheochromocytoma
   a. Si/Sx = hypertension (episodic or chronic), **diaphoresis, palpitations**, tachycardia, headache, nausea/vomit, flushing, dyspnea, diarrhea

b. **Rule of 10**: 10% malignant, 10% bilateral, 10% extra-adrenal (occurs in embryologic cells that reactivate outside the adrenal gland)

c. Dx = ↑ urinary catecholamines, CT scan of adrenal showing neoplasm

d. Tx

    1) Surgical excision after preop administration of α-blockers

    2) Ca^{2+} channel blockers for hypertensive crisis

    3) Phenoxybenzamine or phentolamine (α-blockers) for inoperable disease

IV. Gonadal Disorders

A. MALE GONADAL AXIS [SEE OB-GYN FOR FEMALE AXIS]

TABLE 1-29 Differential Diagnosis of Male Gonadal Disorders

DISEASE	CHARACTERISTICS	TX
Klinefelter's syndrome	• XXY chromosome inheritance, variable expressivity • Often not Dx until puberty when ↓ virilization is noted • Si/Sx = tall, eunuchoid, with small testes & gynecomastia, ↓ testosterone, ↑ LH/FSH from lack of feedback • **Dx = buccal smear analysis for presence of Barr bodies**	Testosterone supplements
XYY syndrome	• Si/Sx = may have mild mental retardation, severe acne, ↑ incidence of violence & antisocial behavior • Dx = karyotype analysis	None
Testicular feminization syndrome	• Defect in the dihydrotestosterone receptor → female external genitalia with sterile, undescended testes • Si/Sx = appear as females but are sterile & the vagina is blind-ended, testosterone, estrogen & LH are all ↑ • Dx = H&P, genetic testing	None
5-α-reductase deficiency	• Si/Sx = ambiguous genitalia until puberty, then a burst in testosterone overcomes lack of dihydrotestosterone → external genitalia become masculinized, **testosterone & estrogen are normal** • Dx = genetic testing	Testosterone supplements

B. HYPOGONADISM OF EITHER SEX

TABLE 1-30 Genetic Hypogonadism

DISEASE	CHARACTERISTICS	TX
Congenital adrenal hyperplasia (CAH)	• Defects in steroid synthetic pathway causing either virilization of females or failure to virilize males • 21-α-hydroxylase deficiency causes 95% of all CAH • Severe dz presents in infancy with ambiguous genitalia & salt loss (2° to ↓↓ aldosterone) • Less severe variants → minimal virilization & salt loss, & can have Dx delayed for several years	Tx = replacement of necessary hormones
Prader-Willi syndrome	• Paternal imprinting (only gene from dad is expressed) • Si/Sx = presents in infancy with floppy baby, **short limbs**, obesity due to gross hyperphagia, nasal speech, retardation, **classic almond-shaped eyes with strabismus** • Dx = clinical or genetic analysis	None

TABLE 1-30   *Continued*

DISEASE	CHARACTERISTICS	TX
Laurence-Moon-Biedl syndrome	• Autosomal recessive inheritance • Si/Sx = obese children, **normal craniofacies**, may be retarded, **are not short, have polydactyly** • Dx = clinical or genetic	None
Kallmann's syndrome	• Autosomal dominant hypogonadism with anosmia (can't smell) • Due to ↓ production/secretion of GnRH by hypothalamus • Dx by lack of circulating LH & FSH	Pulsatile GnRH → virilization

V. Thyroid

A. HYPERTHYROIDISM

1. Causes = Graves' dz, Plummer's dz, adenoma, subacute thyroiditis
2. Si/Sx of hyperthyroidism = tachycardia, **isolated systolic hypertension**, tremor, a-fib, anxiety, diaphoresis, weight loss with increased appetite, insomnia/**fatigue**, diarrhea, **exophthalmus, heat intolerance**
3. Graves' disease
   a. Diffuse toxic goiter, causes 90% of US hyperthyroid cases
   b. Seen in young adults, & is 8x more common in females than males
   c. **Si/Sx include 2 findings only seen in hyperthyroid due to Graves': infiltrative ophthalmopathy & pretibial myxedema**
   d. **Infiltrative ophthalmopathy** = exophthalmus not resolving when thyrotoxicosis is cured, due to autoantibody-mediated damage
   e. **Pretibial myxedema**
      1) Brawny, pruritic, nonpitting edema usually on the shins
      2) Often spontaneously remits after months to years
   f. Dx confirmed with thyroid stimulating immunoglobulin test
4. Plummer's disease (toxic multinodular goiter)
   a. Due to multiple foci of thyroid tissue that cease responding to T4 feedback inhibition, more common in older people
   b. Dx = multiple thyroid nodules felt in gland, confirm with radioactive iodine uptake tests → hot nodules with cold background
5. Thyroid adenoma due to overproduction of hormone by tumor in the gland
6. Subacute thyroiditis (giant cell or de Quervain's thyroiditis)
   a. Gland inflammation with spilling of hormone from the damaged gland
   b. **Presents with hyperthyroidism, later turns into hypothyroidism**
7. Tx for all
   a. Propylthiouracil or methimazole induces remission in 1 mo to 2 yr (up to 50% of time), lifelong Tx not necessary unless relapses
   b. Radioiodine is first line for Graves': radioactive iodine is concentrated in the gland & destroys it, resolving the diffuse hyperthyroid state
   c. If the above fail → surgical excision (of adenoma or entire gland)
8. Thyroid storm is the most extreme manifestation of hyperthyroidism
   a. Due to exacerbation of hyperthyroidism by surgery or infection
   b. Si/Sx = high fever, dehydration, cardiac arrhythmias, high output cardiac failure, coma & 25% mortality

c. Tx
1) β-blockers and IV fluids are first priority to restore hemodynamic stability
2) Give propylthiouracil (PTU) to inhibit iodination of more thyroid hormone
3) After PTU on board, give iodine-containing product which will feedback inhibit further thyroid hormone release—make sure the PTU is on board first, or the iodine can cause an initial INCREASE in hormone release before it feedback suppresses release

B. HYPOTHYROIDISM

1. Causes include Hashimoto's & subacute thyroiditis
2. Si/Sx = **cold intolerance**, weight gain, **low energy**, husky voice, mental slowness, constipation, thick/coarse hair, puffiness of face/eyelids/hands (**myxedema**), prolonged relaxation phase of deep tendon reflexes
3. Hashimoto's disease
   a. Autoimmune lymphocytic infiltration of the thyroid gland
   b. **8:1 ratio in women to men**, usually between ages of 30 and 50
   c. **Dx confirmed by antithyroid peroxidase (TPO) antibodies**
   d. Tx = lifelong Synthroid
4. Subacute thyroiditis
   a. Seen following flu-like illness with sore throat & fevers
   b. Si/Sx = **jaw/tooth pain**, can be confused with dental dz, ↑ ESR
   c. Early on looks like hyperthyroidism as damaged gland spills T4
   d. Tx with aspirin, only with cortisol in very severe disease
   e. Usually self-limiting, resolves after weeks to months
5. Myxedema coma
   a. **The only emergent hypothyroid condition**—spontaneous onset or precipitated by cold exposure, infection, analgesia, sedative drug use, respiratory failure, or other severe illness
   b. Si/Sx = stupor, coma, seizures, hypotension, hypoventilation
   c. Tx = IV levothyroxine, cortisone, mechanical ventilation

VI. Thyroid Malignancy

1. Terms *hot* & *cold* used to describe nodules, refer to whether or not the nodules take up iodine (i.e., are they functionally active or not)
2. Hot nodules are rarely cancerous, usually seen in elderly, soft to palpation, ultrasound (Utz) shows cystic mass, thyroid scan shows autonomously functioning nodule
3. Cold nodule
   a. Has a greater potential of being malignant
   b. More common in women
   c. Nodule is firm to palpation, often accompanied by vocal cord paralysis. Utz shows solid mass
4. Papillary CA
   a. The most common cancer of thyroid
   b. Good Px, 85% 5-yr survival, spread is indolent, via lymph nodes
   c. Pathologically distinguished by ground glass Orphan Annie nucleus & psammoma bodies (other psammoma body dz = serous papillary cystadenocarcinoma of ovary, mesothelioma, meningioma)
5. Medullary CA
   a. Has intermediate prognosis

b. Cancer of parafollicular "C" cells that are derived from the ultimobranchial bodies (cells of branchial pouch 5)

c. Secretes calcitonin, can Dx & follow dz with this blood assay

6. Follicular CA

a. Good Px, commonly blood-borne metastases to bone & lungs

7. Anaplastic CA has one of the poorest Px of any cancer (0% survival at 5 yr)

a. Note: Thyroid Nodule—fine needle aspirate, surgical excison

VII.

TABLE 1-31   The Multiple Endocrine Neoplasia Syndromes

Type I (Wermer's syndrome)	**The 3(4) Ps: P**ituitary (**P**rolactinoma most common), **P**arathyroid, **P**ancreatoma
Type IIa (Sipple's syndrome)	Pheochromocytoma, medullary thyroid CA, parathyroid hyperplasia or tumor
Type IIb (Type III)	Pheochromocytoma, medullary thyroid CA, mucocutaneous neuromas, particularly of the GI tract

Musculoskeletal

I. Metabolic Bone Diseases

A. OSTEOPOROSIS

1. Due to **postmenopausal (↓estrogen)**, physical inactivity, high cortisol states (e.g., Cushing's, exogenous), hyperthyroidism, Ca^{2+} deficiency

2. Si/Sx = typically aSx until fracture occurs, particularly of hip & vertebrae

3. Dx = **DEXA scan** showing ↓ bone density compared to general population

4. Tx

a. Estrogens are first line, only Tx shown to stimulate new bone growth

b. Bisphosphonates are second line, like estrogen proven to ↓ risk of fracture & slow or stop bone degeneration

c. Calcitonin particularly useful for treating bone pain but its effects wear off after chronic use

d. Raloxifene & tamoxifen (selective estrogen receptor modulators) ↑ bone density but also ↑ risk for thromboembolism—role unclear currently

5. **Every osteoporosis pt should take Ca to keep dietary intake ≥ 1.5 g/day**

B. RICKETS/OSTEOMALACIA

1. Vitamin D deficiency in children = rickets, in adults = osteomalacia

2. Si/Sx in kids (rickets) = **craniotabes** (thinning of skull bones), **rachitic rosary** (costochondral thickening looks like string of beads), **Harrison's groove** (depression along line of diaphragmatic insertion into rib cage), **Pigeon breast** = pectus carinatum (sternum protrusion)

3. In adults the dz mimics osteoporosis

4. Dx = x-ray → radiolucent bones, can confirm with vitamin D level

5. Tx = vitamin D supplementation

C. SCURVY

1. Vitamin C deficiency → ↓ osteoid formation

2. Si/Sx = subperiosteal hemorrhage (painful), **bleeding gums**, multiple ecchymoses, osteoporosis, **"woody leg"** from soft tissue hemorrhage

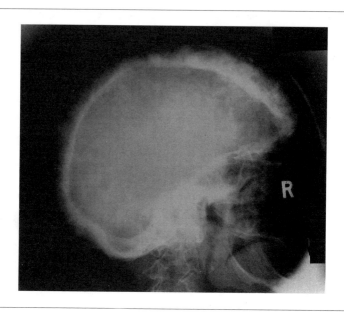

FIGURE 1-14   Radiograph showing Paget's bone disease.

3. Dx = clinical
4. Tx = Vitamin C supplementation

D. PAGET'S BONE DISEASE (OSTEITIS DEFORMANS)
 1. Idiopathic ↑ activity of both osteoblasts & osteoclasts, usually in elderly
 2. Si/Sx = **diffuse fractures & bone pain**, most commonly involves spine, pelvis, skull, femur, tibia, **high output cardiac failure, ↓ hearing**
 3. Dx = ↑↑ **alkaline phosphatase**, ⊕ bone scans, x-rays → sclerotic lesions
 4. Tx = bisphosphonates first line, calcitonin second line
 5. Complications = pathologic fractures, hypercalcemia & kidney stones, spinal cord compression in vertebral disease, osteosarcoma in long-standing disease

II. Nonneoplastic Bone Diseases

A. FIBROUS DYSPLASIA
 1. Idiopathic replacement of bone with fibrous tissue
 2. 3 types = a) monostotic, b) polystotic, c) McCune-Albright's
 3. McCune-Albright's syndrome
    a. Syndrome of hyperparathyroidism, hyperadrenalism & acromegaly
    b. **Dx = polystotic fibrous dysplasia, precocious puberty, café-au-lait spots** (See Color Plate 1)
 4. Tx = supportive surgical debulking of deforming defects

B. PYOGENIC OSTEOMYELITIS
 1. *S. aureus* most common cause, also *S. epidermidis* & *Strep.* spp.
 2. **Sickle cell patients get *Salmonella*, IV drug abusers get *Pseudomonas***

3. Si/Sx = painful inflammation of bone, striking skin changes include hyperpigmentation, ulceration, erythema
4. Dx = **x-ray → periosteal elevation, can lag onset of dz by weeks**, MRI is gold standard, can confirm with cultures of deep bone biopsy
5. Tx = 6–8 weeks of antibiotics, fluoroquinolones empirically, then narrow as cultures come back, surgical débridement as needed

III. Bone Tumors

1.

TABLE 1-32   Diagnosis[a] and Treatment of Primary Bone Neoplasms

TUMOR	PT AGE[b]	CHARACTERISTICS	TX
Osteochondroma	<25	• Benign, usually in males • Seen at distal femur & proximal tibia	Excision
Giant cell	20–40	• Benign, epiphyseal ends of long bones (>50% in knee) • X-ray → **soap bubble** sign • Often recurs after excision	Excision & local irradiation
Osteosarcoma	10–20	• #1 primary bone malignancy, in males • Seen at distal femur & proximal tibia • 2–3 fold ↑ alkaline phosphatase • **X-ray → Codman's triangle** = periosteal elevation due to tumor & **"sun-burst" sign** = lytic lesion with surrounding spiculated periostitis (See Figure 1-15)	Excision & local irradiation
Ewing's sarcoma	<15	• Young boys, metastasizes very early • Si/Sx mimic osteomyelitis (See Figure 1-15)	Chemotherapy

[a] Diagnoses all confirmed with bone biopsy.
[b] Peak age of onset.

2. Multiple myeloma
   a. Malignant clonal neoplasm of plasma cells producing whole Abs (e.g., IgM, IgG, etc.), light chains only, or very rarely no Abs (just ↑ B cells)
   b. Seen in pts >40, African Americans have 2 : 1 incidence
   c. **Si/Sx = bone pain worse with movement, lytic bone lesions on x-ray** (See Figure 1-16), pathologic fractures, **hypercalcemia**, renal failure, anemia, frequent infections by encapsulated bacteria, ↓ **anion gap** (Abs positively charged, unseen cations make anion gap appear ↓)
   d. **Hyperviscosity syndrome** = stroke, retinopathy, CHF, **ESR > 100**
   e. **Bence-Jones proteinuria**
      1) **Urine dipsticks do NOT detect light chains**, can use sulfosalicylic acid test in lieu of dipstick to screen
      2) Dx = 24-hr urine collection → protein electrophoresis
      3) Light chain deposition causes renal amyloidosis
   f. Dx
      1) Serum/urine protein electrophoresis (SPEP/UPEP)
         a) Both → tall electrophoretic peak called "M-spike" due to ↑ Ab
         b) SPEP → M-spike if clones make whole Ab

      c) UPEP → spike if clones make light chains only

      d) **Either SPEP or UPEP will almost always be** ⊕

   2) Dx = ⊕ SPEP/UPEP & any of **1)**↑ plasma cells in bone marrow, **2)** osteolytic bone lesions, **3)** Bence-Jones proteinuria

g. Tx

   1) Radiation given for isolated lesions, chemotherapy for metastatic dz

   2) Bone marrow transplantation may prolong survival

   3) Palliative care important for pain

h. Px poor despite Tx

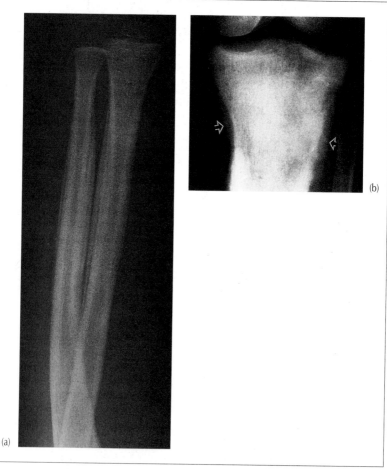

FIGURE 1-15   Different types of periosteal reactions. (a) Smooth lamellar periosteal reaction on the radius and ulna in a case of nonaccidental injury. (b) Spiculated (sunray) periosteal reaction in a case of osteogenic sarcoma (arrows). (c) Onion skin periosteal reaction in a case of Ewing's sarcoma (arrows). Here the periosteal new bone consists of several distinct layers. (d) Codman's triangle in a case of osteogenic sarcoma. At the edge of the lesion the periosteal new bone is lifted up to form a cuff (arrow).

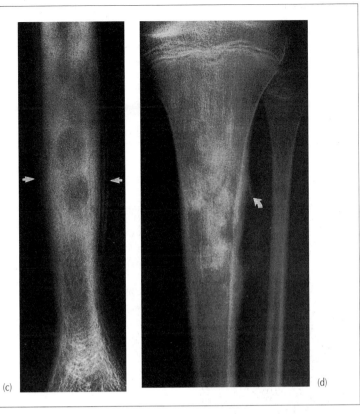

(c)

(d)

FIGURE 1-15   *Continued*

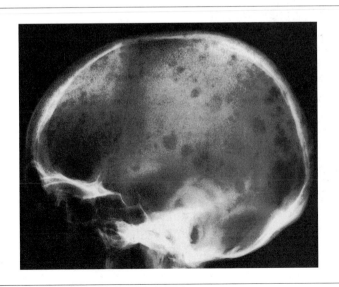

FIGURE 1-16   Myeloma.

IV. Arthropathies and Connective Tissue Disorders

A. RHEUMATOID ARTHRITIS (RA)

1. Autoimmune dz of unknown etiology → **symmetric inflammatory arthritis**
2. Female-male = 3:1, patients are commonly **HLA-DR4⊕**
3. Si/Sx = **symmetric arthritis worse in morning** affecting knees, feet, metacarpopha-
   langeal (**MCP**) & proximal interphalangeal (**PIP**) joints, pleural effusions (serositis),
   anemia of chronic dz, flexion contractures → ulnar deviation of digits, subQ nodules
   (present in <50% of pts)
4. Labs
   a. Rheumatoid factor (RF) = IgM anti-IgG
      1) Present in >70% of RA pts, but may appear late in dz course
      2) **Not specific for RA,** can be ⊕ in any chronic inflammatory state & may be
         present in 5–10% of healthy geriatric patients
   b. ESR is elevated in >90% cases, but is not specific for RA
5. **Dx = clinical,** no single factor is sufficient
6. Tx
   a. NSAIDs are first line, selective cyclooxygenase-2 inhibitors may be preferable
   b. Hydroxychloroquine second line, refractory pts → prednisone, gold salts, penicil-
      lamine, all of which cause severe side effects
   c. TNF antagonists markedly improve symptoms, even in patients refractory to
      standard therapy

B. SYSTEMIC LUPUS ERYTHEMATOSUS

1. Systemic autoimmune disorder, female-male = 9:1
2. Si/Sx = fever, polyarthritis, skin lesions, splenomegaly, hemolytic anemia, thrombocytopenia, serositis (e.g., pleuritis & pericarditis), Libman-Sacks endocarditis, renal dz,
   skin rashes, thrombosis, neurologic disorders
3. Labs
   a. **Antinuclear antibody (ANA) sensitive (>98%) but not specific**
   b. **Anti-double-stranded-DNA (anti-ds-DNA) antibodies 99% specific**
   c. Anti-Smith (anti-Sm) antibodies are highly specific but not sensitive
   d. Anti-Ro antibodies are ⊕ in 50% of ANA negative lupus
   e. Antiribosomal P & antineuronal antibodies correlate with risk for cerebral
      involvement of lupus (lupus cerebritis)
   f. Antiphospholipid autoantibodies cause false-positive lab tests in SLE
      1) **SLE pts frequently have false ⊕ RPR/VDRL tests for syphilis**
      2) **SLE pts frequently have ↑ PTT (lupus anticoagulant antibody)**
         a) PTT is falsely ↑ because the lupus anticoagulant antibody binds to
            phospholipid that initiates clotting in the test tube
         b) **Despite the PTT test & the name lupus anticoagulant antibody, SLE**
            patients are THROMBOGENIC, because antiphospholipid antibodies
            cause coagulation in vivo
4. Mnemonic for SLE diagnosis: **DOPAMINE RASH**
   a. **D**iscoid lupus = circular, erythematous macules with scales
   b. **O**ral aphthous ulcers (can be nasopharyngeal as well)
   c. **P**hotosensitivity

d. Arthritis (typically hands, wrists, knees)

e. Malar rash = classic butterfly macule on cheeks

f. Immunologic criteria = anti-ds-DNA, anti-Sm Ab, anti-Ro Ab, anti-La

g. Neurologic changes = psychosis, personality change, seizures

h. ESR rate ↑ (NOT 1 of the 11 criteria, but it is a frequent lab finding)

i. Renal disease → nephritic or nephrotic syndrome

j. ANA⊕

k. Serositis (pleurisy, pericarditis)

l. Hematologic dz = hemolytic anemia, thrombocytopenia, leukopenia

5. Drug-induced SLE

a. Drugs = procainamide, hydralazine, Dilantin, sulfonamides, INH

b. **Lab → antihistone antibodies**, differentiating from idiopathic SLE

6. Tx = NSAIDs, hydroxychloroquine, prednisone, cyclophosphamide depending on severity of dz

7. Px = variable, 10-yr survival is excellent, **renal dz is a poor Px indicator**

C. SJÖGREN'S SYNDROME (SS)

1. An autoinflammatory disorder associated with **HLA-DR3**

2. Si/Sx = **classic triad of keratoconjunctivitis sicca** (dry eyes), **xerostomia** (dry mouth), **arthritis**, usually less severe than pure RA

3. Systemic Si/Sx = pancreatitis, fibrinous pericarditis, CN V sensory neuropathy, renal tubular acidosis, 40-fold ↑ in lymphoma incidence

4. Dx = Concomitant presence of 2 of the triad is diagnostic

5. Lab → ANA⊕, anti-Ro/anti-La Ab⊕ ("SSA/SSB Abs"), 70% are RF⊕

6. Tx = steroids, cyclophosphamide for refractory disease

D. BEHÇET'S SYNDROME

1. Multisystem inflammatory disorder that chronically recurs

2. Si/Sx = painful oral & genital ulcers, also arthritis, vasculitis, neurologic dz

3. Tx = prednisone during flare-ups

E. SERONEGATIVE SPONDYLOARTHROPATHY

1. Osteoarthritis

a. **A noninflammatory arthritis** caused by joint wear & tear

b. The most common arthritis, results in wearing away of joint cartilage

c. Si/Sx = pain & crepitation upon joint motion, ↓ range of joint motion, can have radiculopathy due to cord impingement

d. **X-ray → osteophytes (bone spurs) & asymmetric joint space loss**

e. Physical exam → **Heberden's nodes** (DIP swelling 2° to osteophytes) & **Bouchard's nodes** (PIP swelling 2° to osteophytes)

f. **Note: RA affects MCP & PIP joints, osteoarthritis affects PIP & DIP**

g. Tx = NSAIDs, muscle relaxants, joint replacement (third line)

h. **Isometric exercise to strengthen muscles around joint has been shown to improve Sx**

2. Ankylosing spondylitis

a. Rheumatologic dz usually in **HLA-B27⊕** males (male-female = 3 : 1)

b. Si/Sx = sacroiliitis, spinal dz → complete fusion of adjacent vertebral bodies causing **"bamboo spine"** (See Figures 1-17 and 1-18), uveitis, heart block

c. **If sacroiliac joint is not affected, it is not ankylosing spondylitis!**

d. Dx = x-ray signs of spinal fusion & negative rheumatoid factor

e. Tx = NSAIDs & strengthening of back muscles

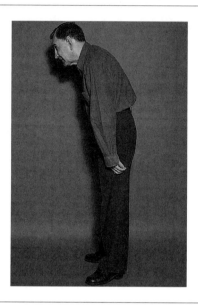

FIGURE 1-17   Spine. AS can cause a marked thoracic kyphosis with increased wall-to-tragus measurement.

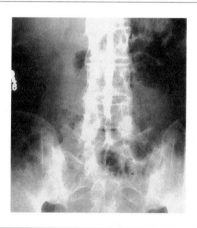

FIGURE 1-18   Radiograph of the lumbar spine (anteroposterior view). This patient has what is known as a "bamboo spine." There is syndesmophyte formation causing fusion of the vertebral bodies and there is also calcification of the interspinus ligament. The sacroiliac joints are also fused.

3. Reiter's syndrome
   a. Usually seen in males, **about 3/4 of these patients are HLA-B27⊕**
   b. Presents as nongonococcal **urethritis** (often chlamydial), **conjunctivitis, reactive arthritis** & **uveitis**
   c. Classic dermatologic Sx = **circinate balanitis** (serpiginous, moist plaques on glans penis) & **keratoderma blennorrhagicum** (crusting papules with central erosion, **looks like mollusk shell**)
   d. Tx = erythromycin (for *Chlamydia* coverage) + NSAIDs for arthritis
4. Psoriatic arthritis
   a. Presents with **nail-pitting** & **DIP** joint involvement
   b. Occurs in up to 10% of patients with psoriasis
   c. Psoriatic flares may exacerbate arthritis, & vice versa
   d. Tx = UV light for psoriasis & gold/penicillamine for arthritis
5. Inflammatory bowel disease can cause seronegative arthritis
6. Disseminated gonococcal infection can cause **monoarticular** arthritis

F. SCLERODERMA (PROGRESSIVE SYSTEMIC SCLEROSIS = PSS)
1. Systemic fibrosis affecting virtually every organ, female-male = 4 : 1
2. Can be diffuse disease (PSS), or more benign CREST syndrome
3. **Si/Sx of CREST syndrome**
   a. **C**alcinosis = subcutaneous calcifications, often in fingers (See Figure 1-19)
   b. **R**aynaud's phenomenon, often the initial symptom (See Figure 1-20)
   c. **E**sophagitis due to lower esophageal sphincter sclerosis → reflux
   d. **S**clerodactyly = fibrosed skin causes immobile digits & rigid facies (See Figure 1-21)
   e. **T**elangiectasias occur in mouth, on digits, face & trunk (See Figure 1-22)
4. Other Sx = flexion contractures, biliary cirrhosis, lung/cardiac/renal fibrosis
5. Lab = ⊕ ANA in 95%, anti-Scl-70 has ↓ sensitivity but ↑ specificity, anticentromere is 80% sensitive for CREST syndrome
6. Dx = clinical
7. Tx = immunosuppressives for palliation, none are curative

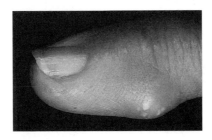

FIGURE 1-19   Subcutaneous and periarticular calcium deposits may occur and can be extremely painful.

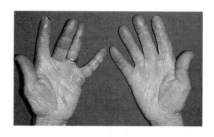

FIGURE 1-20   Raynaud's disease. Cyanosis of the fingers due to arterial vasoconstriction, which in this patient has resulted in an area of infarction of the left forefinger.

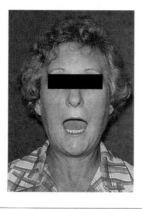

FIGURE 1-21   Scleroderma may cause thickening of the skin around the mouth and an inability to open the jaw fully.

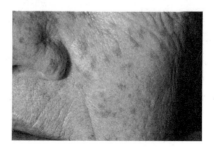

FIGURE 1-22   Telangiectasia in a patient with systemic sclerosis.

G. SARCOIDOSIS

1. Idiopathic, diffuse dz presenting in 20s to 40s, **African Americans are 3x more likely to develop than Caucasians**
2. Si/Sx = **50% of pts present with incidental finding on CXR & are aSx**, other presentations include fevers, chills, night sweats, weight loss, cough, dyspnea, rash, arthralgia, blurry vision (uveitis)
3. **CXR → bilateral hilar adenopathy** (See Figure 1-23)
4. Can affect ANY organ system
    a. CNS → CN palsy, classically CN VII (can be bilateral)
    b. **Eye → uveitis (can be bilateral), requires aggressive Tx**
    c. Cardiac → heart blocks, arrhythmias, constrictive pericarditis
    d. Lung → typically a restrictive defect
    e. GI → ↑ AST/ALT, CT → granulomas in liver, cholestasis
    f. Renal → nephrolithiasis due to hypercalcemia
    g. Endocrine → diabetes insipidus
    h. Hematologic → anemia, thrombocytopenia, leukopenia
    i. Skin → various rashes, including erythema nodosum
5. Dx is clinical, **noncaseating granulomas on biopsy is very suggestive**
6. Lab → 50% pts have ↑ angiotensin converting enzyme level
7. Tx = prednisone (first line), but 50% pts spontaneously remit, so only Tx if 1) eye/heart involved, 2) dz does not remit after months

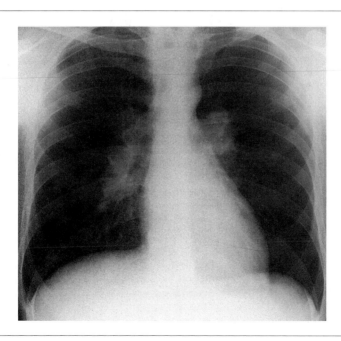

FIGURE 1-23   Bilateral hilar lymphadenopathy.

H. Mixed Connective Tissue Disease (MCTD)

1. Commonly onsets in women in teens & 20s
2. Si/Sx = overlapping SLE, scleroderma & polymyositis, but **characterized by ⊕ anti-U1 RNP antibody that defines the dz**
3. Dx = anti-U1RNP antibody
4. Tx = steroids, azathioprine

I. Gout

1. **Monoarticular arthritis** due to urate crystal deposits in joint
2. **Gout develops after 20–30 yrs of hyperuricemia, often precipitated by sudden changes in serum urate levels** (gout in teens → 20s likely genetic)
3. **Most people with hyperuricemia never get gout**
4. ↑ production of uric acid can be genetic or acquired (e.g., alcohol, hemolysis, neoplasia, psoriasis)
5. Underexcretion of urate via kidney (<800 mg/dL urine urate) can be idiopathic or due to kidney dz, drugs (aspirin, diuretics, alcohol)
6. Si/Sx of gout = painful monoarticular arthritis affecting distal joints (often first metatarsophalangeal joint = **podagra** [See Figure 1-24a]), **overlying skin erythema** (See Figure 1-24b)
7. Dx = **clinical triad of monoarticular arthritis, hyperuricemia, ⊕ response to colchicine** (see below), confirm with needle tap of joint → crystals
8. Acute Tx = colchicine & NSAIDs (not aspirin!)
9. Px = some people never suffer more than 1 attack, those that do → chronic tophaceous gout, with significant joint deformation (**classic rat-bite appearance to joint on x-ray**) & toothpaste-like discharge from joint
10. Maintenance Tx
    a. Do not start unless patient has more than 1 attack
    b. Over-producers → allopurinol (inhibits xanthine oxidase)
    c. Under-excreters → probenecid/sulfinpyrazone
    d. **Always start while pt still taking colchicine, because sudden ↓ in serum urate precipitates an acute attack**
11. Pseudogout
    a. Caused by calcium pyrophosphate dihydrate (CPPD) crystal deposition in joints & articular cartilage (chondrocalcinosis)
    b. Mimics gout very closely, seen in persons age 60 or older, often affects larger, more proximal joints
    c. Can be 1° or 2° to metabolic dz (hyperparathyroidism, Wilson's dz, diabetes, hemochromatosis)
    d. Dx → microscopic analysis of joint aspirate
    e. Tx = colchicine & NSAIDs
12. Microscopy
    a. Gout → **needle-like negatively birefringent crystals** (See Color Plate 2)
    b. **"P"seudogout → "P"ositively birefringent crystals** (See Color Plate 3)

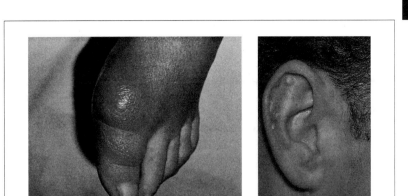

FIGURE 1-24   Gout. (a) Acute gouty arthritis affecting the big toe. This is extremely painful. (b) Urate crystal deposition in the cartilage of the ear.

V. Muscle Diseases

A. GENERAL
1. Diseases of muscle are divided into 2 groups: neurogenic & myopathic
2. Neurogenic diseases → **distal weakness, no pain, fasciculations present**
3. Myopathic diseases → **proximal weakness, ± pain, no fasciculations**

B. DUCHENNE'S MUSCULAR DYSTROPHY
1. **X-linked** lack of dystrophin
2. Si/Sx commence at 1 yr of age with **progressive proximal weakness & wasting,** ↑ CPK, **calf hypertrophy,** waddling gait, Gower's maneuver (pts pick themselves off the floor by using arms to help legs)
3. Tx = supportive
4. Px = death occurs in 10s–20s, most often due to pneumonia
5. Becker's dystrophy is similar but less severe disease

C. POLYMYOSITIS
1. Autoinflammatory dz of muscles & sometimes skin (dermatomyositis)
2. Female-male = 2 : 1, occurs in young children & geriatric populations
3. Si/Sx = symmetric weakness/atrophy of proximal limb muscles, muscle aches, dysphonia (laryngeal muscle weakness), dysphagia
4. Dermatomyositis presents with periorbital heliotropic red to purple rash
5. Dx = ANA⊕, ↑ creatine kinase, muscle biopsy → inflammatory changes
6. Tx = steroids, methotrexate or cyclophosphamide for resistant disease

D. MYASTHENIA GRAVIS (MG)
1. Autoantibodies block the postsynaptic acetylcholine receptor
2. Most common in women in 20s–30s or men in 50s–60s
3. **Associated with thymomas, thyroid & other autoimmune dz (e.g., lupus)**
4. Sx = **muscle weakness worse with use,** diplopia, dysphagia, proximal limb weakness, can progress to cause respiratory failure

5. Dx = trial of edrophonium → immediate ↑ in strength, confirm with electromyelography → repetitive stimulation ↓ action potential
6. DDx
   a. **Lambert-Eaton syndrome**
      1) AutoAb to **pre**synaptic Ca channels seen with small cell lung CA
      2) Differs from MG in that Lambert-Eaton → ↓ reflexes, autonomic dysfunction (xerostomia, impotence) & **Sx improve with muscle use (action potential strength ↑ with repeated stimulation)**
   b. Aminoglycosides worsen MG, or induce mild MG Sx in normal people
7. Tx = anticholinesterase inhibitors (e.g., pyridostigmine) first line
   a. Steroids, cyclophosphamide, azathioprine for ↑ severe dz
   b. Plasmapheresis temporarily alleviates Sx by removing the Ab
   c. Resection of thymoma can be curative

Hematology (See Figure 1-25)

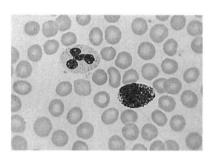

FIGURE 1-25 Normal blood films.

I. Anemia

A. MICROCYTIC ANEMIAS (≡ MCV <80)
1. **Result from ↓ hemoglobin (Hgb) production or impaired Hgb function**
2. Iron deficiency anemia
   a. **NOT a Dx, must find the cause of iron deficiency!!!**
   b. Epidemiology
      1) #1 anemia in the world, hookworms the #1 cause in the world
      2) ↑ incidence in women of childbearing age 2° to menses
      3) **In the elderly it is colon cancer until proven otherwise!**
      4) Dietary deficiency **virtually impossible in adults, seen in kids**
   c. Si/Sx = tachycardia, fatigue, pallor all from anemia, smooth tongue, brittle nails, esophageal webs & pica all from iron deficiency
   d. Dx = ↓ **serum iron**, ↓ serum ferritin, ↑ **total iron binding capacity (TIBC)**, peripheral smear → target cells
   e. Tx = iron sulfate, should achieve baseline hematocrit within 2 mo

3. Sideroblastic anemia
   a. Ineffective erythropoiesis due to disorder of porphyrin pathway
   b. Etiologies = chronic alcoholism, drugs (commonly isoniazid), genetic
   c. Si/Sx as per any anemia
   d. Labs: ↑ **iron**, N/↑ TIBC, ↑ ferritin
   e. Dx = ringed sideroblasts on iron stain of bone marrow
   f. Tx = sometimes responsive to pyridoxine (vitamin B_6 supplements)
4. Lead poisoning
   a. Si/Sx = anemia, encephalopathy (worse in children), seizures, ataxic gait, **wrist/foot drops**, renal tubular acidosis
   b. Classic findings
      1) **Bruton's lines** = blue/gray discoloration at gumlines
      2) **Basophilic stippling of red cells (blue dots in red cells)**
   c. Dx = serum lead level
   d. Tx = chelation with dimercaprol (BAL) &/or EDTA
5. Thalassemias
   a. Hereditary dz of ↓ production of globin chains → ↓ Hgb production
   b. Differentiation through gel-electrophoresis of globin proteins
   c. α-Thalassemia (↓ α-globin chain synthesis, there are 4 α alleles)
      1) Seen commonly in Asians, less so in Africans & Mediterraneans
      2)

TABLE 1-33   α-Thalassemia

#ALLELES AFFECTED/DZ		CHARACTERISTIC	BLOOD SMEAR
4	Hydrops fetalis	Fetal demise, total body edema	Bart's β_4 Hgb precipitations
3	Hgb H disease	Precipitation of β-chain tetramers	Intraerythrocytic inclusions
2	α-Thalassemia minor	Usually clinically silent	Mild microcytic anemia
1	Carrier state	No anemia, asymptomatic	No abnormalities

   d. β-Thalassemia (↓ β-globin chain synthesis, there are 2 β alleles)
      1) Usually of Mediterranean or African descent
      2)

TABLE 1-34   β-Thalassemia

	THALASSEMIA MAJOR (β–/β–)	THALASSEMIA MINOR (β+/β–)
Si/Sx	Anemia develops at 6 mo old (due to switch from fetal γ Hgb to adult β), splenomegaly, frontal bossing due to extramedullary hematopoiesis, iron overload (2° to transfusions)	Typically asymptomatic carriers
Dx	**Electrophoresis** ↓↓↓ Hgb A, ↑ Hgb A2, ↑ **Hgb F**	**Electrophoresis** ↓ Hgb A, ↑ Hgb A2(γ), **N Hgb F**
Tx	Folate supplementation, splenectomy for hypersplenism, transfuse only for severe anemia	Avoid oxidative stress

6. Sickle cell anemia (See Figure 1-26)
   a. HgS tetramer polymerizes, causing sickling of deoxygenated RBCs
   b. Si/Sx
      1) Vaso-occlusion → pain crisis, myocardiopathy, infarcts of bone/CNS/lungs/kidneys & autosplenectomy due to splenic infarct → ↑susceptible to encapsulated bacteria
      2) **Intravascular hemolysis → gallstones in children or teens**
      3) ↑ risk of aplastic anemia from parvovirus B19 infections
   c. Dx = hemoglobin electrophoresis → HgS phenotype
   d. Tx
      1) O_2 (cells sickle when Hgb desaturates), transfuse as needed
      2) Hydroxyurea → ↓ incidence & severity of pain crises
      3) Pneumococcal vaccination due to ↑ risk of infection

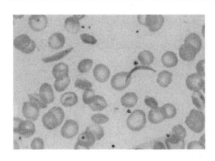

FIGURE 1-26   Sickle cell anemia.

B. MEGALOBLASTIC ANEMIAS (≡ MCV >100)

1. **Results from ↓ DNA synthesis with normal RNA/protein synthesis**
2. **Pathognomonic blood smear → hypersegmented neutrophils** (See Figure 1-27)
3. Vitamin B_{12} deficiency
   a. Pernicious anemia is most common cause
      1) Antibody to gastric parietal cells → ↓ production of intrinsic factor (necessary for uptake of B_{12} in the terminal ileum)
      2) Accompanied by achlorhydria & atrophic gastritis
   b. Other causes = malabsorption due to gastric resection, resection of terminal ileum, or intestinal infection by *Diphyllobothrium latum*
   c. Si/Sx = megaloblastic anemia **with neurologic signs** = peripheral neuropathy, paresthesias, ↓ balance & position sense, **worse in legs**
   d. **Dx = ↑serum methylmalonic acid & ↑ homocysteine levels**—more sensitive than B_{12} levels, which may or may not be ↓
   e. Tx = Vitamin B_{12}, high-dose oral Tx proven equivalent to parenteral
4. Folic acid deficiency
   a. Folic acid derived from green, leafy vegetables ("foliage")

b. Causes = dietary deficiency (most common), pregnancy or hemolytic anemia (↑ requirements), methotrexate or prolonged Bactrim Tx (inhibits reduction of folate into tetrahydrofolate)

c. Si/Sx = megaloblastic anemia, no neurologic signs

d. Dx = **Nml serum methylmalonic acid but ↑ homocysteine levels**—more sensitive than folate levels, which may or may not be ↓

e. Tx = oral folic acid supplementation

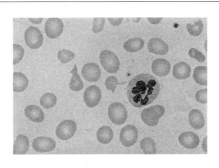

FIGURE 1-27 Hypersegmented neutrophil in severe pernicious anemia; also see ovalocytes.

C. NORMOCYTIC ANEMIAS
1.

TABLE 1-35 Hypoproliferative Anemias

DISEASE	CHARACTERISTICS	TX
Anemia of renal failure	• ↓ erythropoietin production by kidney • Indicates chronic renal failure	Erythropoietin IM 3x per week
Anemia of chronic dz	• Seen in chronic inflammation (e.g., cancer, TB or fungal infxn, collagen-vascular dz) • Dx = ↓ **serum iron**, Nml/↑ ferritin, ↓**TIBC**	Tx underlying inflammatory dz, supportive
Aplastic anemia	• Bone marrow failure, usually idiopathic, or due to parvovirus B19 (especially in sickle cell), hepatitis virus, radiation, drugs (e.g., chloramphenicol) • Dx = bone marrow Bx → hypocellular marrow	BMT[a] for severe dz, ATG[b] & cyclosporin may help for mild dz

[a] BMT = bone marrow transplantation.
[b] ATG = antithymocyte globulin.

2.

TABLE 1-36   Hemolytic Anemias

DISEASE	CHARACTERISTICS	TX
Intrinsic Hemolysis (RBC defects)		
Spherocytosis	• Autosomal dominant membrane protein defect (fibrillin) → spherical, stiff RBCs trapped in the spleen • Si/Sx = childhood jaundice & gallstones, indirect hyperbilirubinemia, Coombs negative • Dx = clinical ⊕ peripheral smear → spherocytes	Folic acid, splenectomy for severe dz
Extrinsic Hemolysis		
Autoimmune hemolysis (IgG-mediated)	• Etiologies = idiopathic (most common), lupus, drugs (e.g., penicillin), leukemia, lymphoma • Si/Sx = rapid-onset, **spherocytes on blood smear**, ↑ indirect bilirubin, jaundice, **↓ haptoglobin, ↑ urine hemosiderin** • Dx = ⊕ direct Coombs' test	First line = prednisone +/– splenectomy, cyclophosphamide for refractory dz
Cold-agglutinin disease (IgM-mediated)	• Most commonly idiopathic, can be due to *Mycoplasma pneumoniae* & mononucleosis (CMV, EBV infxns) • Si/Sx = anemia on exposure to cold or following URI • Dx = cold-agglutinin test & indirect Coombs' test	Prednisone for severe dz, supportive for mild
Mechanical destruction	• Causes = disseminated intravascular coagulation (DIC), thrombotic thrombocytopenic purpura (TTP), hemolytic-uremic syndrome (HUS) & artificial heart valve • Peripheral smear → schistocytes (See Figure 1-28)	Tx directed at underlying disorder

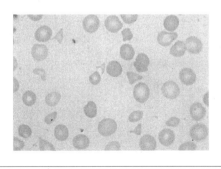

FIGURE 1-28   Schistocytes in patient with malfunctioning aortic valve.

II. Coagulation Disorders

A. THROMBOCYTOPENIA

1. Caused by splenic sequestration, stem-cell failure, or ↑ destruction
2. Si/Sx = bleeding time ↑ at counts < 50,000, clinically significant bleeds start at counts < 20,000, CNS bleeds occur when counts < 10,000
3. ↓ production seen in leukemia, aplastic anemia & alcohol (even minimal)
4.

TABLE 1-37   Causes of Platelet Destruction (Thrombocytopenia)

DISEASE	CHARACTERISTICS	TX
Idiopathic thrombocytopenic purpura (ITP)	• Autoantibody-mediated platelet destruction • **In children follows URI & is self-limiting, in adults it is chronic**	Steroids (first line), splenectomy (second line) or cyclophosphamide
Thrombotic thrombocytopenic purpura (TTP)	• Idiopathic dz, often seen in HIV, can be fatal • **Pentad** = hemolytic anemia, renal failure, thrombocytopenia, fever, neurologic dz	Plasma exchange or IVIG until dz abates, dz is fatal without Tx
Hemolytic-uremic syndrome (HUS)	• Usually in kids, often due to E. coli O157:H7 • Si/Sx = acute renal failure, bloody diarrhea & abdominal pain, seizures, **fulminant thrombocytopenia with hemolytic anemia**	Dialysis helps children, but adult Px is much poorer
Disseminated intravascular coagulation (DIC)	• Seen in adenocarcinoma, leukemia, sepsis, trauma • ↑ fibrin-split products, ↓ fibrinogen, ↑ PT/PTT	Directed at underlying cause
Drug-induced	• Causes = heparin, sulfonamides, valproate • Reverses within days of ceasing drug intake	Stop drug

5.

TABLE 1-38   Labs in Platelet Destruction

STUDY	AUTOANTIBODY	DIC	TTP/HUS
Blood smear	Microspherocytes	Schistocytes (+)	**Schistocytes (+++)**
Coombs' test	⊕	–	–
PT/PTT	Nml	↑↑↑	Nml/↑

B. INHERITED DISORDERS

1. von-Willebrand factor (vWF) deficiency
   a. **Most common inherited bleeding dz**
   b. Si/Sx = **episodic ↑ bleeding time & ecchymoses, normal PT/PTT**
   c. Dx = vWF levels & ristocetin-cofactor test
   d. Tx = DDAVP (↑ vWF secretion) or cryoprecipitate for acute bleeding
2. Hemophilia
   a. X-linked deficiency of factor VIII (hemophilia A) or autosomal recessive defect of factor IX (hemophilia B = Christmas disease)
   b. Si/Sx = hemarthroses (bleeding into joint), ecchymoses with minor trauma, **↑ PTT, normal PT, normal bleeding time**
   c. Dx = ↓ factor levels
   d. Tx = recombinant factor VIII or factor IX concentrate

C. Hypercoagulable Diseases

TABLE 1-39   Hypercoagulable Diseases

PRIMARY (INHERITED)	SECONDARY (ACQUIRED)	
Antithrombin III deficiency	Prolonged immobilization	L-asparaginase
Protein C deficiency	Pregnancy	Hyperlipidemia
Protein S deficiency	Surgery/Trauma	Anticardiolipin Ab
Factor V Leiden deficiency	Oral contraceptives	Lupus anticoagulant
Dysfibrinogenemia	Homocystinuria	DIC
Plasminogen (activator) deficiency	Malignancy (adenocarcinoma)	Vitamin K deficiency
Heparin cofactor II deficiency	Smoking	
Homocystinemia	Nephrotic syndrome	
Factor II (prothrombin) mutation		

III. Myeloproliferative Diseases

1. Caused by clonal proliferation of a myeloid stem cell → excessive production of mature, differentiated myeloid cell lines
2. All can transform into acute leukemias
3.

TABLE 1-40   Myeloproliferative Diseases

DISEASE	CHARACTERISTICS	TX
Polycythemia vera	• Rare, peak onset at 50–60 yr, male predominance • Si/Sx = headache, diplopia, retinal hemorrhages, stroke, angina, claudication (all due to vascular sludging), early satiety, splenomegaly, gout, **pruritus after showering, plethora, basophilia** • **5% progress to leukemia, 20% to myelofibrosis**	Phlebotomy, hydroxyurea to keep blood counts low
Essential thrombocythemia	• Si/Sx = platelet count >5 × 10⁵ cells/μL, splenomegaly, ecchymoses • Dx = rule out 2° thrombocytosis (due to iron deficiency, malignancy, etc.) • 5% progress to myelofibrosis or acute leukemia	Platelet exchange (apheresis), hydroxyurea or anagrelide
Idiopathic myelofibrosis	• Typically affects patients ≥ 50 yr • Si/Sx = massive hepatosplenomegaly, blood smear → **teardrop cells** • Dx = hypercellular marrow on biopsy • Poor Px, median 5 yr before marrow failure	Supportive (splenectomy, antibiotics, allopurinol for gout)

Chronic myelogenous leukemia—see below.

4. Thrombocytosis
   a. 1° (essential) versus 2° (reactive)
   b. 1° can be Essential Thrombocythemia, but can also see a thrombocytosis in polycythemia rubra vera or chronic myelogenous leukemia
   c. 2° or reactive thrombocytosis can be seen in any chronic inflammatory disorder, serious infection, acute bleed, iron-deficiency anemia (mechanism unclear), or following splenectomy

IV. Leukemias

A. Acute Lymphoblastic Leukemia
1. **Peak age 3–4 yr**, most common neoplasm in children

2. Si/Sx = fever, fatigue, anemia, pallor, petechiae, infections
3. Lab → leukocytosis, anemia, ↓ platelets, marrow bx → ↑ blasts, peripheral blood blasts are **PAS +, CALLA +, TdT +**
4. Tx = chemotherapy: induction, consolidation, maintenance—CNS radiation or intrathecal chemotherapy during consolidation
5. Px = 80% cure in children (much worse in adults)

B. Acute Myelogenous Leukemia (AML)

1. **Most common leukemia in adults**
2. Si/Sx = fever, fatigue, pallor, petechiae, infections, lymphadenopathy
3. Lab → thrombocytopenia, peripheral blood & marrow bx → myeloblasts that are **myeloperoxidase +, Sudan Black +, Auer Rods +**
4. Tx
   a. Chemotherapy → induction, consolidation (no maintenance)
   b. All-trans retinoic acid used for a subtype of AML, causes differentiation of blasts, beware of onset of disseminated intravascular coagulation in these patients
5. Px = overall 30% cure, bone marrow transplant improves outcomes

C. Chronic Myelogenous Leukemia

1. Presents most commonly in the 50s, can be any age
2. Si/Sx = anorexia, early satiety, diaphoresis, arthritis, bone tenderness, leukostasis (WBC $\geq 1 \times 10^5$) → dyspnea, dizzy, slurred speech, diplopia
3. Labs → **Philadelphia chromosome** ⊕ (see below), **peripheral blood → cells of all maturational stages**, ↓ leukocyte alkaline phosphatase
4. Philadelphia (Ph) chromosome is pathognomonic, seen in > 90% of CML pts, due to translocation of *abl* gene from chromosome 9 to *bcr* on 22
5. Tx in chronic phase = reduction of WBC count with hydroxyurea or interferon (IFN)-α, or brand new Tx with the drug-designed tyrosine kinase inhibitor, signal transduction inhibitor (STI)-571, which specifically blocks the oncogenic tyrosine kinase protein formed by the *bcr:abl* translocation
6. **Blast crisis = acute phase, invariably develops causing death in 3–6 mo, mean time to onset = 3–4 yr, only BMT can prevent**

D. Chronic Lymphocytic Leukemia

1. Increasing incidence with age, causes 30% of leukemias in US
2. Si/Sx = organomegaly, hemolytic anemia, thrombocytopenia, blood smear & marrow → normal morphology lymphocytosis of blood & marrow, **lymphocytes almost always express CD5 protein**
3. **Tx = palliative, early therapy does NOT prolong life**
4. Other presentations of similar leukemias
   a. Hairy cell leukemia (B-cell subtype)
      1) Si/Sx = characteristic hairy cell morphology, pancytopenia
      2) Tx = interferon-α, splenectomy
   b. T-cell leukemias tend to involve skin, often present with erythematous rashes, some are due to human T-cell leukemia virus (HTLV)

Most Common Leukemias by Age:
Up to age 15 = ALL; age 15–39 = AML; age 40–59 = AML & CML;
60 & over = CLL

V. Lymphoma

A. NON-HODGKIN'S LYMPHOMA (NHL)

1. Commonly seen in HIV, often in brain, teenagers get in head & neck
2. Burkitt's lymphoma
    a. Closely related to Epstein-Barr virus (EBV) infections
    b. African Burkitt's involves jaw/neck, US Burkitt's involves abdomen
3. Cutaneous T-cell lymphoma (CTCL, mycosis fungoides)
    a. Si/Sx = often in elderly, diffuse scaly rash or erythroderma (total body erythema), precedes clinically apparent malignancy by years
    b. **Stained cells have cerebriform nuclei** (looks like cerebral gyri)
    c. Leukemic phase of this disease is called "Sézary syndrome"
    d. Tx = UV light therapy, consider systemic chemotherapy
4. Angiocentric T-cell lymphoma
    a. 2 subtypes = nasal T-cell lymphoma (lethal midline granuloma) & pulmonary angiocentric lymphoma
    b. Si/Sx = large mass, biopsy often non-Dx due to diffuse necrosis
    c. Tx = palliative radiation therapy, Px very poor

B. HODGKIN'S LYMPHOMA

1. Occurs in a bimodal age distribution, young men & the elderly
2. EBV infection is present in up to 50% of cases
3. Si/Sx = **Pel-Epstein fevers** (fevers wax & wane over weeks), chills, night sweats, weight loss, pruritus, **Sx worsen with alcohol intake**
4. Reed-Sternberg (RS) cells seen on biopsy, **appear as binucleated giant cells ("owl eyes")** or **mononucleated giant cell (lacunar cell)** (See Figure 1-29)
5. Tx depends on clinical staging
    a. Stage I = 1 lymph node involved → radiation
    b. Stage II = ≥ 2 lymph nodes on same side of diaphragm → radiation
    c. Stage III = involvement on both sides of diaphragm → chemo
    d. Stage IV = disseminated to organs or extranodal tissue → chemo
    e. Chemo regimens
        1) MOPP = **m**eclorethamine, **o**ncovin (vincristine), **p**rocarbazine, **p**rednisone
        2) ABVD = **a**driamycin, **b**leomycin, **v**incristine, **d**acarbazine

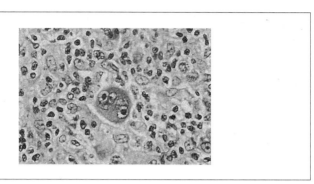

FIGURE 1-29 Reed-Sternberg cell in patient with Hodgkin's disease.

VI. Acid/base and Electrolytes

Disorder	pH	PCO_2	HCO_3-
Respiratory acidosis			
Acute	↓	↑	↑
Chronic	N	↑	⬆
Respiratory alkalosis			
Acute	↑	↓	↓
Chronic	N	↓	⬇
Metabolic acidosis			
Acute	↓	N	↓
Chronic	N	⬇	↓
Metabolic alkalosis	↑	↑	⬆

FIGURE 1-30 Acid/base disorders.

DETERMINATION OF PRIMARY ACID-BASE DISORDER

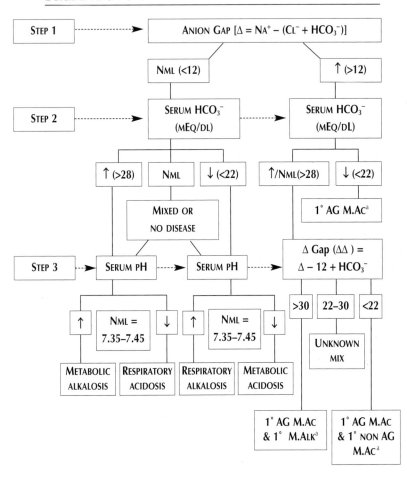

STEP 1 ----→ ANION GAP [$\Delta = NA^+ - (CL^- + HCO_3^-)$]

NML (<12)   ↑ (>12)

STEP 2 ----→ SERUM HCO_3^- (MEQ/DL) ----→ SERUM HCO_3^- (MEQ/DL)

↑ (>28)   NML   ↓ (<22)   ↑/NML(>28)   ↓ (<22)

MIXED OR NO DISEASE   1° AG M.Ac[a]

STEP 3 ---→ SERUM PH ---→ SERUM PH ----→ Δ Gap ($\Delta\Delta$) = $\Delta - 12 + HCO_3^-$

>30   22–30   <22

↑   NML = 7.35–7.45   ↓   ↑   NML = 7.35–7.45   ↓   UNKNOWN MIX

METABOLIC ALKALOSIS   RESPIRATORY ACIDOSIS   RESPIRATORY ALKALOSIS   METABOLIC ACIDOSIS

1° AG M.Ac & 1° M.Alk[a]   1° AG M.Ac & 1° NON AG M.Ac[a]

[a] AG = anion gap. M.Alk = metabolic alkalosis. M.Ac = metabolic acidosis.

METABOLIC ACIDOSIS

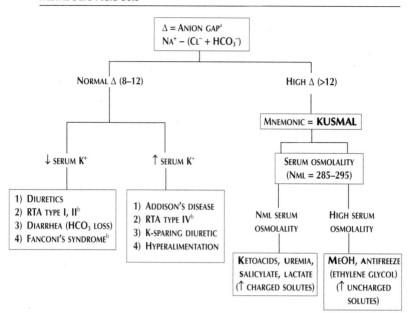

$\Delta = \text{ANION GAP}^a$
$\text{NA}^+ - (\text{CL}^- + \text{HCO}_3^-)$

NORMAL Δ (8–12)   HIGH Δ (>12)

MNEMONIC = **KUSMAL**

↓ SERUM K⁺   ↑ SERUM K⁺   SERUM OSMOLALITY (NML = 285–295)

1) DIURETICS
2) RTA TYPE I, II[b]
3) DIARRHEA (HCO₃ LOSS)
4) FANCONI'S SYNDROME[b]

1) ADDISON'S DISEASE
2) RTA TYPE IV[b]
3) K-SPARING DIURETIC
4) HYPERALIMENTATION

NML SERUM OSMOLALITY   HIGH SERUM OSMOLALITY

KETOACIDS, UREMIA, SALICYLATE, LACTATE (↑ CHARGED SOLUTES)

MeOH, ANTIFREEZE (ETHYLENE GLYCOL) (↑ UNCHARGED SOLUTES)

Check for compensation or the presence of a mixed disorder. Winter's formula predicts the CO_2 if there is compensation: $CO_2 = 1.5 * HCO_3^- + 8 \pm 2$. If the CO_2 is higher than expected, there is an additional acidotic process occurring. If the CO_2 is lower than expected, there is an additional alkalotic process occurring.

---

[a] Calculate Δ in *all* patients, regardless of pH or HCO_3^-. Mixed acidosis and alkalosis can cancel each other out, causing neutral pH. Perform the following steps to search for a mixed disorder.
1) Calculate Δ: if $\Delta \geq 12$, the disorder is a 1° anion gap acidosis
2) Calculate $\Delta\Delta = [\Delta - 12 + HCO_3^-]$: if $\Delta\Delta \geq 31$, there is also a 1° metabolic alkalosis
       if $\Delta\Delta \leq 21$, there is also a 1° *non*anion gap acidosis
Example: A diabetic in ketoacidosis who is vomiting can have a 1° anion gap acidosis from the ketoacidosis and a 1° metabolic alkalosis from the vomiting. In this case, the $\Delta > 12$, the $\Delta\Delta \geq 31$. A diabetic with renal failure who presents with ketoacidosis can have a 1° anion gap and nonanion gap acidosis, with a $\Delta > 12$ and a $\Delta\Delta \leq 21$. Note that this patient may also be vomiting and either tachypneic or bradypneic from obtundation. Thus the patient may have three 1° metabolic acid-base disorders (1° AG acidosis, 1° nonAG acidosis, 1° metabolic alkalosis) and a respiratory disorder. In this case, the disorders must be discriminated clinically or by changes in status in response to therapy.
     Our thanks to Dr. Arian Torbati for his assistance with the $\Delta\Delta$ algorithm.
[b] See Section III.F for description of RTA and Fanconi's syndrome.

METABOLIC ALKALOSIS

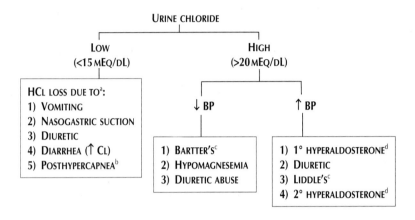

---

[a] These conditions are all known as "contraction alkaloses," or "chloride-responsive alkaloses." The contraction in extracellular volume creates a hypochloremic state. The kidney resorbs extra bicarbonate from the tubules due to the loss of chloride anion (tubules need a different anion to maintain electrical neutrality). Administration of chloride anion in the form of normal saline will correct the alkalosis.

[b] Patients who are hypercapnic undergo renal compensation, with resorption of extra bicarb from the tubules to offset the respiratory acidosis. When the hypercapnia is corrected (e.g., via intubation) the kidneys must adjust and resorb less bicarb. Until they adjust, the patient will have a posthypercapnic metabolic alkalosis.

[c] See Appendix B for Bartter's & Liddle's.

[d] 1° hyperaldosteronism is known as Conn's syndrome. See Endocrinology, Section III.D.1. 2° hyperaldosteronism can be caused by renal artery stenosis (see Nephrology, Section V), Cushing's syndrome (see Endocrine, Section III.B), congestive heart failure, and hepatic cirrhosis.

RESPIRATORY ACID-BASE DIFFERENTIAL

RESPIRATORY ALKALOSIS
• CNS LESION
• PREGNANCY
• HIGH ALTITUDE
• SEPSIS/INFECTION
• SALICYLATE TOXICITY
• LIVER FAILURE
• ANXIETY (HYPERVENTILATION)
• PAIN/FEAR (HYPERVENTILATION)
• CONGESTIVE HEART FAILURE
• PULMONARY EMBOLUS
• PNEUMONIA
• HYPERTHYROIDISM
• COMPENSATION FOR A 1° ACIDOSIS

RESPIRATORY ACIDOSIS
• MORPHINE/SEDATIVES
• STROKE IN BULBAR AREA OF BRAIN STEM
• ONDINE'S CURSE (CENTRAL SLEEP APNEA)
• COPD (EMPHYSEMA, ASTHMA, BRONCHITIS)
• ADULT RESPIRATORY DISTRESS SYNDROME
• CHEST WALL DISEASE (POLIO, KYPHOSCOLIOSIS, MYASTHENIA GRAVIS, MUSCULAR DYSTROPHY)
• OBESITY
• HYPOPHOSPHATEMIA (DIAPHRAGM REQUIRES LOTS OF ATP DUE TO HIGH ENERGY DEMAND)
• SUCCINYLCHOLINE (PARALYSIS FOR INTUBATION)
• PLEURAL EFFUSION
• PNEUMOTHORAX

Check for the presence of a mixed disorder by comparing the change in CO_2 and HCO_3 from normal (normal CO_2 = 40, normal HCO_3 = 24).

Acute respiratory acidosis: HCO_3^- increases by 1 for every 10 the CO_2 increases.
Acute respiratory alkalosis: HCO_3^- decreases by 2 for every 10 the CO_2 decreases.
Chronic respiratory acidosis: HCO_3^- increases by 3.5 for every 10 the CO_2 increases.
Chronic respiratory alkalosis: HCO_3^- decreases by 5 for every 10 the CO_2 decreases.

It's easy to remember the compensations by organizing them in the following table.

	ACIDOSIS	ALKALOSIS
Acute	1	2
Chronic	3–4 (3.5)	5
Change in HCO_3^- per 10 change in CO_2. Just remember = 1 : 2 : 3–4 : 5!		

As usual, if the CO_2 is higher than predicted, there is a mixed acidotic process. If the CO_2 is lower than predicted, there is a mixed alkalotic process.

EVALUATION OF HYPONATREMIA

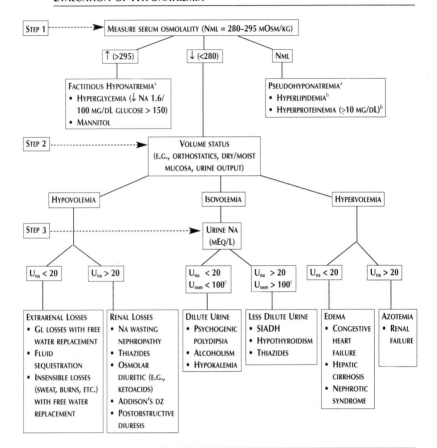

STEP 1 ┄┄┄┄> MEASURE SERUM OSMOLALITY (NML = 280–295 MOSM/KG)

↑ (>295)   ↓ (<280)   NML

FACTITIOUS HYPONATREMIA[a]
• HYPERGLYCEMIA (↓ NA 1.6/ 100 MG/DL GLUCOSE > 150)
• MANNITOL

PSEUDOHYPONATREMIA[a]
• HYPERLIPIDEMIA[b]
• HYPERPROTEINEMIA (>10 MG/DL)[b]

STEP 2 ┄┄┄┄> VOLUME STATUS
(E.G., ORTHOSTATICS, DRY/MOIST MUCOSA, URINE OUTPUT)

HYPOVOLEMIA   ISOVOLEMIA   HYPERVOLEMIA

STEP 3 ┄┄┄┄> URINE NA
(MEQ/L)

$U_{na} < 20$ $U_{na} > 20$ $U_{na} < 20$ $U_{osm} < 100$[c] $U_{na} > 20$ $U_{osm} > 100$[c] $U_{na} < 20$ $U_{na} > 20$

EXTRARENAL LOSSES
• GI LOSSES WITH FREE WATER REPLACEMENT
• FLUID SEQUESTRATION
• INSENSIBLE LOSSES (SWEAT, BURNS, ETC.) WITH FREE WATER REPLACEMENT

RENAL LOSSES
• NA WASTING NEPHROPATHY
• THIAZIDES
• OSMOLAR DIURETIC (E.G., KETOACIDS)
• ADDISON'S DZ
• POSTOBSTRUCTIVE DIURESIS

DILUTE URINE
• PSYCHOGENIC POLYDIPSIA
• ALCOHOLISM
• HYPOKALEMIA

LESS DILUTE URINE
• SIADH
• HYPOTHYROIDISM
• THIAZIDES

EDEMA
• CONGESTIVE HEART FAILURE
• HEPATIC CIRRHOSIS
• NEPHROTIC SYNDROME

AZOTEMIA
• RENAL FAILURE

[a] Pseudohyponatremia is a lab artifact due to serum volume occupation by lipid or protein, resulting in an apparent decrease in the amount of Na per given volume of serum. Factitious hyponatremia is a true decrease in serum Na concentration (but normal total body Na) caused by glucose or mannitol osmotically drawing water into the serum.
[b] These disorders are characterized by ≥ 10 mOsm/kg gap between the calculated & and the measured serum osmolarity. Serum osmolarity is calculated by (2*Na) + (BUN/2.8) + (glucose/18). The gap is due to the presence of solutes detected by the lab but not accounted for in the osmolality calculation.
[c] U_{osm} = urine osmolality.

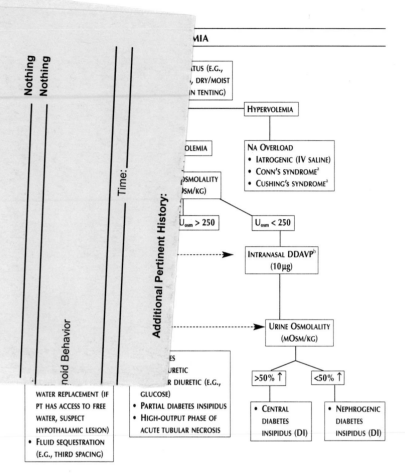

...MIA

Nothing
Nothing

...TUS (E.G.,
..., DRY/MOIST
...IN TENTING)

HYPERVOLEMIA

...OLEMIA

NA OVERLOAD
• IATROGENIC (IV SALINE)
• CONN'S SYNDROME[a]
• CUSHING'S SYNDROME[a]

Time:

...OSMOLALITY
...)SM/KG)

$U_{osm} > 250$ | $U_{osm} < 250$

INTRANASAL DDAVP[b]
(10 µg)

Additional Pertinent History:

URINE OSMOLALITY
(mOSM/KG)

...noid Behavior

>50% ↑ | <50% ↑

...ES
...URETIC
...R DIURETIC (E.G.,
  GLUCOSE)
• PARTIAL DIABETES INSIPIDUS
• HIGH-OUTPUT PHASE OF
  ACUTE TUBULAR NECROSIS

• CENTRAL
  DIABETES
  INSIPIDUS (DI)

• NEPHROGENIC
  DIABETES
  INSIPIDUS (DI)

WATER REPLACEMENT (IF
PT HAS ACCESS TO FREE
WATER, SUSPECT
HYPOTHALAMIC LESION)
• FLUID SEQUESTRATION
  (E.G., THIRD SPACING)

[a] See Endocrinology, Section III.B.1 and III.D.1 for Cushing's syndrome and Conn's syndrome.
[b] DDAVP = long-acting antidiuretic hormone analogue. Patients with central DI respond by successfully increasing the concentration of their urine by 50%. Patients with nephrogenic DI are unable to concentrate their urine in the presence of DDAVP. Patients with DI tend to be only mildly hypernatremic.

TABLE 1-41   Hypokalemia

1. For urgent K$^+$ replacement give iv and oral K$^+$ simultaneously.
   - Give iv at 10 meq/h through peripheral line or 20 meq/h through central line (more rapid administration causes vessel necrosis).
   - Give oral K$^+$ at up to 40 meq/h
   - Contrary to popular belief, oral K$^+$ increases serum K$^+$ much faster than iv (because you can't give iv quickly)
   - Each 10 meq oral or iv should ↑ serum K$^+$ by 0.1 mmol/l

2. If K$^+$ repeatedly falls or remains low
   - Check pts meds for diuretics or toxins (e.g., amphotericin) that cause K$^+$-wasting
   - Replete serum magnesium, normal Mg is required for maintenance of serum K$^+$ levels
   - Start K$^+$ sparing diuretic (e.g., spironolactone) or ACE inhibitor to help maintain K$^+$ levels
   - Advise to eat high K$^+$ food (e.g., banana)

3. Peri-MI the K$^+$ should be kept > 4.0 to suppress arrhythmias—be aggressive!

4. In renal failure small doses of oral or iv K$^+$ will dramatically ↑ serum K$^+$ so be careful!

EVALUATION OF HYPOKALEMIA

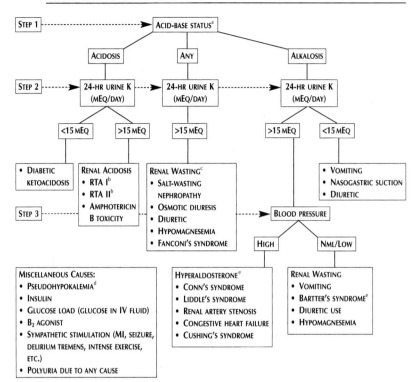

---

[a] Metabolic acidosis or alkalosis. Please see Acid-Base algorithms to determine acid-base status.

[b] RTA = Renal Tubular Acidosis. See Nephrology, Section III.F for a full description.

[c] Salt wasting nephropathies are tubulointerstitial disorders (e.g., pyelonephritis, renal medullary dz, acute tubular necrosis & allergic interstitial nephritis). For Fanconi's syndrome, see Nephrology, Section III.F.2.

[d] Pseudohypokalemia is seen in conditions with very high white blood cell counts (e.g., leukemia). The white cells take up potassium while they are sitting in the blood draw tube, creating spurious results.

[e] See Endocrinology, Sections III.B & D for Cushing's & Conn's syndromes, IV.C for congenital adrenal hyperplasia, Nephrology, Section V for renal artery stenosis, and Appendix B for Liddle's & Bartter's syndromes.

EVALUATION OF HYPERKALEMIA

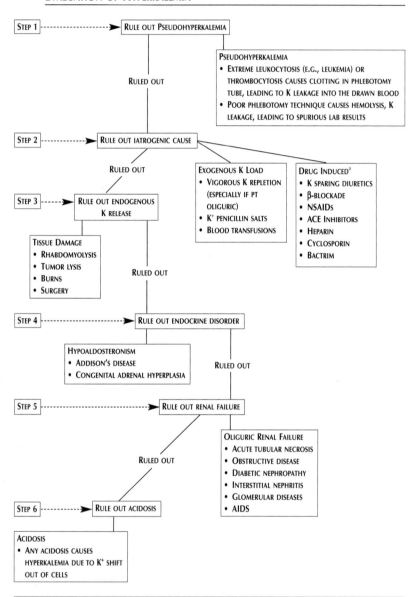

STEP 1 ------------------> RULE OUT PSEUDOHYPERKALEMIA

PSEUDOHYPERKALEMIA
- EXTREME LEUKOCYTOSIS (E.G., LEUKEMIA) OR THROMBOCYTOSIS CAUSES CLOTTING IN PHLEBOTOMY TUBE, LEADING TO K LEAKAGE INTO THE DRAWN BLOOD
- POOR PHLEBOTOMY TECHNIQUE CAUSES HEMOLYSIS, K LEAKAGE, LEADING TO SPURIOUS LAB RESULTS

RULED OUT

STEP 2 -------------> RULE OUT IATROGENIC CAUSE

RULED OUT

EXOGENOUS K LOAD
- VIGOROUS K REPLETION (ESPECIALLY IF PT OLIGURIC)
- K^+ PENICILLIN SALTS
- BLOOD TRANSFUSIONS

DRUG INDUCED[a]
- K SPARING DIURETICS
- β-BLOCKADE
- NSAIDS
- ACE INHIBITORS
- HEPARIN
- CYCLOSPORIN
- BACTRIM

STEP 3 ------> RULE OUT ENDOGENOUS K RELEASE

TISSUE DAMAGE
- RHABDOMYOLYSIS
- TUMOR LYSIS
- BURNS
- SURGERY

RULED OUT

STEP 4 ------------------> RULE OUT ENDOCRINE DISORDER

HYPOALDOSTERONISM
- ADDISON'S DISEASE
- CONGENITAL ADRENAL HYPERPLASIA

RULED OUT

STEP 5 -----------------> RULE OUT RENAL FAILURE

OLIGURIC RENAL FAILURE
- ACUTE TUBULAR NECROSIS
- OBSTRUCTIVE DISEASE
- DIABETIC NEPHROPATHY
- INTERSTITIAL NEPHRITIS
- GLOMERULAR DISEASES
- AIDS

RULED OUT

STEP 6 ----------> RULE OUT ACIDOSIS

ACIDOSIS
- ANY ACIDOSIS CAUSES HYPERKALEMIA DUE TO K^+ SHIFT OUT OF CELLS

[a] **NSAIDs** = nonsteroidal anti-inflammatories, inhibit prostaglandins → ↓ renal perfusion → ↓ K delivery to nephron. **ACE inhibitors** block efferent arteriole constriction → ↓ GFR → ↓ K delivery to the nephron. **Heparin** blocks aldosterone production, while **cyclosporine** blocks aldosterone activity. **Bactrim** (trimethoprim) has K-sparing diuretic effect on tubules.

TABLE 1-42   Hyperkalemia

Diagnosis
Plasma potassium >6.5 mmol/liter.
Dangerous level of K⁺ depends on if acute (7 ≈ 5 mmol/liter) or chronic (7 ≈ 6.5 mmol/liter).
May be associated with muscle weakness and ECG abnormalities (e.g., widening of QRS complexes, peaked T waves, loss of the P wave).
Predominantly occurs inpatients with renal failure or muscle breakdown.

Emergency treatment: hyperkalemia associated with ECG abnormalities
Give:
10 ml of 10% calcium gluconate bolus intravenously repeated if necessary (up to 100 ml/24 hours) to stabilize myocardial cell membranes.
It does not lower potassium.
Then:
Glucose + insulin: give 50 ml of dextrose 50% with 10 units of short-acting insulin. This will lower plasma potassium for several hours (4–6 hours).
±50 ml 8.4% sodium bicarbonate if ph <7.4.
±Kayexelate oral or per rectum (↓ K⁺ for 24 h).

Longer-term treatment
Remove the cause.
Diet (≤60 mmol K⁺/day).
Regular dialysis in renal failure.

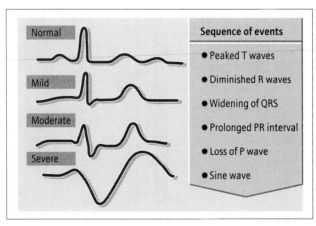

FIGURE 1-31   Hyperkalemia related EKG changes.

2. Surgery

Ming-Sing Si
Eric Daniels

I. Fluid and Electrolytes

A. Physiology (See Figure 2-1)
1. 50–70% of lean body weight is water, most of it is in skeletal muscle
2. Total body water (TBW) is divided into extracellular (1/3) & intracellular (2/3) compartments
3. Extracellular water
   a. Comprises 20% of lean body weight
   b. 25% intravascular & 75% extravascular (interstitial)
4. Intracellular water comprises 40% of lean body weight

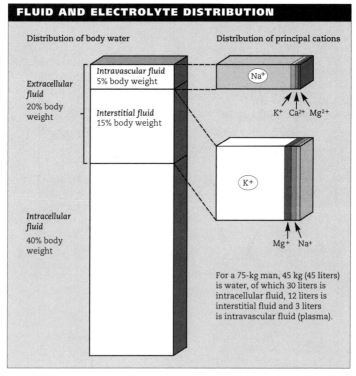

FLUID AND ELECTROLYTE DISTRIBUTION

Distribution of body water

Distribution of principal cations

Extracellular fluid
20% body weight

Intravascular fluid
5% body weight

Interstitial fluid
15% body weight

Na^+

K^+ Ca^{2+} Mg^{2+}

K^+

Intracellular fluid
40% body weight

Mg^+ Na^+

For a 75-kg man, 45 kg (45 liters) is water, of which 30 liters is intracellular fluid, 12 liters is interstitial fluid and 3 liters is intravascular fluid (plasma).

Figure 2-1   Distribution of fluid and electrolytes within the body.

B. Fluid Management

1. **3 for 1 rule**
   a. By 1–2 hours after a 1 L infusion of isotonic saline or lactated Ringer's, only 300 mL remains in the intravascular compartment
   b. **Thus 3–4 times the vascular deficit should be administered** if isotonic crystalloid solutions are used for resuscitation
2. Colloid solutions (contain high molecular weight molecules, e.g., albumin, hetastarch & dextrans) stay in the intravascular space longer
3. Colloids are more expensive than crystalloids & are most useful in the edematous patient where, for instance, 100 mL of 1% albumin solution will be able to draw about 400 mL from the extravascular compartment, thus decreasing edema

C. Hydration of Surgical Patients

1. Pts are commonly NPO (Nothing Per Oral) & require IV fluid hydration
2. An uncomplicated pt without oral intake loses ≥1 L of fluid a day from sweat, urine, feces & respiration
3. Adequate fluid hydration is indicated by **urine output ≥$\frac{1}{2}$ cc/kg/hr (for typical patient ≥30 cc/hr)** & by measuring daily weight changes
4. Electrolytes should be replaced as necessary
   a. Salivary & colon secretions are high in K^+
   b. Stomach, ileum & bile secretions are high in Cl^-
   c. Salivary, ileum, pancreas & bile secretions are high in HCO_3^-

D. Common Electrolyte Disorders

TABLE 2-1   Common Electrolyte Disorders

Disorder	DDx	Si/Sx	Tx
↑ Na^+	• Fluid loss • Steroid use • Hypertonic fluids	• Lethargy, weakness, irritability • Can be severe → seizures & coma	• Normal saline IV • Correct 1/2 the deficit in first 24 hr & the second 1/2 over 2–3 days
↓ Na^+	• Copious bladder irrigation s/p TURP* • High output ileostomy • Adrenal insufficiency	• Severe (<115 mmol/L) → seizures, nausea, vomiting, stupor, or coma	• Water restriction • Hypertonic saline IV & loop diuretics
↑ K^+	• Acidosis • ↓ insulin • Leukocytosis • Burns • Crush injury	• Neuromuscular & cardiac sequelae (heart block, v-fib & asystole) • EKG → peaked T waves, flattened P waves, wide QRS, eventually a sinusoidal pattern	• Stabilize cardiac membranes with IV calcium gluconate • Glucose & insulin infusion • Albuterol & loop diuretics • Binding resins (Kayexalate) & dialysis longer term
↓ K^+	• Diarrhea, NG suction & vomiting • Diuretics, met. alk. • Cushing's, burns, β-agonists, ↓ Mg++	• Ectopy, T-wave depression, prominent U waves • Also V-Tach & increased sensitivity to digoxin	• Oral supplements unless the patient is NPO • Infusion of K^+ over ≤ 10 mEq/hr • Correction of hypomagnesemia • K^+ sparing diuretics

TABLE 2-1   *Continued*

DISORDER	DDX	SI/SX	TX
↑ Ca⁺⁺	• Malignancy (#1 cause in inpatients) • Disorders involving bone, parathyroid, or kidneys	• Altered mental status, muscle weakness, ileus, constipation, nausea & vomiting • Nephrolithiasis • QT interval shortening	• Calcium restriction • Hydration & loop diuretics • Calcitonin, pamidronate • Dialysis
↓ Ca⁺⁺	• Acute pancreatitis • Blood transfusion • Parathyroid resection • ↓ Mg⁺⁺ • Renal failure	• Chvostek's & Trousseau's signs • Paresthesias, tetany, seizures, weakness & mental status changes • QT interval prolonged	• Calcium gluconate • Vitamin D supplement
↑ Mg⁺⁺	• Overzealous Mg⁺⁺ supplements in patients with renal failure	• Lethargy, weakness, ↓ deep tendon reflexes • Paralysis, ↓ BP & HR • Prolonged PR & QT intervals	• Calcium gluconate • Normal saline infusion with a loop diuretic • Dialysis
↓ Mg⁺⁺	• Diarrhea, malabsorption • Vomiting • Aggressive diuresis, alcoholism, chemoTx	• Torsades des pointes, • v-fib, atrial tach & atrial fib • Hyperreflexia & tetany • T wave & QRS widening PR & QT intervals prolonged	• MgSO₄
↑ Phos	• Usually iatrogenic • Rhabdomyolysis • Hypoparathyroid • Hypocalcemia • Villous adenoma • Refeeding syndrome	• Can cause soft-tissue calcification • Heart block	• Decrease dietary phosphorus • Aluminum hydroxide • Hydration & acetazolamide • Dialysis
↓ Phos	• Excessive IV glucose • Hyperparathyroidism • Osmotic diuresis	• Diffuse weakness & flaccid paralysis (all due to decreased ATP production)	• Potassium phosphate or sodium phosphate

*TURP = transurethral resection of prostate.

Note: Refeeding syndrome caused by a large glucose load too soon after prolonged NPO status-see decrease in Mg⁺⁺, K⁺, and Phos

II. Blood Product Replacement

A. NORMAL HEMOSTASIS

1. Coagulation involves endothelium, platelets & coagulation factors
2. Endothelial damage allows platelets to bind to subendothelium, inducing platelet release of ADP, 5-HT, PDGF, which promote platelet aggregation
3. Initial thrombus stabilized by fibrin laid down by coagulation factors
4. Coagulation cascades
   a. The two coagulation pathways share factors I, II, V & X
   b. Extrinsic pathway
      1) Tissue thromboplastin (tissue factor) activates factor VII, which then activates factor X
      2) Measured in vitro by prothrombin time (PT)
   c. Intrinsic pathway

      1) Factor XII → XI → IX → VIII, activated factor VIII causes activation of the common factor X

      2) Measured in vitro by partial thromboplastin time (PTT)

   d. Factor I = fibrin, which cross-links platelets to provide the tensile strength needed to stabilize the thrombus

5. Vitamin K is fat soluble, derived from leafy vegetables & colonic flora

   a. Cofactor for γ-carboxylation of factors II, VII, IX, X & the anticoagulation factors, proteins C & S, enables them to interact with Ca^{2+}

   b. Deficiency caused by malabsorption, prolonged parenteral feeding, prolonged oral antibiotics, or ingestion of oral anticoagulants

   c. First sign is prolonged PT, due to the short half-life of factor VII

B. PREOPERATIVE EVALUATION OF BLEEDING DISORDERS

1. Si/Sx = Hx or FHx of ↑ bleeding following minor cuts, dental procedures, menses, or past surgeries, ecchymoses or sequelae of liver dz

2. Ask about NSAID or herbal medicine intake the week of surgery

3. Bleeding time

   a. Evaluates platelet function

   b. ↑ bleeding time indicates quantitative or qualitative platelet dz

   c. Also ↑ in von Willebrand's dz & vasculitis

4. Thrombin time (TT)

   a. Measures the time to clot after the addition of thrombin, which is responsible for conversion of fibrinogen to fibrin

   b. ↑ TT may be due to ↑ fibrin, dysfibrinogenemia, DIC, or heparin

5. **Routine preoperative lab screening is not warranted without Si/Sx suggestive of underlying disorder**

C. TRANSFUSIONS

1. Packed red blood cells (pRBCs)

   a. Type & screen = pt's RBCs tested for A, B & Rh antigens & donor's serum screened for antibodies to common RBC antigens

   b. Cross-match = when the pt's serum checked for preformed antibodies against the donor's RBCs

   c. In trauma situations, type O negative blood is given while additional units are being typed & crossed

   d. **1 unit pRBCs should ↑ hemoglobin by 1 g/dL & ↑ hematocrit 3%**

   e. Complications

      1) Acute rejection

         a) Due to preformed antibodies against the donor RBCs

         b) Si/Sx = anxiety, flushing, tachycardia, renal failure, shock

         c) **The most common cause is clerical error**

         d) Recheck all paperwork & repeat cross-match

         e) Tx = stop transfusion, IV fluids to maintain urine output

      2) Infectious diseases

         a) HCV is by far the most common cause of hepatitis in pts who received prior transfusions, although risk of new HCV infection is now lower with blood bank screening

         b) Current risks

TABLE 2-2   Risk of Viral Infection from Blood Transfusions

DISEASE	ESTIMATED RISK*
Hepatitis B	1 case per 50,000 units transfused
Hepatitis C	1 case per 50,000 units transfused
HIV	1 case per 300,000 units transfused

*Mean estimates from *New Engl J Med* 1999, 340:438–47.

2. Platelet transfusions
    a. Pts do not bleed significantly until platelets <50,000/µL, so transfusion should be given only to maintain this level
    b. If pt is anticipated to experience severe blood loss intraoperatively or the pt is actively bleeding transfuse to maintain even higher
    c. Most common complication is alloimmunization
        1) Platelet counts fail to rise despite continued transfusion
        2) Caused by induction of antibodies against the donor's MHC type
        3) Single donor, HLA-matched platelets may overcome problem
3. Plasma component transfusion
    a. Plasma products do not require cross-matching but donor & recipient should be ABO compatible
    b. Fresh frozen plasma (FFP)
        1) Contains all the coagulation factors
        2) Used to correct all clotting factor deficiencies
    c. Cryoprecipitate is rich in factor VIII, fibrinogen & fibronectin

III. Perioperative Care

A. PREOPERATIVE CARE
1. All pts require detailed history & physical
2. Laboratory tests
    a. CBC for pts undergoing procedure that may incur large blood loss
    b. Electrolytes, BUN & creatinine in pts over 60 yr or who have illnesses (e.g., diarrhea, liver & renal dz) or take medications (e.g., diuretics) that predispose them to electrolyte disorders
    c. UA in pts with urological Sx or those having urologic procedures
    d. PT & PTT in pts with bleeding diathesis, with liver disease, or who are undergoing neurosurgery or cardiac surgery
    e. Liver function tests in pts with liver disease
    f. CXR in pts with ↑ risk of pulmonary complications (e.g., obesity or thoracic procedures) & those with preexisting pulmonary problems
    g. EKG in males >40, females >50, or young pts with preexisting cardiac dz

B. PERIOPERATIVE REVIEW OF SYSTEMS
1. Neurological
    a. Cerebrovascular disease
        1) Strokes usually occur postop & are caused by hypotension or emboli from atrial fibrillation

2) Patients with a recent history of strokes should have their surgical procedure delayed 6 wk

3) Anticoagulation should stop 2 weeks prior to surgery if possible

2. Cardiovascular

   a. Most postop complications are cardiac related

   b. Goldman cardiac risk index stratifies the operative risk of noncardiac surgery pts & helps in the decision of pursuing further Dx testing

   c.

TABLE 2-3   Goldman Cardiac Risk Index

CONDITION	POINTS	CONCERN
S3 gallop, JVD	11	CHF
MI within 6 mo	10	Cardiac injury
Abnormal EKG rhythm	7	Diseased cardiac conduction
>5 PVCs/min	7	Cardiac excitability
Age > 70	5	Increased comorbidity
General poor health	3	Increased morbidity
Aortic stenosis	3	Left ventricular outflow obstruction
Peritoneal/thoracic/aortic surgery	3	Major surgery
Emergency	3	Emergency surgery
>26 points warrants life-saving procedures only due to ↑↑↑ risk of cardiac-related death		

3. Pulmonary

   a. Pulmonary complications rarely occur in healthy pts

   b. COPD is the most important & significant risk factor to consider

   c. Obesity, abdominal, & intrathoracic procedures predispose pts to pulmonary complications in the postoperative period

   d. Smoking Hx, independent of COPD, is also an important risk factor

4. Renal

   a. Postop acute renal failure → ≥50% mortality despite hemodialysis

   b. Chronic renal failure is a significant risk factor not only because of the ↑ risk of developing acute failure, but because of the associated metabolic disturbances & underlying medical conditions

   c. Azotemia, sepsis, intraoperative hypotension, nephrotoxic drugs & radiocontrast agents are risk factors for postoperative renal failure

   d. Preventive measures include expanding the intravascular volume with IV fluids & use of diuretics after administration of radiocontrast dye

5. Infection/Immunity

   a. Infection risk depends upon patient characteristics & surgery

   b. Advanced age, diabetes, immunosuppression, obesity, preexisting infection & pre-existing illness all increase risk

   c. Surgical risk factors include GI surgery, prosthetic implantation, preoperative wound contamination & duration of the operation

   d. Prophylaxis

1) To prevent surgical wound infections, antibiotics should be administered before the skin incision is made
2) Appropriate choice of the antibiotics depends on the procedure
3) Give all patients with prosthetic heart valves antibiotic prophylaxis to prevent bacterial endocarditis

6. Hematologic
   a. Deep venous thrombosis (DVT) prevented by early ambulation & mechanical compression stockings
   b. Subcutaneous heparin may be substituted for compression stockings
   c. Pulmonary embolus should always be considered as a cause of postop acute onset dyspnea

7. Endocrinology
   a. Adrenal insufficiency
      1) Surgery creates stress for the body, normally the body reacts to stress by secreting more corticosteroids
      2) Response may be diminished in pts taking corticosteroids for ≥ 1 week preoperatively & pts with primary adrenal insufficiency
      3) Hence, for these patients, steroid replacement is needed, & **hydrocortisone is given before, during & after surgery to approximate the response of the normal adrenal gland.** If these measures are not taken, then adrenal crisis may occur.
      4) Adrenal crisis
         a) A life-threatening complication of adrenal insufficiency
         b) **Si/Sx = unexplained hypotension & tachycardia despite fluid & vasopressor administration**
         c) Tx = corticosteroids dramatically improve BP

C. FEVER

1. Intraoperative fever
   a. DDx = transfusion reaction, malignant hyperthermia, or prior infxn
   b. Malignant hyperthermia
      1) Triggered by several anesthetic agents, e.g., halothane, isoflurane & succinylcholine
      2) Tx = dantrolene, cooling measures, ICU monitoring
2. Postoperative fever
   a. **Mnemonic for causes: the 5 Ws**
      1) Wind (lungs)
      2) Water (urinary tract)
      3) Wound
      4) Walking (DVT)
      5) Wonder drug (drug reaction)
   b. Immediate postoperative fever includes atelectasis, *Streptococcus* & *Clostridium* wound infections & aspiration pneumonia
   c. 1–2 days postoperatively look for indwelling vascular line infection, aspiration pneumonia & infectious pneumonia
   d. Tx = encourage early postoperative ambulation, incentive spirometry use postoperatively, treat infections with appropriate antibiotics

IV. Trauma

A. GENERAL
1. Trauma is the major cause of death in those under age 40
2. Management broken into primary & secondary surveys

B. PRIMARY SURVEY = ABCDE
1. **A** = **A**irway
   a. All pts immobilized due to ↑ risk of spinal injury
   b. Maintain airway with jaw thrust or mandible/ tongue traction, protecting cervical spine
   c. If pt is likely to vomit, position them in a slightly lateral & head-down position to prevent aspiration
   d. If airway cannot be established, 2 large bore (14-gauge) needles can be inserted into the cricothyroid membrane
   e. Do not perform tracheotomy in the field or ambulance
   f. Unconscious patients need endotracheal (ET) tube!
2. **B** = **B**reathing
   a. Assess chest expansion, breath sounds, respiratory rate, rib fractures, sub-Q emphysema & penetrating wounds
   b. Life-threatening injuries to the lungs or thoracic cavity are:
      1) Tension pneumothorax → contralateral mediastinal shift, distended neck veins (↑ CVP), hypotension, ↓ breath sounds on 1 side & hyperresonance on the other side, Tx = immediate chest tube or 14-gauge needle puncture of affected side
      2) Open pneumothorax → Tx = immediate closure of the wound with dressings & placement of a chest tube
      3) Flail chest → caused by multiple rib fractures that form a free-floating segment of chest wall that moves paradoxically to the rest of the chest wall, resulting in an inability to generate sufficient inspiratory or expiratory pressure to drive ventilation, Tx = intubation with mechanical ventilation
      4) Massive hemothorax → injury to the great vessels with subsequent hemorrhage into the thoracic cavity, Tx = chest tube, surgical control of the bleeding site
3. **C** = **C**irculation
   a. 2 large bore IVs placed in upper extremities (if possible)
   b. For severe shock, place a central venous line
   c. O-negative blood on stand-by for any suspected significant hemorrhage
4. **D** = **D**isability
   a. Neurologic disability assessed by history, careful neurologic examination (Glasgow Coma Scale), laboratory tests (blood alcohol level, blood cultures, blood glucose, ammonia, electrolytes & urinalysis) & skull x-rays
   b. Loss of consciousness
      1) DDx = **AEIOU TIPS** = **A**lcohol, **E**pilepsy, **E**nvironment (temp), **I**nsulin(+/−), **O**verdose, **U**remia (electrolytes), **T**rauma, **I**nfection, **P**sychogenic, **S**troke
      2) Tx = Coma cocktail = dextrose, thiamine, naloxone & O_2
   c. ↑ ICP → HTN, bradycardia & bradypnea = Cushing's triad
   d. Tx = ventilation to keep $PaCO_2$ at 30–40 mm Hg, controlling fever, administration of osmotic diuretics (mannitol), corticosteroids & even bony decompression (burr hole)

5. **E** = **E**xposure
   a. Remove all clothes without moving pt (cut off if necessary)
   b. Examine all skin surfaces & back for possible exit wounds
   c. Ensure patient not at risk for hypothermia (small children)

C. SECONDARY SURVEY

1. Identify all injuries, examine all body orifices
2. Periorbital & mastoid hematomas ("raccoon eyes" & Battle's sign), hemotympanum & CSF otorrhea/rhinorrhea → basilar skull fractures
3. The Glasgow Coma Scale should be performed

TABLE 2-4   Glasgow Coma Scale

FINDING	POINTS	FINDING	POINTS
Eye Opening		**Motor Response**	
Spontaneous	4	To command	6
To voice	3	Localizes	5
To stimulation (pain)	2	Withdraws	4
No response	1	Abnormal flexion	3
Verbal Response		Extension	2
Oriented	5	No response	1
Confused	4		
Incoherent	3		
Incomprehensible	2		
No response	1		
GCS < 8 indicates severe neurologic injury, intubation must be performed to secure airway.			

4. Deaths from abdominal trauma are usually from sepsis due to hollow viscus perforation or hemorrhage if major vessels are penetrated
5. Diagnostic peritoneal lavage, abdominal Utz, or CT scan (if pt stable) suggests abdominal injury, if pt unstable Dx is by surgical laparotomy, Tx = surgical hemostasis
6. If blood noted at urethra perform retrograde urethrogram before placement of a bladder catheter, hematuria suggests significant retroperitoneal injury & requires CT scan for evaluation, take pt to OR for surgical exploration if unstable
7. Check for compartment syndrome of extremities, Si/Sx = tense, pale, paralyzed, paresthetic & painful extremity, Tx = fasciotomy

D. SHOCK

1.

TABLE 2-5   Differential Diagnosis of Shock

TYPE	CARDIAC OUTPUT	PULMONARY CAPILLARY WEDGE PRESSURE	PERIPHERAL VASCULAR RESISTANCE
Hypovolemic	↓	↓	↑
Cardiogenic	↓	↑	↑
Septic	↑	↓	↓

2.

TABLE 2-6 Correction of Defect in Shock

TYPE	DEFECT	FIRST-LINE TREATMENT
Hypovolemic	↓ preload	2 large bore IVs, crystalloid or colloid infusions [see Fluids and Electrolytes above], replace blood losses with the **3 for 1** rule = give 3 L of fluid per liter of blood loss
Cardiogenic	Myocardial failure	Pressors—dobutamine first line, can add dopamine &/or norepinephrine, supplemental O_2
Septic	↓ peripheral vascular resistance	Norepinephrine to vasoconstrict peripheral arterioles, prevent progression to multiple organ dysfunction syndrome (MODS), give IV antibiotics as indicated, supplemental O_2

3. Shock in trauma can be neurogenic or hypovolemic
4. Neurogenic due to blood pooling in splanchnic bed & muscle from loss of autonomic innervation
5. Tx = usually self-limiting, can be managed by placing pt in supine or Trendelenburg position

V. Burns

A. PARTIAL THICKNESS

1. 1° & 2° burns are limited to epidermis & superficial dermis
2. Si/Sx = skin is red, blistered, edematous, skin underneath blister is pink or white in appearance, very painful
3. Infection may convert to full-thickness burns

B. FULL THICKNESS

1. 3° & 4° burns affect all layers of skin & subcutaneous tissues
2. Si/Sx = skin is initially painless, dry, white, charred, cracked, insensate
3. 4° burns also involve muscle & bone
4. All full-thickness burns require surgical treatment
5. % of body surface area (BSA) affected (See Figure 2-2)

TABLE 2-7 Body Surface Area in Burns

Palm of hand	1%	Upper extremities*	9%
Head & neck*	9%	Lower extremities*	18%
Anterior trunk*	18%	Genital area*	1%
Posterior trunk*	18%		

* In adults.

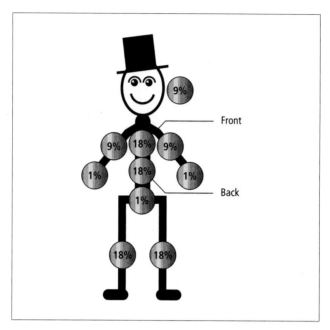

FIGURE 2-2   Rule of nines.

6. Tx = resuscitation, monitor fluid status, remove eschars
  a. Consider any facial burns or burning of nasal hairs as a potential candidate for ARDS & airway compromise
  b. Fluid resuscitation
    1) Parkland formula = % BSA × weight (kg) × 4, formula used to calculate volume of crystalloid needed
    2) Give $\frac{1}{2}$ of fluid in first 8 hr, remainder given over the next 16 hr
  c. CXR to r/o inhalation injury
  d. Labs → PT/PTT, CBC, type & cross, ABGs, electrolytes, UA
  e. Irrigate & débride wound, IV & topical antibiotics (silver sulfadiazine, mafenide, Polysporin), tetanus prophylaxis & stress ulcer prophylaxis
  f. Transfer to burn center if pt is very young or old, burns >20% BSA, full-thickness burns >5% BSA, coexisting chemical or electrical injury, facial burns, or preexisting medical problems
  g. Make pt NPO until bowel function returns, pt will have extremely ↑ protein & caloric requirements with vitamin supplementation
  h. Excision of eschar to level of bleeding capillaries & split thickness skin grafts
  i. **Marjolin's ulcer = squamous cell carcinoma arising in an ulcer or burn**

VI. Neck Mass Differential

TABLE 2-8   Neck Mass Differential Diagnosis

DISEASE	CHARACTERISTICS	DX FINDINGS	TX
Congenital			
Torticollis	• Lateral deviation of head due to hypertrophy of unilateral sternocleidomastoid • Can be congenital, neoplasm, infection, trauma, degenerative disease, or drug toxicity (particularly D_2 blockers = phenothiazines)	Rock hard knot in the sternocleido-mastoid that is easily confused with the hyoid bone upon palpation	Muscle relaxants &/or surgical repair
Thyroglossal duct cyst	• **Midline** congenital cysts, which usually present in childhood	**Cysts elevate upon swallowing**	Surgical removal
Branchial cleft cyst	• **Lateral** congenital cysts, which usually do not present until adulthood, when they become infected or inflamed	**Do not elevate upon swallowing** Aspirate contains cholesterol crystals	Surgical excision
Cystic hygroma	• Occluded lymphatics, which usually present within first 2 years of life • **Lateral or midline**	Translucent, benign mass painless, soft & compressible	Surgical excision
Dermoid cyst	• **Lateral or midline** • Soft, fluctuant mass composed of an overgrowth of epithelium	**No elevation with swallowing**	Surgical excision
Carotid body tumor = paraganglioma	• Palpable mass at bifurcation of common carotid artery • Not a vascular tumor, but originate from neural crest cells in the carotid body within the carotid sheath • Rule of 10: 10% malignant, 10% familial, 10% secrete catecholamines	**Pressure on tumor can cause bradycardia & dizziness**	Surgical excision
Acquired-Inflammatory			
Cervical lymphadenitis	• Bilateral lymphadenopathy is usually viral, caused by EBV, CMV, or HIV • Unilateral is usually bacterial, caused by *S. aureus*, group A & B Strep Other Causes • Cat scratch fever (*Bartonella henselae*), transmitted via scratch of young cats • Scrofula due to miliary tuberculosis • *Actinomyces israelii* → sinuses drain pus containing "sulfur granules" • Kawasaki's syndrome • Hodgkin's lymphoma	Fine-needle aspirate & culture	Per cause: Viral → supportive, bacteria → IV antibiotics, Kawasaki's → aspirin, Lymphoma → chemotherapy
Thyroid			
Goiter	• Enlargement of thyroid gland • Usually 2° to decreased iodine intake, inflammation or use of goitrogens	Fine-needle aspirate, TSH, T4 levels	Treat underlying condition

TABLE 2-8   *Continued*

DISEASE	CHARACTERISTICS	DX FINDINGS	TX
Malignancy	• Papillary CA ◊ **most common cancer of thyroid** ◊ good Px, 85% 5-yr survival • Medullary CA ◊ intermediate Px ◊ **secretes calcitonin**, can use it to Dx & follow dz • Follicular CA ◊ has good Px ◊ commonly metastasizes to bone & lungs • Anaplastic CA ◊ has terrible Px (0% survival at 5 yr)	Fine-needle aspirate	Surgical excision

VII. Surgical Abdomen (See Figure 2-3)

A. RIGHT UPPER QUADRANT (RUQ)

TABLE 2-9A   RUQ Differential Diagnosis

DISEASE	CHARACTERISTICS
Biliary colic	• Si/Sx = constant RUQ to epigastric pain • Utz → gallstones but no gallbladder wall thickening or pericholecystic fluid
Cholecystitis	• Si/Sx = fever, RUQ tenderness, **Murphy's sign** (inspiratory arrest upon deep palpation of RUQ) • Labs → moderate to severe leukocytosis, ↑ LFTs, ↑ bilirubin • Utz → gallstones, pericholecystic fluid, thickened gallbladder wall
Choledocholithiasis	• Si/Sx = RUQ pain worse with fatty meals, jaundice • Utz → common bile duct dilatation • Labs → ↑ LFTs, ↑ bilirubin
Pneumonia*	• Si/Sx = pleuritic chest pain & fever • CXR → infiltrate, labs → leukocytosis
Fitz-Hugh-Curtis syndrome*	• Syndrome of perihepatitis caused by ascending *Chlamydia* or *N. gonorrhoeae* salpingitis • Si/Sx = RUQ pain, fever, Hx or Si/Sx of salpingitis • Labs → leukocytosis but normal bilirubin & LFTs • Utz → normal gallbladder & biliary tree but fluid around the liver & gallbladder
Cholangitis	• Life threatening • Si/Sx ◊ **Charcot's triad** = fever, jaundice & RUQ pain ◊ **Reynolds' pentad**: add hypotension & mental status change • Labs → leukocytosis, blood Cx → enteric organisms, ↑ LFTs, ↑ bilirubin • Utz & CT → biliary duct dilatation from obstructing gallstones • Dx with ERCP or percutaneous transhepatic cholangiography (PTC)
Hepatitis*	• Si/Sx = RUQ pain/tenderness, jaundice, fever • Labs → ↑ LFTs, ↑ bilirubin, leukocytosis, ⊕ hepatitis virus serologies • Utz rules out other causes of RUQ pain

*Medical treatment indicated unless patient absolutely requires surgery for cure.

B. Right Lower Quadrant (RLQ)

TABLE 2-9B   RLQ Differential Diagnosis

DISEASE	CHARACTERISTICS
Appendicitis	• Si/Sx = RLQ pain/tenderness originally diffuse & then migrating to **McBurney's point** (1/3 the distance from the anterior superior iliac spine to the umbilicus), fever, diarrhea • Perform rectal exam to rule out retroperitoneal appendicitis • Labs → leukocytosis, fecalith on plain film or abdominal CT • Decision to take to OR based mostly on clinical picture
Yersinia enterocolitis*	• Si/Sx = fever, diarrhea, severe RLQ pain make it hard to distinguish from appendicitis • Labs → leukocytosis, plain films negative for fecalith
Ectopic pregnancy	• Si/Sx = crampy to constant lower abdominal pain, vaginal bleeding, tender adnexal mass & menstrual irregularity • Labs → anemia, ↑ hCG, culdocentesis reveals blood
Salpingitis/ Tubo-ovarian abscess (TOA)	• Si/Sx = lower abdominal/pelvic pain (constant to crampy, sharp to dull), purulent vaginal discharge, cervical motion tenderness, adnexal mass • Labs → leukocytosis, wet smear → WBCs, endocervical Cx ⊕ for N. gonorrhoeae or Chlamydia • Utz → TOA. CT scan can help r/o appendicitis
Meckel's diverticulum	• **1-10-100 rule: 1**–2% prevalence, 1–**10** cm in length, 50–**100** cm proximal to ileocecal valve, or rule of 2's: **2% of the population, 2% are symptomatic (usually before age 2), remnants are roughly 2 in, found 2 ft from ileocecal valve & found 2x as common in males** • Si/Sx = GI bleed (melena, hematochezia), small bowel obstruction (intussusception, Littre's hernia), Meckel's diverticulitis (similar presentation to appendicitis) • Nuclear medicine gastric scan to detect gastric mucosa present in 50% of Meckel's diverticula or tagged RBC scan to detect bleeding source
Ovarian torsion	• Si/Sx = acute onset, sharp unilateral lower abdominal/pelvic pain, pain may be intermittent due to incomplete torsion, pain related to change in position, nausea & fever present, tender adnexal mass • Utz & laparoscopy confirm Dx
Intussusception	• Most common in infants 5–10 mo • Si/Sx = infant crying with pulling legs up to abdomen, dark, red stool (**currant jelly**), vomiting, shock • Barium or air contrast enema → diagnostic "coiled spring" sign

*Medical treatment indicated unless patient absolutely requires surgery for cure.

C. Left Upper Quadrant (LUQ)

TABLE 2-9C   LUQ Differential Diagnosis

DISEASE	CHARACTERISTICS
Peptic ulcer*	• Si/Sx = epigastric pain relieved by food or antacids • Perforated ulcers present with sudden upper abdominal pain, shoulder pain & GI bleed (See Figure 2-3) • Labs → endoscopy or upper GI series
Myocardial infarction*	• Si/Sx = chest pain, dyspnea, diaphoresis, nausea • Labs → EKG, troponins, CK-MB
Splenic rupture	• Si/Sx = tachycardia, broken ribs, Hx of trauma, & hypotension • **Kehr's sign** = left upper quadrant pain & referred left shoulder pain • Labs → leukocytosis • X-ray → fractured ribs, medially displaced gastric bubble • CT scan of abdomen preferred method of Dx

*Medical treatment indicated unless patient absolutely requires surgery for cure.

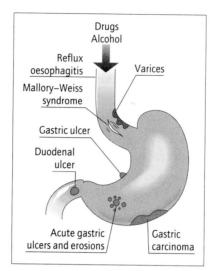

FIGURE 2-3   Common causes of acute upper gastrointestinal bleeding.

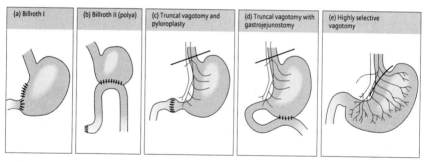

FIGURE 2-4   Operations for peptic ulceration. (a) Partial gastrectomy with Billroth I anastomosis. The ulcer and the ulcer-bearing portion of the stomach are resected. (b) Partial gastrectomy with creation of a duodenal loop (Billroth II, polya). (c) Truncal vagotomy and pyloroplasty. The main nerves are divided to eliminate nervous stimulation of the stomach, reducing the acid secretory capacity, and gastric emptying is maintained with pyloroplasty. (d) Truncal vagotomy with gastrojejunostomy. The main nerves are divided and gastric emptying maintained with gastrojejunostomy. (e) Highly selective vagotomy. Innervation of the acid-producing area of the stomach is interrupted, leaving the nerve supply to the antrum and pylorus intact. This does not affect gastric emptying so a drainage procedure is not required.

D. LEFT LOWER QUADRANT (LLQ)

TABLE 2-9D   LLQ Differential Diagnosis

DISEASE	CHARACTERISTICS
Diverticulitis*	• Si/Sx = LLQ pain & mass, fever, urinary urgency • Labs → leukocytosis • CT scan & Utz → thickened bowel wall, abscess—do not do contrast enema
Sigmoid volvulus	• Si/Sx = elderly, chronically constipated patient, abdominal pain, distention, obstipation • X-ray → **inverted-U**, contrast enema → **bird's beak deformity**
Pyelonephritis*	• Si/Sx = high fever, rigors, costovertebral angle tenderness, Hx of UTI • Labs → pyuria & ⊕ urine culture
Ovarian torsion	• See RLQ above
Ectopic pregnancy	• See RLQ above
Salpingitis	• See RLQ above

*Medical treatment indicated unless patient absolutely requires surgery for cure.

E. MIDLINE

TABLE 2-9E   Midline Differential Diagnosis

DISEASE	CHARACTERISTICS
Pancreatitis	• Si/Sx = severe epigastric pain radiating to the back, nausea/vomiting, signs of hypovolemia because of "third spacing," ↓ bowel sounds • In hemorrhagic pancreatitis, there are ecchymotic appearing skin findings in the flank (**Grey Turner's** sign) or periumbilical area (**Cullen's sign**) • Labs → leukocytosis, ↑ serum & urine amylase, ↑ lipase • X-ray → dilated small bowel or transverse colon adjacent to the pancreas, called **"sentinel loop"** • CT → phlegmon, pseudocyst, necrosis, or abscess
Pancreatic pseudocyst	• Si/Sx = sequelae of pancreatitis, if pancreatitis Sx do not improve, may present with fever or shock in infected or hemorrhagic cases • CT & Utz → fluid-filled cystic mass
Abdominal aortic aneurysm (AAA)	• Si/Sx = usually aSx, rupture presents with back or abdominal pain & shock, compression on duodenum or ureters can cause obstructive Sx, palpable pulsatile periumbilical mass • X-ray (cross-table lateral films), Utz, CT & aortography reveal aneurysm
Gastroesophageal reflux disease*	• Si/Sx = position dependent (supine worse) substernal or epigastric burning pain, regurgitation, dysphagia, hoarse voice • Dx by barium swallow, manometric or pH testing & esophagoscopy
Myocardial infarction*	• See LUQ above
Peptic ulcer*	• See LUQ above
Gastroenteritis*	• Si/Sx = diarrhea, vomiting, abdominal pain, fever, malaise, headache • Labs → stool studies not usually indicated except in severe cases

*Medical treatment indicated unless patient absolutely requires surgery for cure.

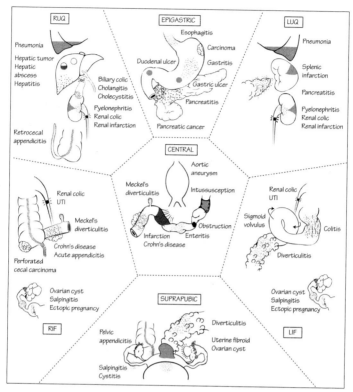

Figure 2-5 Acute abdominal pain.

F. Treatment

1. Generally all above surgical conditions will require **NPO, NG tube, IV fluids, cardiac monitoring**
2. IV antibiotics as needed
3. Surgery for hemostasis, & life-threatening conditions, consulting appropriate surgical service (O.B., pediatric surgery, etc.) as indicated

VIII. Esophagus

A. Hiatal Hernia

1. The majority of patients with reflux have hiatal hernia (80%)
2. Si/Sx = same as GERD
3. Dx = barium swallow to identify anatomic variations
4. There are two types of hiatal hernias
   a. Type I
      1) Sliding hiatal hernia, is more common than the type II hernia
      2) It is the movement of the gastroesophageal junction & stomach up into the mediastinum
      3) Tx = medical as per GERD (see above) according to the degree of Sx present

b. Type II
1) Herniation of the stomach fundus through the diaphragm parallel to the esophagus
2) Tx = mandatory surgical repair due to ↑ risk of strangulation

B. ACHALASIA

1. The most common motility disorder, affects 70% of pts with scleroderma
2. Loss of esophageal motility & failure of lower esophageal sphincter (LES) relaxation, may be caused by ganglionic degeneration or Chagas' disease, results in the dilatation of the proximal esophagus
3. Si/Sx = dysphagia of both solids & liquids, weight loss & repulsion of undigested foodstuffs that may produce a foul odor
4. May ↑ risk of esophageal CA because stasis promotes development of Barrett's esophagus
5. Dx
   a. Barium swallow → dilatation of the proximal esophagus with subsequent narrowing of the distal esophagus, studies may also reveal esophageal diverticula
   b. Manometry → ↑ LES pressure & diffuse esophageal spasm
6. Tx
   a. Endoscopic dilation of LES with balloon cures 80% of pts
   b. Alternative is a myotomy with a modified fundoplication
   c. Surgical Tx may be used for palliation in patients with scleroderma, who may experience dysphagia or severe reflux

C. ESOPHAGEAL DIVERTICULA (ZENKER'S DIVERTICULUM)

1. Proximal diverticula are usually Zenker's
2. Pulsion diverticula involving only the mucosa, located between the thyropharyngeal & cricopharyngeus muscle fibers (condition associated with muscle dysfunction/spasms)
3. Si/Sx = dysphagia, regurgitation of solid foods, choking, left-sided neck mass & bad breath
4. Dx = clinically + barium swallow
5. Tx = myotomy of cricopharyngeus muscle & removal of diverticulum

D. ESOPHAGEAL TUMORS

1. Squamous cell carcinoma
   a. Most common esophageal cancer, alcohol & tobacco synergistically ↑ risk of development
   b. Most commonly seen in men in the sixth decade of life
2. Adenocarcinoma
   a. Seen in pts with chronic reflux → Barrett's esophagus = squamous to columnar metaplasia
   b. 10% of Barrett's patients will develop adenocarcinoma
3. Si/Sx for both = **dysphagia**, weight loss, hoarseness, tracheoesophageal fistula, recurrent aspiration & may include symptoms of metastatic disease
4. Dx = barium study demonstrates **classic apple-core lesion**, Dx confirmed with endoscopy with biopsy to confirm diagnosis, CT of abdomen & chest is also performed to determine extent of spread

5. Tx = esophagectomy with gastric pull-up or colonic interposition with or without chemotherapy/radiation
6. Px poor unless resected prior to spread (very rare); however, palliation should be attempted to restore effective swallowing

IX. Gastric Tumors

1. Benign tumors comprise <10% of all gastric tumors, most commonly are polyps & leiomyoma
2. Stomach CA most common after 50 yr, ↑ incidence in men
3. Linked to blood group A (suggesting genetic predisposition), immunosuppression & environmental factors
4. Nitrosamines, excess salt intake, low fiber intake, *H. pylori*, achlorhydria, chronic gastritis are all risk factors
5. Almost always adenocarcinoma, usually involves antrum, rarely fundus, aggressive spread to nodes/liver
6. Rarer gastric tumors = lymphoma & leiomyosarcoma
7. Several classic physical findings in metastatic gastric cancers
   a. **Virchow's node = large rock-hard supraclavicular node**
   b. **Krukenberg tumor = mucinous, signet-ring cells that metastasize from gastric CA to bilateral ovaries, so palpate for ovarian masses in women**
   c. **Sister Mary Joseph sign = metastasis to umbilicus, feel for hard nodule there, associated with poor prognosis**
   d. **Blumer's shelf = palpable nodule superiorly on rectal exam, caused by metastasis of GI cancer**
8. Linitis plastica
   a. Infiltrating, diffuse CA, invariably fatal within months
   b. **This is the most deadly form of gastric cancer**
9. Lymphoma causes 4% of gastric cancers, better Px than adenocarcinoma, associated with *H. pylori* infection
10. Si/Sx for all = weight loss, anemia, anorexia, GI upset
11. Dx = biopsy
12. Tx = mostly palliative, combination surgery & chemotherapy when tolerated
13. Px = about 5% survival at 5 yr

X. Hernia

A. INGUINAL HERNIAS

1. Most common hernia, more common in men
2. Direct type = viscera protrudes directly through abdominal wall at Hesselbach's triangle (inferior epigastric artery, rectus sheath & inguinal ligament), medial to inferior epigastric artery
3. Indirect type is more common (2/3 are indirect), pass lateral to inferior epigastric artery into spermatic cord covered by cremasteric muscle
4. Si/Sx = intermittent groin mass with bowel sounds that appear during Valsalva maneuvers
5. DDx = femoral hernias, which protrude below the inguinal ligament
6. Dx = physical exam, some unable to completely differentiate until surgery
7. Tx = surgical repair with mesh placement

B. FEMORAL HERNIAS

1. More common in women
2. Si/Sx = bulge above or below the inguinal ligament, ↑ risk of incarceration
3. Dx = clinical &/or surgical
4. Tx = surgical repair should not be delayed

C. VISCERAL HERNIAS

1. Cause intestinal obstruction
2. Si/Sx = as per bowel obstruction (e.g., obstipation, abdominal pain, etc.)
3. X-ray → no gas in rectum, distended bowel, air–fluid levels
4. DDx = other causes of bowel obstruction such as adhesions, external hernia, malignancy, etc.
5.

TABLE 2-10   Hernia Definitions

Combined (pantaloon)	Concurrent direct & indirect hernias
Sliding	Part of the hernia sac wall is formed by a visceral organ
Richter's	Part of the bowel is trapped in the hernia sac
Littre's	Meckel's diverticulum contained inside hernia
Reducible	Able to replace herniated tissue to its usual anatomic location
Incarcerated	Hernias that are not reducible
Strangulated	Incarcerated hernia with vascular compromise → ischemia
Incisional	Herniation through surgical incision, commonly 2° to wound infection

6. Dx = clinical or surgical
7. Tx = surgical repair if hernia is not reducible

XI. Hepatic Tumors

A. BENIGN TUMORS

1. Hemangioma is most common benign tumor of the liver
2. Hepatic adenoma incidence related to oral contraceptives
3. Adenomas may rupture → severe intraperitoneal bleed
4. Dx = Utz, CT scan
5. Tx = Surgery only indicated if danger of rupture, patient symptomatic, or large amount of liver involved

B. MALIGNANT TUMORS

1. Metastases are the most common malignant hepatic tumors
2. Hepatocellular CA is the most common 1° hepatic malignancy
   a. Note also called "hepatoma," incorrectly implying benign tumor (historical misnomer)
   b. Most common malignancy in the world, endemic in Southeast Asia & sub-Saharan Africa due to vertical transmission of HBV
   c. Associated with cirrhosis, HBV & HCV infection, alcoholism, hemochromatosis, Wilson's disease
   d. Si/Sx = weight loss, jaundice, weakness, dull & constant RUQ or epigastric pain, hepatomegaly, palpable mass or bloody ascites may also be present

    e. Labs → ↑ serum alkaline phosphatase, ↑ bilirubin, ⊕ hepatitis B or C virus serologies, commonly causes ↑ α-fetoprotein (AFP) level

    f. Dx = Utz or CT scan

    g. Tx = surgical resection & its variations is the treatment modality that offers the greatest survival rates

  3. Hemangiosarcoma

    a. Associated with toxic exposure to polyvinyl chloride, Thorotrast, & arsenic

    b. Dx = Utz or CT scan

    c. Tx = surgical resection, may be curative if liver function is normal; in presence of cirrhosis, usually not effective

XII. Gallbladder

A. Cholelithiasis = Gallstones

  1. Higher incidence in women, multiple pregnancies, obesity **(the 4 Fs = female, forty, fertile, fat)**

  2. 10% of US population has gallstones, complications of the disorder are what necessitate intervention

  3. Pts ≤20 yr with gallstones should be worked up for congenital spherocytosis or hemoglobinopathy

  4. Si/Sx = asymptomatic by definition

  5. Dx = Utz, often incidental finding that does not require therapy

  6. Tx

    a. Asymptomatic pts with gallstones do not require cholecystectomy unless there is an ↑ risk for developing cancer

    b. Pts with a porcelain gallbladder (calcified gallbladder walls) & those of Native American descent with gallstones are at ↑ risk of developing gallbladder cancer & should receive a cholecystectomy

B. Biliary Colic

  1. Due to gallstone impaction in cystic or common bile duct

  2. **The vast majority of people who have asymptomatic gallstones WILL NEVER progress to biliary colic** (2–3% progress per year, lifelong risk = 20%)

  3. Sx = sharp colicky pain made worse by eating, particularly fats

  4. May have multiple episodes that resolve, but eventually this condition will lead to further complications so surgical resection of the gallbladder is required

  5. Dx = Utz, ERCP

  6. Tx = cholecystectomy to prevent future complications

C. Cholecystitis

  1. Cholecystitis is due to 2° infection of obstructed gallbladder

    a. The EEEK! bugs: *Escherichia coli, Enterobacter cloacae, Enterococcus, Klebsiella* spp.

    b. Si/Sx = sudden onset, severe, steady pain in RUQ/epigastrium; muscle guarding/rebound; ⊕ **Murphy's sign** (RUQ palpation during inspiration causes sharp pain & sudden cessation of inspiration)

    c. Labs → leukocytosis (may be over 20,000 in emphysematous cholecystitis = presence of gas in gallbladder wall), ↑ AST/ALT, ↑ bilirubin

d. Dx = Utz → gallstones, pericholecystic fluid & thickened gallbladder wall, if results equivocal can confirm with radionuclide cholescintigraphy (e.g., HIDA scan)—CT scan is usually not the test of choice to diagnose cholecystitis

e. Tx
1) NPO, IV hydration & third-generation cephalosporins or mezlocillin +/– aminoglycoside & Flagyl
2) Demerol better for pain as morphine causes spasm of the sphincter of Oddi
3) Surgical resection if unresponsive or worsening

D. CHOLEDOCHOLITHIASIS
1. Passage of stone through the cystic duct, can obstruct common bile duct (CBD)
2. Si/Sx = obstructive jaundice, ↑ conjugated bilirubin, hypercholesterolemia, ↑ alkaline phosphatase
3. Dx = ultrasound (Utz) → CBD > 9 mm diameter (Utz first line for Dx)
4. **Passage of stone to CBD can cause acute pancreatitis if the ampulla of Vater is obstructed by the stone**
5. Tx = laparoscopic cholecystectomy

E. ASCENDING CHOLANGITIS
1. Results from 2° bacterial infection of obstructed CBD, facilitated by obstructed bile flow
2. Obstruction usually due to choledocholithiasis, but can be 2° to strictures, foreign bodies (e.g., surgical clips from prior abdominal surgery) & parasites
3. **Charcot's triad = jaundice, RUQ pain, fever (85% sensitive for cholangitis)—for Reynold's pentad add altered mental status & hypotension**
4. Dx = Utz or CT → common bile duct dilation, definitive Dx requires endoscopic retrograde pancreaticoduodenoscopy (ERCP) or percutaneous transhepatic cholangiography (PTC)
5. This is a life-threatening emergency!
6. Tx
   a. NPO, IV hydration, IV ampicillin/gentamicin/Flagyl or mezlocillin/Flagyl
   b. ERCP or PTC to decompress the biliary tree & remove obstructing stones

F. CANCER
1. Very rare, usually occurs in seventh decade of life
2. More commonly seen in females, gallstones are risk factors for developing cancer
3. Most common 1° tumor of gallbladder is adenocarcinoma
4. Frequently seen in Far East, associated with *Clonorchis sinensis* (liver fluke) infestation
5. When the tumor occurs at the confluence of the hepatic ducts forming the common duct, the tumor is called **"Klatskin's tumor"** (mean survival = 9–12 mo, no Tx, invariably lethal)
6. **Courvoisier's law** = gallbladder enlarges when CBD is obstructed by pancreatic CA but not enlarged when CBD is obstructed by stone
7. Courvoisier's sign is a palpable gallbladder
8. Si/Sx = as for biliary colic but persistent
9. Dx = Utz or CT to show tumor, but preoperative Dx of gallbladder CA is often incorrect

10. Tx = palliative stenting of bile ducts, can consider surgical resection for palliation only
11. Px = terminal, almost all pts are dead within 1 yr of Dx

XIII. Exocrine Pancreas

A. ACUTE PANCREATITIS

1. Pancreatic enzymes autodigest pancreas → hemorrhagic fat necrosis, calcium deposition & sometimes formation of pseudocysts (cysts not lined with ductal epithelium)
2. Most common causes in US = gallstones & alcohol
3. Other causes include infection, trauma, radiation, drug (thiazides, AZT, protease inhibitors), hyperlipidemia, hypercalcemia, vascular events, tumors, scorpion sting
4. Si/Sx = severe abdominal pain, prostration (fetal position opens up retroperitoneal space & allows more room for swollen pancreas), hypotension (due to retroperitoneal fluid sequestration), tachycardia, fever, ↑ serum amylase (90% sensitive)/ lipase, hyperglycemia, hypocalcemia
5. Dx = clinically &/ or abdominal CT, **classic x-ray finding = sentinel loop or colon cut-off sign** (loop of distended bowel adjacent to pancreas)
6. **Classic physical findings = Grey Turner's sign (discoloration of flank) & Cullen's sign (periumbilical discoloration)**
7. Tx is aimed at decreasing stress to pancreas
   a. NPO until symptoms/amylase subside; TPN if NPO for >7–10 days
   b. Demerol to control pain
   c. IV fluid resuscitation
   d. Alcohol withdrawal prophylaxis
   e. May require ICU admission if severe
8. Complications = abscess, pseudocysts, duodenal obstruction, shock lung & acute renal failure
9. Repeated bouts of pancreatitis cause chronic pancreatitis, resulting in fibrosis & atrophy of the organ with early exocrine & later endocrine insufficiency
10. Prognosis of acute pancreatitis determined by **Ranson's criteria:**

TABLE 2-11   Ranson's Criteria

ON ADMISSION	WITHIN 24–48 HRS
Age > 55, WBCs > 16,000/mL, AST > 250 IU/dL, LDH > 350, blood glucose > 200, base deficit > 4 mEq/L	↓ HCT > 10%, BUN rise > 5 mg/dL, serum calcium < 8 mg/dL, arterial pO_2 < 60 mm Hg, fluid sequestration > 6 L

Risk of mortality: 20% if 3–4 signs, 40% if 5–6 signs, 100% if 7 or more signs

B. PANCREATIC PSEUDOCYST

1. Collection of fluid in pancreas surrounded by a fibrous capsule, no communication with fibrous ducts
2. **Suspect anytime a patient is readmitted with pancreatitis complaints within several weeks of being discharged after a bout of pancreatitis**
3. 2° to pancreatitis or trauma as in steering wheel injury
4. Dx = Abd Utz/CT (See Figure 2-6)

5. Tx = percutaneous surgical drainage or pancreaticogastrostomy (creation of surgical fistula to drain cyst into the stomach), but small cysts will resorb on their own

6. New cysts contain blood, necrotic debris, leukocytes; old cysts contain straw-colored fluid

7. Can become infected with purulent contents, causing peritonitis after rupture

C. PANCREATIC CANCER (See Figure 2-7)

1. Epid = 90% are adenocarcinoma with 60% of these arising in the head of pancreas

2. More common in African Americans, cigarette smokers & males, linked to chronic pancreatitis & diabetes mellitus

3. Si/Sx = jaundice, weight loss, abdominal pain, **classic sign is Trousseau's syndrome = migratory thrombophlebitis, occurs in 10% of patients**

4. Frequently invades duodenum, ampulla of Vater, common bile duct & can also cause biliary obstruction

5. Dx = Labs: $\uparrow$ bilirubin, $\uparrow$ alk phos, $\uparrow$ CA 19-9 (not diagnostic), **CT scan** (See Figure 2-8)

6. Tx = Whipple's procedure, resection of pancreas, part of small bowel, stomach, gallbladder

7. Site of cancer & extent of disease at time of diagnosis determines Px: usually very poor, 5-yr survival rate after palliative resection is 5%

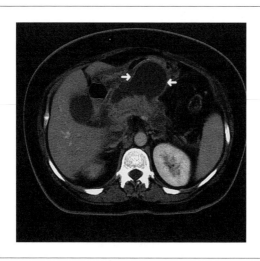

FIGURE 2-6   CT scan showing a well-defined, low-density pseudocyst (arrows).

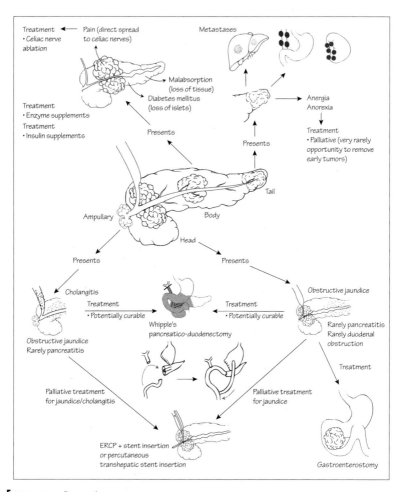

FIGURE 2-7   Pancreatic tumors.

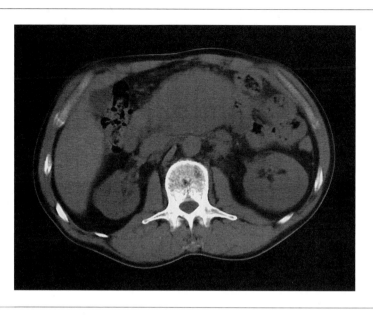

FIGURE 2-8   CT scan showing an upper abdominal mass: pancreatic carcinoma.

D. ENDOCRINE PANCREATIC NEOPLASM
1. Insulinoma due to hyperplasia of insulin producing β-cells
2. Hyperglucagonemia = α cell tumor → hyperglycemia & exfoliative dermatitis
3. Zollinger-Ellison syndrome
    a. Dx = clinically, elevated serum levels of insulin, glucagon, or gastrin
    b. Tx = surgical resection of the tumor

XIV. Small Intestine

A. SMALL BOWEL OBSTRUCTION (SBO)
1. **Most common surgical condition of the small bowel**
2. Causes = peritoneal adhesions, hernias & neoplasms in order of occurrence in the adult population
3. Other causes include Crohn's, Meckel's, radiation enteritis, gallstone ileus & inflammation
4. Si/Sx = crampy abdominal pain, nausea, vomiting, lack of flatus, abdominal tenderness, abdominal distention & hyperactive, high-pitched bowel sounds
5. DDx = paralytic ileus (similar Si/Sx)
6. Numerous etiologies including abdominal surgery, hypokalemia, narcotics, anticholinergics, acute pancreatitis, gastroenteritis & cholecystitis
7. Dx = abdominal series → distended loops of small bowel proximal to the obstruction, upright film → air–fluid levels or free air beneath the diaphragm on a PA chest film

8. Tx
   a. Conservative Tx = IV fluids, NG tube decompression & Foley catheter, partial obstructions may be successfully treated with conservative therapy
   b. Surgical candidates receive antibiotics to include both anaerobic & gram-negative coverage
   c. Objective of surgery is to remove obstruction & resect nonviable bowel

B. Small Bowel Neoplasms

1. Leiomyoma is most common benign tumor of the small bowel
2. Si/Sx = pain, anemia, weight loss, nausea & emesis, common complication is obstruction that is caused primarily by leiomyomas
3. Carcinoid tumors (small bowel is the second most common location, appendix is first) → cutaneous flushing, diarrhea & respiratory distress
4. Malignant neoplasms in order of decreasing incidence: **adenocarcinoma, carcinoid, lymphoma & sarcomas**
5. Dx = biopsy, not necessarily reliable
6. Tx = surgical resection of primary tumor along with lymph nodes & liver metastases if possible

XV. Colon

A. Colonic Polyps

1. Classified as **neoplastic, hamartomas, inflammatory, or miscellaneous**
2. Neoplastic polyps are most commonly adenomas & can be classified as either tubular adenoma (smallest malignant potential), tubulovillous adenoma, or villous adenoma (greatest malignant potential)
3. The mean age of patients with polyps is 55, incidence ↑ with age
4. 50% of polyps occur in the sigmoid or rectum
5. Si/Sx = intermittent rectal **bleeding** is most common presenting complaint
6. Dx = colonoscopy, sigmoidoscopy, always consider family Hx
7. Tx
   a. Colonoscopic polypectomy or laparotomy
   b. If invasive adenocarcinoma is found, a colectomy is not mandatory if gross & microscopic margins are clear, if tissue is well-differentiated without lymphatic or venous drainage & polyp stalk does not invade

B. Familial Polyposis Syndromes [see Appendix A for more]

1. Familial adenomatous polyposis (FAP)
   a. Si/Sx = autosomal dominant inheritance of APC gene, abundant polyps throughout the colon & rectum beginning at puberty
   b. Gardner's syndrome consists of polyposis, desmoid tumors, osteomas of mandible or skull, & sebaceous cysts
   c. Turcot's syndrome is polyposis with medulloblastoma or glioma
   d. Dx = family Hx, colonoscopy, presence of congenital hypertrophy of retinal pigment epithelium predicts FAP with 97% sensitivity
   e. Tx = colectomy & upper GI endoscopy to rule out gastroduodenal lesions—a favored operation is an abdominal colectomy, mucosal proctectomy & ileoanal anastomosis
2. Peutz-Jeghers syndrome

    a. Si/Sx = autosomal dominant inheritance, nonneoplastic hamartomatous polyps in stomach, small intestine & colon, skin & mucous membrane hyperpigmentation, **particularly freckles on lips**

    b. ↑ **risk of developing CA in other tissues** (e.g., breast, pancreas)

    c. Dx = clinical & family Hx

    d. Tx = careful, regular monitoring for malignancy

  3. Juvenile polyposis syndromes

    a. Examples include juvenile polyposis coli, generalized juvenile gastrointestinal polyposis & Cronkhite-Canada syndrome

    b. Si/Sx = hamartomatous polyps & thus carry decreased malignant potential, similar to Peutz-Jeghers, patients with familial juvenile polyposis carry increased risk of gastrointestinal cancer

    c. Dx = clinical & family Hx

    d. Tx = polypectomy is generally reserved for symptomatic polyps

C. DIVERTICULAR DISEASE

  1. General characteristics

    a. ≅ 50% of people will have diverticula, ↑ incidence between fifth & eighth decade of life in Western countries, but **only 10–20% cause Sx**

    b. True diverticula = herniations involving the full bowel wall thickness

    c. True diverticula are rare, often found in cecum & ascending colon

    d. False diverticula = only mucosal herniations through muscular wall

    e. False diverticula are common, >90% found in sigmoid colon

    f. It is believed that ↑ intraluminal pressure (perhaps promoted by ↓ fiber diet) causes herniation

  2. Diverticulosis

    a. Presence of multiple false (acquired) diverticula

    b. Si/Sx = 80% are aSx & are found incidentally, can cause recurrent abdominal pain in left lower quadrant & changes in bowel habits, 5–10% of pts present with lower GI hemorrhage that can be massive

    c. Dx = colonoscopy or barium enema to reveal herniations

    d. Tx

      1) aSx pts should ↑ fiber content of diet, ↓ fatty food intake & avoid foods that exacerbate diverticular obstruction (e.g., seeds)

      2) Surgical therapy for uncomplicated diverticulosis is **rare**

      3) See below for management of GI hemorrhage

  3. Diverticulitis

    a. Diverticular infxn & macroperforation resulting in inflammation

    b. The inflammation may be limited to the bowel, extend to pericolic tissues, form an abscess, or result in peritonitis

    c. Si/Sx

      1) Left lower quadrant pain, diarrhea or constipation, fever, anorexia & leukocytosis—**bleeding is more consistent with diverticulosis, not diverticulitis**

      2) **Life-threatening complications from diverticulitis include large perforations, abscess or fistula formation & obstruction**

      3) The most common fistula associated with diverticular dz is colovesicular (presenting with recurrent urinary tract infections)

d. Dx

1) CT scan may demonstrate edema of the bowel wall & the presence/location of formed abscesses

2) Barium enema & colonoscopy are generally contraindicated for the acute pt, but if the pt's Sx point to obstruction or to the presence of a fistula, a contrast enema is warranted

e. Tx

1) Majority of pts respond to conservative Tx with IV hydration, antibiotics with anaerobic coverage & NPO orders

2) Abscess requires CT- or Utz-guided percutaneous drainage

3) If pt suffers recurrent bouts after acute resolution, a sigmoid colectomy is usually considered on an elective basis

4) Perforation or obstruction → resection of affected bowel & construction of a temporary diverting colostomy & a Hartman pouch—reanastomosis performed 2–3 months postop

D. GI HEMORRHAGE

1. **Bright-red blood per rectum** (BRBPR) usually points to bleeding in the **distal small bowel or colon**, although a proximal bleeding site must be considered

2. Massive lower GI hemorrhage is usually caused by diverticular disease, angiodysplasia, ulcerative colitis, ischemic colitis, or a solitary ulcer

3. Chronic rectal bleed is usually due to hemorrhoids, fissures, CA, or polyps

4. Dx

a. Digital rectal exam (DRE) & visualization with an anoscope & sigmoidoscope to locate & Tx obvious bleeding site

b. Endoscopy to evaluate for an upper gastrointestinal bleed

c. Angiography if pt continues to bleed despite r/o upper GI source

d. If bleeding is minimal/stopped or angiography is indeterminate & the pt is stable, the bowel should be prepped & colonoscopy performed

e. Tagged RBC scan or barium enema if colonoscopy is non-Dx

5. Tx

a. IV fluids & transfusions as needed to maintain hemodynamic stability

b. Surgery is fortunately rarely required & should be considered only if bleeding persists (over 90% of bleeding ceases spontaneously) despite intervention

E. LARGE INTESTINE OBSTRUCTION

1. Accounts for 15% of obstructions—most common site is sigmoid colon

2. 3 most common causes are **adenocarcinoma**, **scarring 2° to diverticulitis** & **volvulus—consider adhesions if pt had previous abdominal surgery**

3. Other causes are fecal impaction, inflammatory disorders, foreign bodies & other benign tumors

4. Si/Sx = abdominal distention, crampy abdominal pain, nausea/vomiting

5. **X-ray → distended proximal colon, air–fluid levels, no gas in rectum**

6. Dx = clinical + x-ray, consider barium enema if x-rays are equivocal—**DO NOT GIVE BARIUM ORALLY WITH SUSPECTED OBSTRUCTION**

7. Tx = emergency laparotomy if cecal diameter >12 cm or for severe tenderness, peritonitis, sepsis, free air

8. Pseudo-obstruction **(Ogilvie's syndrome)**

a. The presence of massive right-sided colon dilatation with no evidence of obstruction

b. Tx = colonoscopy & rectal tube for decompression

F. VOLVULUS

1. Rotation of the large intestine along its mesenteric axis—twisting can promote ischemic bowel, gangrene & subsequent perforation
2. Most common site is **sigmoid** (70%) followed by **cecum** (30%)
3. **Commonly occurs in elderly individuals**
4. Si/Sx = obstructive symptoms, including distention, tympany, rushes & high-pitched bowel sounds
5. Dx = clinical, confirmed by radiographic studies
   a. X-ray → dilated loops of bowel with loss of haustra with **a kidney bean appearance**
   b. Barium enema → a narrowing mimicking a **"bird's beak" or "ace of spades"** picture, with point of beak pointing to site of bowel rotation
6. Tx
   a. Sigmoidoscopy or colonoscopy for decompression
   b. If not successful, laparotomy with a two-stage resection & anastomosis is necessary
   c. Cecal volvulus is treated with cecopexy (attachment of mobile cecum to peritoneal membrane) or right hemicolectomy

G. COLON CANCER

1. Epidemiology
   a. Second leading cause of cancer deaths
   b. Low-fiber, high-fat diet may contribute to risk of development—**while this has been classically taught it remains controversial & recent data suggest otherwise [see *N Engl J Med* 1999, 340:169–76]**
   c. Genetic influences include tumor suppressor & proto-oncogenes
   d. Lynch syndromes I & II or hereditary nonpolyposis colorectal cancer (HNPCC)
      1) **Lynch syndrome I** is an autosomal dominant predisposition to colorectal cancer with right-sided predominance (70% proximal to the splenic flexure)
      2) **Lynch syndrome II** shows all of the features of Lynch syndrome I & also causes extracolonic cancers, particularly endometrial carcinoma, carcinoma of the ovary, small bowel, stomach & pancreas, & transitional cell CA of the ureter & renal pelvis
2. Screening
   a. >40 yr of age without risk factors (strong family Hx, ulcerative colitis, etc.) → yearly stool occult blood tests, flexible sigmoidoscopy q 3–5 yr or colonoscopy q 10 yr or barium enema q 5–10 yr
   b. Colonoscopy/barium enema if polyps found
   c. Pts with risk factors require more frequent & full colonoscopies
3. Dx
   a. Endoscopy or barium enema—biopsy not essential
   b. Obtain preoperative carcinoembryonic antigen (CEA) to follow disease, these levels will be elevated before any physical evidence of disease
4. Surgical = resection and regional lymph node dissection

5. Adjuvant Tx for metastatic dz = 5-fluorouracil ⊕ leucovorin or levamisole → 30% improvement in survival
6. Follow-up
   a. Hx & physical & CEA level q 3 mo for 3 yr then follow up every 6 mo for 2 yr
   b. Colonoscopy at 6 mo, 12 mo & yearly for 5 yr
   c. CT & MRI for suspected recurrences

XVI. Rectum and Anus (See Figure 2-9)

A. HEMORRHOIDS
1. A varicosity in the lower rectum or anus caused by congestion in the veins of the hemorrhoidal plexus
2. Si/Sx = anal mass, bleeding, itching, discomfort
3. The presence or absence of pain depends on the location of the hemorrhoid: internal hemorrhoid is generally not painful whereas an external hemorrhoid can be extremely painful
4. **Thrombosed external hemorrhoid**
   a. Not a true hemorrhoid, but subcutaneous external hemorrhoidal veins of the anal canal
   b. It is classically **painful**, tense, bluish elevation beneath the skin or anoderm
5. Hemorrhoids are classified by degrees
   a. 1° = no prolapse
   b. 2° = prolapse with defecation, but returns on its own
   c. 3° = prolapse with defecation or straining, require manual reduction
   d. 4° = not capable of being reduced
6. Dx = H&P, inspection of the perianal area, digital rectal exam, anoscopy & sigmoidoscopy
7. Tx = conservative therapy consists of a high-fiber diet, Sitz baths, stool bulking agents, stool softeners, cortisone cream, astringent medicated pads
8. Definitive Tx = sclerotherapy, cryosurgery, rubber band ligation & surgical hemorrhoidectomy

B. FISTULA-IN-ANO
1. Communication between the rectum to the perianal skin, usually secondary to anal crypt infection
2. Infection in the crypt forms abscess then ruptures & a fistulous tract is formed, can be seen in Crohn's disease
3. Si/Sx = intermittent or constant discharge, may exude pus, incontinence
4. Dx = physical exam
5. Tx = fistulotomy
6. Factors that predispose to maintenance of fistula patency = **FRIEND** = **F**oreign body, **R**adiation, **I**nfection, **E**pithelialization, **N**eoplasm, **D**istal obstruction

C. ANAL FISSURE
1. Epithelium in the anal canal denuded 2° to passage of irritating diarrhea & a tightening of the anal canal related to nervous tension
2. Si/Sx = **classic** presentation, a severely painful bowel movement associated with bright-red bleeding
3. Dx = anoscopy

4. Tx = stool softeners, dietary modifications & bulking agents
5. Surgical Tx = lateral internal sphincterotomy if pain is unbearable & fissure persists

D. RECTAL CANCER

1. More common in males
2. Si/Sx = **rectal bleeding**, obstruction, altered bowel habits & tenesmus
3. Dx = colonoscopy, sigmoidoscopy, biopsy, barium enema
4. Tx = sphincter-saving surgery, adjuvant Tx for rectal cancer with positive nodal metastasis or transmural involvement includes radiation therapy & 5-FU chemotherapy

E. ANAL CANCER

1. Most commonly squamous cell CA, others include transitional cell, adenocarcinoma, melanoma & mucoepidermal
2. Risk factors include fistulas, abscess, infections & Crohn's disease
3. Si/Sx = **anal bleeding**, pain & mucus evacuation
4. Dx = biopsy
5. Tx = chemotherapy & radiation

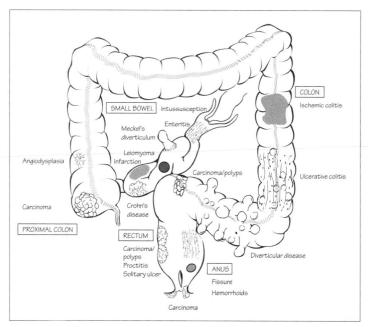

FIGURE 2-9   Rectal bleeding.

XVII. Breast

A. CANCER RISKS

1. Risk increased by
   a. #1 factor is gender (1% of breast cancers are in men)

    b. Age (#1 factor in women)

    c. Young first menarche (<11 yr)

    d. Old first pregnancy (>30 yr)

    e. Late menopause (>50 yr)

    f. Family history defined as 1° relatives with cancer at a young age (95% of cancers are not familial)

2. Risk NOT increased by caffeine, sexual orientation (lesbian)

3. Vitamin E does NOT protect against breast cancer

4. While breast cancers can be asymptomatic, others can present with nipple discharge (unilateral), pain, nipple retraction, dimpling & nipple rash

5. Remember, **most breast cancers develop in the upper outer quadrants**

6. Most common types of cancer are invasive ductal carcinoma (majority), invasive lobular CA & inflammatory CA

B. MASTALGIA

1. Cyclical or noncyclical breast pain NOT due to lumps

2. Pain worse with respiration may be due to Tietze syndrome (costochondritis)

3. Mondor's disease = thoracoepigastric vein phlebitis → skin retraction along vein course

4. Dx = clinical

5. Tx = danazol, works by inducing amenorrhea (hirsutism & weight gain side effects)

C. FIBROADENOMA (FA)

1. Most common tumor in teens & young women (peak in 20s)

2. FAs grow rapidly, no increased risk for developing CA

3. Dx = clinical

4. Tx NOT required, often will resorb within several weeks, reevaluation after a month is standard

D. CYSTS

1. Most common tumor in 35–50-yr-olds, rarely postmenopausal, arise in terminal ductal lobular unit

2. Cysts can arise overnight

3. No clinical significance, can be easily drained

4. Si/Sx = pain & tenderness that varies with the menstrual cycle

5. Dx = history, breast exam & aspiration of any suspected cystic lesions, fluid that is drawn from a cyst is usually straw- or green-colored

6. If aspirated fluid is bloody, send for cytology to rule out cystic malignancy

7. Tx = drainage of cyst

E. DUCTAL CARCINOMA IN SITU (DCIS)

1. Usually nonpalpable, seen as irregularly shaped ductal calcifications on mammography

2. This is a true premalignancy, will lead to invasive ductal CA

3. Dx = core or excisional biopsy

4. Tx = excision of mass, ensure clean margins on excision (if not, excise again with wider margins) & add postop radiation that reduces rate of recurrence

F. INVASIVE DUCTAL CARCINOMA (IDC)

1. Most common breast cancer, occurs commonly in mid-30s to late 50s, forms solid tumors

2. **Tumor size is the most important Px factor,** node involvement is also important for Px
3. Dx = core or excisional biopsy—all breast masses in women >35 yr require a tissue diagnosis, regardless of mammographic findings (i.e., even if mammography is not suspicious)
4. Tx = **either** modified radical mastectomy or lumpectomy with postop radiation, both give equivalent outcomes
5. Adjuvant tamoxifen or raloxifene can be added to reduce the risk of metastasis depending on the size of the primary tumor

G. INVASIVE LOBULAR CARCINOMA
1. Only 3–5% of invasive CA is lobular, present at age 45–56, vague appearance on mammogram
2. Patients have increased frequency of bilateral cancer
3. Dx = core or excisional biopsy
4. Tx = **either** prophylactic bilateral mastectomy at time of diagnosis, or mastectomy plus very close follow-up

H. PAGET'S BREAST DISEASE (NOT BONE DISEASE!)
1. Presents with dermatitis/macular rash over nipple or areola
2. Underlying ductal CA almost always present
3. Dx = biopsy
4. Tx = excision + radiation

I. INFLAMMATORY CARCINOMA
1. Breast has classic Sx of inflammation: redness, pain & heat
2. Rapidly progressive breast cancer, almost always widely metastatic at presentation
3. Dx = physical exam & biopsy
4. Tx = chemotherapy + radiation, Px poor

J. MAMMOGRAPHY
1. Highly effective screening tool in all but young women
2. Dense breast tissue found in young women interferes with the test's sensitivity & specificity
3. All women over age 50 should have yearly mammograms (proven to ↓ mortality in these patients)
4. Women over age 40 recommended to have yearly or biannual mammograms (efficacy less clear in this group)
5. Women with 1° relatives who have cancer should begin mammogram screenings **10 yr prior to the age at which the relative developed cancer**

WORK-UP OF A BREAST MASS

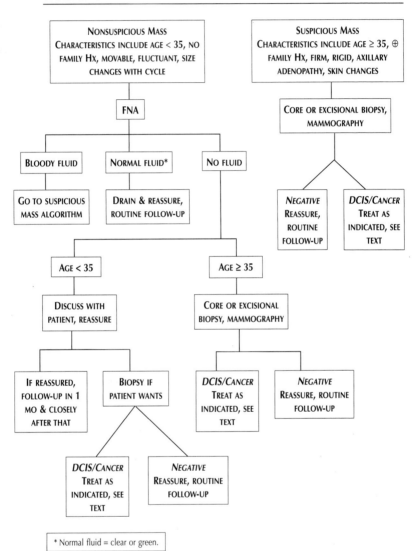

* Normal fluid = clear or green.

XVIII. Urology

A. SCROTAL EMERGENCIES

1. Testicular torsion
   a. Usually peripubertal patient
   b. Si/Sx = acute onset testicular pain & edema, nausea & vomiting, tender, swollen testicle with transverse lie, **absent cremasteric reflex on affected side**
   c. Dx = Doppler Utz to assess testicular artery flow
   d. Tx = emergent surgical decompression, with excision of testicle if it infarcts
2. Epididymitis
   a. Si/Sx = unilateral testicular pain, dysuria, occasional urethral discharge, fever, leukocytosis in severe cases, painful & swollen epididymis
   b. Dx = history & physical, labs → UA can be negative or show pyuria, urine Cx should be obtained, swab for *N. gonorrhoeae* & *Chlamydia*
   c. Tx = antibiotics & NSAIDs
3. Appendix testis (torsion of testicular appendage)
   a. Si/Sx = similar to testicular torsion, severe tenderness over superior pole of testicle, **"blue dot" sign** of ischemic appendage, normal position & lie, **cremasteric reflex present,** testicle & epididymis not tender
   b. Dx = Utz, perfusion confirmed with nuclear medicine scan
   c. Tx = supportive, should resolve in 2 wk
4. Fournier's gangrene
   a. Necrotizing fasciitis of the genital area
   b. Si/Sx = acute pruritus, rapidly progressing edema, erythema, tenderness, fever, chills, malaise, necrosis of skin & subcutaneous tissues, crepitus caused by gas-forming organisms
   c. Dx = history of diabetes mellitus, or immunocompromise, physical exam, labs → leukocytosis, positive blood & wound cultures (polymicrobial); x-ray → subcutaneous gas
   d. Tx emergently with wide surgical débridement & antibiotics

B. PROSTATE CANCER

1. Si/Sx = advanced dz causes obstructive Sx, UTI, urinary retention, pts may also present with Sx due to metastases (bone pain, weight loss & anemia), rock-hard nodule in prostate
2. Dx = labs → anemia, azotemia, elevated serum acid phosphatase & PSA—note that use of these tests for screening is controversial due to relatively low sensitivity & specificity
3. Transrectal Utz, CT scan, MRI, plain films for metastatic work-up, biopsy to confirm Dx
4. Bone scan helpful to detect bony metastases (See Figure 2-10)
5. Tx
   a. May not require Tx, most are indolent cancers, but note that some are very aggressive & may warrant Tx depending on pt's wishes
   b. Modalities include finasteride, local irradiation, nerve sparing or radical prostatectomy—risks of surgery include impotence & incontinence
   c. Aggressiveness of Tx depends on extent of disease & age of patient

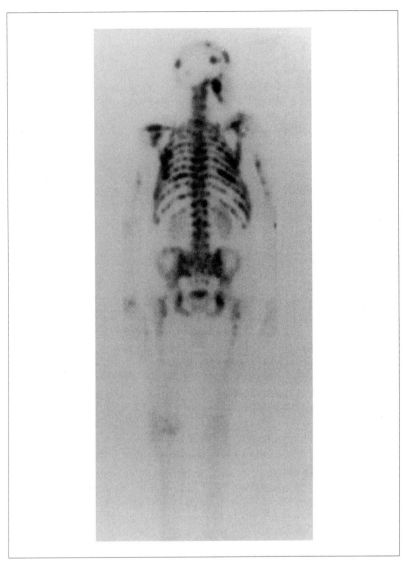

FIGURE 2-10   Bone scan showing multiple metastases secondary to prostatic cancer.

XIX. Orthopedics

A. Wrist Injuries

1. Fractures
   a. Distal radius fracture (**Colles'**) occurs after fall on outstretched hand (See Figure 2-11)
   b. Ulnar fracture occurs after direct blow, commonly seen in hockey, lacrosse or martial arts
   c. Dx = x-rays, history & physical
   d. Tx for both = cast immobilization for 2–4 wk followed by bracing
   e. Scaphoid fracture
      1) Usually 2° to falls, commonly misdiagnosed as a "wrist sprain"
      2) Dx = clinical (pain in anatomical **snuffbox**), x-rays to confirm, bone scan or MRI for athletes that require early definitive diagnosis (See Figure 2-12)
      3) Tx = thumb splint for 10 wk (↑ risk of avascular necrosis)
2. Carpal tunnel syndrome
   a. Si/Sx = pain & paresthesias in fingers worse at night
   b. Dx = **Tinel's sign** (pathognomonic) = tapping median nerve on palmar aspect of wrist producing "shooting" sensation to fingers & **Phalen's test** = wrist flexion to 60° for 30–60 sec reproduces pt's Sx
   c. Tx = avoid causative activities, splint wrist in slight extension, consider steroid injection into carpal canal; surgery for refractory dz
   d. Px = may require up to 1 yr before Sx resolve even after surgery

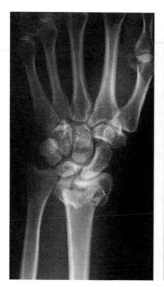
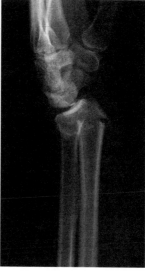

Figure 2-11   Colles' fracture.

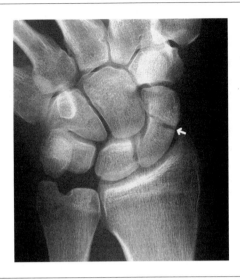

FIGURE 2-12   Scaphoid fracture (arrow).

B. SHOULDER INJURIES
1. Rotator cuff injury (impingement syndrome)
   a. Typically develops over time in pts >45 yr
   b. Si/Sx = pain/tenderness at deltoid & over anterior humeral head, difficulty lying on shoulder, ↓ internal rotation, crepitation, **Neer's sign** (pain elicited with forcible forward elevation of arm), lidocaine injection into subacromial space alleviates pain
   c. Dx = clinical, confirm with MRI
   d. Tx = NSAIDs & stretching, consider steroid injection for refractory dz, arthroscopic surgery for severe dz refractory to steroids
2. Shoulder dislocation
   a. Subluxation = symptomatic translation of humeral head relative to glenoid articular surface
   b. Dislocation = complete displacement out of the glenoid fossa
   c. Anterior instability (about 95% of cases) usually due to subcoracoid dislocation is the most common form of shoulder dislocation (See Figure 2-13)
   d. Si/Sx = pain, joint immobility, arm "goes dead" with overhead motion
   e. Dx = clinical, assess axillary nerve function in neuro exam, look for signs of rotator cuff injury, confirm with x-rays if necessary
   f. Tx = initial reduction of dislocation by various traction–countertraction techniques, 2- to 6-wk period of immobilization (longer for younger patients), intense rehabilitation; rarely is surgery required

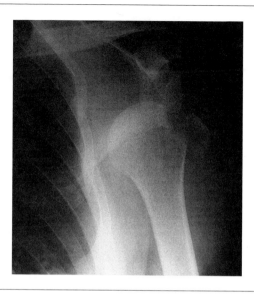

FIGURE 2-13   Anterior dislocation with a fracture of the greater tuberosity.

C. HIP & THIGH INJURIES

1. Dislocations
   a. Requires significant trauma, usually posterior, occur in children
   b. Sciatic nerve injury may be present—do a careful neurologic exam
   c. Dx = x-rays, consider CT scan to assess any associated fractures
   d. Tx
      1) **Orthopedic emergency requiring reduction under sedation (open reduction may be required)**
      2) Light traction for 5 days or longer is strongly recommended
      3) No weight bearing for 3 wk minimum, followed by 3–4 wk of light weight-bearing activities
      4) Follow-up imaging studies required every 3–6 mo for 2 yr
   e. Major complication is avascular necrosis of femoral head
2. Femoral neck fracture (See Figure 2-14)
   a. Like hip dislocation, requires significant force
   b. Si/Sx = severe hip & groin pain worse with movement, leg may be externally rotated
   c. Dx = radiograph is definitive diagnosis
   d. Tx = operative reduction with internal fixation

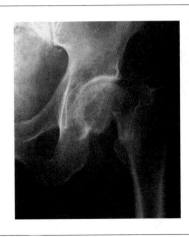

FIGURE 2-14 Femoral neck fracture.

D. KNEE INJURIES

TABLE 2-12 Knee Injuries

INJURY	CHARACTERISTICS	TX
Anterior cruciate ligament tear (ACL)	• Si/Sx = **presents with a "pop" in the knee**, pt may also complain of **knee instability or giving way** • **Lachman test** &/or anterior drawer finds pathologic anterior tibial translation & can Dx without imaging • MRI is most helpful to determine full extent of injury	Conservative or arthroscopic repair of tear
Posterior cruciate ligament tear (PCL)	• Tear seen during falls on flexed knee & dashboard injuries in motor vehicle accidents (MVAs) • X-rays to rule out associated injury or fracture • MRI useful to determine full extent of injury	Conservative or arthroscopic repair of tear
Collateral ligament tear	• **Medial collateral is the most commonly injured knee ligament** (lateral collateral is least commonly injured) • Seen after direct blow to lateral knee • **Commonly pt also injures ACL or PCL** • X-rays to rule out associated injury or fracture • MRI useful to determine full extent of injury	Hinge brace
Meniscus tear	• Acute trauma or more commonly due to degeneration seen with aging • Medial menisci injured 3× more often, male > female • Dx = **McMurray test** = pt supine with hips flexed 90° & knee fully flexed, maneuver foot into abduction-adduction & external-internal rotation while palpating joint line for a click • MRI is standard diagnostic test (See Figure 2-15)	Rest (fails > 50% of time), consider arthroscopy

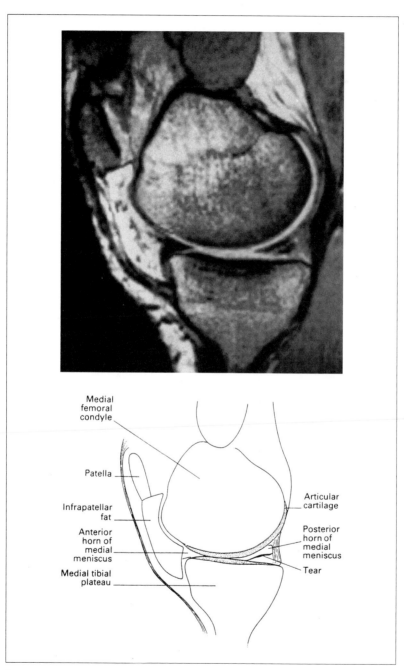

FIGURE 2-15   Tear of medial meniscus. Sagittal MRI through the medial part of the knee joint showing a tear in the posterior horn of the medial meniscus. The anterior horn appears normal.

XX. Neurosurgery

A. HEAD INJURY

   1.

TABLE 2-13   Intracranial Hemorrhage

TYPE	BLEEDING SITE	CHARACTERISTICS	TREATMENT
Epidural	Middle meningeal artery	• **Dx = CT → biconcave disk not crossing sutures** • This is a medical emergency!!! (See Figure 2-16)	Evacuate hematoma via burr holes
Subdural	Cortical bridging veins	• Causes = trauma, coagulopathy, common in elderly • Sx may start 1–2 weeks after trauma • **Dx = CT → crescentic pattern extends across suture lines** • Px worse than epidural due to ↑ risk of concurrent brain injury	Evacuate hematoma via burr holes
Subarachnoid	Circle of Willis, often at MCA branch	• Causes = AV malformation, berry aneurysm, trauma • Berry aneurysms → severe sudden headache, **CN III palsy** • CSF xanthochromia (also seen any time CSF protein > 150 mg/dL or serum bilirubin > 6 mg/dL) • Dx berry aneurysm with cerebral angiogram	Berry aneurysm = surgical excision or fill with metal coil (See Figure 2-15) Nimodipine to prevent vasospasm & resultant 2° infarcts
Parenchymal	Basal ganglia, internal capsule, thalamus	• Causes = hypertension, trauma, AV malformation, coagulopathy • CT/MRI → focal edema, hypodensity	↑ ICP → mannitol, hyperventilate, steroids &/or ventricular shunt

   2. General treatment
      a. Establish ABCs, intubate & ventilate unconscious patients
      b. Maintain cervical spine precautions
      c. ↑ ICP → mannitol, hyperventilate, steroids &/or ventricular shunt

B. FACIAL FRACTURES
   1. LeFort fractures are the classic facial trauma fractures
   2. Look for mobile palate, fractures always involve the pterygoid plates
   3. Dx = clinical + CT
   4. Tx = surgical repair & stabilization

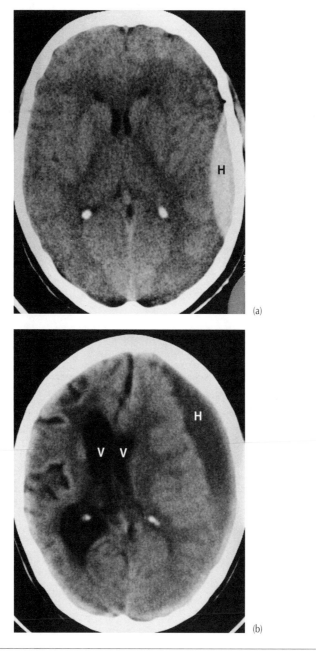

(a)

(b)

FIGURE 2-16 Extracerebral hematoma. (a) CT scan showing a high-density lentiform area typical of an acute epidural hematoma (H). (b) CT scan in another patient taken a month after injury showing a subdural hematoma (H) as a low-density area. Note the substantial ventricular displacement. V = ventricles.

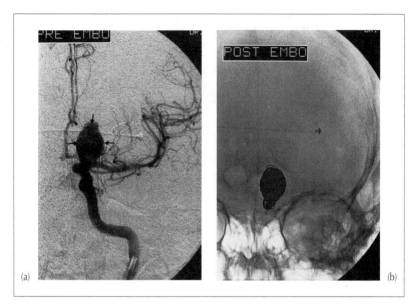

FIGURE 2-17   Aneurysm occlusion. (a) Carotid angiogram showing a large aneurysm (arrows) arising at the termination of the internal carotid artery. (b) Plain film after embolization of the aneurysm that is occluded with metal coils.

C. BASILAR SKULL FRACTURES

1. **Present with 4 classic physical findings: "raccoon's eyes" & Battle's sign, hemotympanum, CSF rhinorrhea & otorrhea**
2. "Raccoon's eyes" are dark circles (bruising) about the eyes, signifying orbital fractures
3. Battle's sign is ecchymoses over the mastoid process, indicating a fracture there
4. Dx = clinical + x-ray or CT
5. Tx = supportive

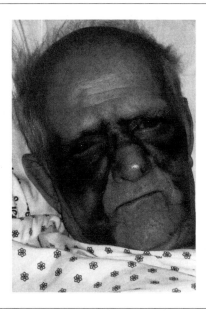

FIGURE 2-18   Racoon eyes-basilar skull fracture.

D. TUMORS

1. Si/Sx
   a. Headache awakening pt at night or is worse in morning after waking
   b. ↑ ICP → nausea/vomit, **bradycardia with hypertension & Cheyne-Stokes respirations (Cushing's triad)** & papilledema
   c. ⊕ focal deficits, frequently of CN III → fixed, dilated pupil
2. DDx

TABLE 2-14   CNS Malignancy

TYPE	CHARACTERISTICS
Metastatic	Small circular lesion, often multiple, at gray/white jnxn—**most common CNS neoplasm**: 1° = lung, breast, melanoma, renal cell, colon, thyroid
Glioblastoma multiforme	Large, irregular, ring enhancing due to central infarction (outgrows blood supply)—**most common 1° CNS neoplasm**
Meningioma	Second most common 1° CNS neoplasm, slow growing & benign
Retinoblastoma	Occurs in children, 60% sporadic, 40% familial (often bilateral)
Craniopharyngioma	Compresses optic chiasm (visual loss) & hypothalamus
Prolactinoma	The most common pituitary tumor, Sx = **bilateral gynecomastia, amenorrhea, galactorrhea, impotence, bilateral hemianopsia**
Lymphoma	The most common CNS tumor in AIDS pts (100× ↑ incidence), **MRI → ring-enhancing lesion difficult to distinguish from toxoplasmosis**
Schwannoma	Usually affects CN VIII (acoustic neuroma) → tinnitus, deafness & ↑ ICP

3. Dx
   a. Bx → definitive diagnosis
   b. Clinical suspicion + CT/MRI can diagnose lymphoma, prolactinoma, meningioma
   c. Demographics important for retinoblastoma
4. Tx = excision for all 1° tumors except prolactinoma & lymphoma
   a. First-line Tx for prolactinoma = bromocriptine (D_2 agonist inhibits prolactin secretion), second line = surgery
   b. Tx for lymphoma is radiation therapy, poor Px
   c. Tx for metastases is generally radiation therapy & support

E. HYDROCEPHALUS

1. Definition = ↑ CSF → enlarged ventricles
2. Si/Sx = ↑ ICP, ↓ cognition, headache, focal findings, in children separation of cranial bones leads to grossly enlarged calvarium
3. **Dx made by finding dilated ventricles on CT/MRI** (See Figure 2-19)
4. Lumbar puncture opening pressure & CT appearance are crucial to determine type of hydrocephalus
5. Normal ICP is always communicating
   a. Hydrocephalus ex vacuo
      1) Ventricle dilation after neuron loss (e.g., stroke, CNS dz)
      2) Sx due to neuron loss, not ventricular dilation in this case
      3) Tx = none indicated
   b. Normal pressure hydrocephalus
      1) Si/Sx = classic triad: bladder incontinence, dementia, ataxia ("wet, wacky, wobbly")
      2) Causes: 50% idiopathic, also meningitis, cerebral hemorrhage, trauma, atherosclerosis
      3) Due to ↓ CSF resorption across arachnoid villi
      4) Dx = clinically, or radionucleotide CSF studies
      5) Tx = diuretic therapy, repeated spinal taps, consider shunt placement
6. ↑ ICP can be communicating or noncommunicating
   a. Pseudotumor cerebri
      1) Communicating spontaneous ↑ ICP
      2) **Commonly seen in obese, young females**, can be idiopathic, massive quantities of vitamin A can cause it
      3) **CT → no ventricle dilation (may even be shrunken)**
      4) Tx = symptomatic (acetazolamide or surgical lumboperitoneal shunt), dz is typically self-limiting
   b. Noncommunicating
      1) Due to block between ventricles & subarachnoid space → CSF outflow obstruction at fourth ventricle, foramina of Luschka/Magendie/Munro/Magnum
      2) Causes = congenital (e.g., Arnold-Chiari syndrome), tumor effacing outflow path, or scarring 2° meningitis or subarachnoid hemorrhage
      3) Dx = CT
      4) Tx = treat underlying cause if possible

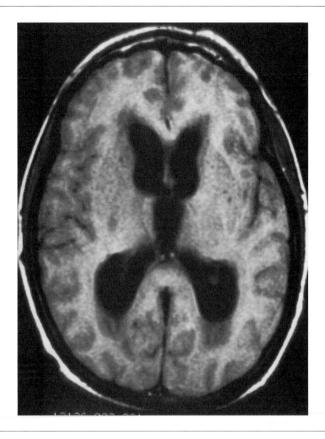

FIGURE 2-19   CT scan showing hydrocephalus.

XXI. Vascular Diseases

A. ANEURYSMS

1. Abnormal dilatation of an artery to **more than twice** its normal diameter
2. Most common cause is atherosclerosis
3. Common sites include abdominal aorta aneurysms (AAAs) & peripheral vessels including femoral & popliteal arteries
4. True aneurysms involve all 3 layers of the vessel wall—caused by atherosclerosis & congenital defects such as Marfan's syndrome
5. False aneurysms are "pulsatile hematomas" covered only by a thickened fibrous capsule (adventitia)—usually caused by traumatic disruption of the vessel wall or at an anastomotic site

6. Si/Sx = mostly asymptomatic; however, patients can present with rupture, thrombosis & embolization, some patients may complain of referred back pain &/or epigastric discomfort

7. Rupture of AAA
   a. **A ruptured AAA is a surgical emergency** & the patient may present with **classic** abdominal pain, pulsatile abdominal mass & hypotension
   b. The rate of rupture for a 5-cm diameter AAA is 6% per yr, rate for 6-cm diameter AAA is 10% per yr
   c. A patient's risk of rupture is increased by large diameter (Laplace's law), recent expansion, hypertension & COPD; as a result, regular follow-up & control of hypertension are critical

8. Dx
   a. Palpation of a pulsatile mass in the abdomen on physical exam, confirmed with abdominal Utz or CT (See Figures 2-20 and 2-21)
   b. CT is the best modality to determine the size of the aneurysm in a stable patient (See Figure 2-22)
   c. A plain film of the abdomen may demonstrate a calcified wall (See Figure 2-23)
   d. Aortogram most definitive diagnosis, also reveals size & extent

9. Tx
   a. BP control & decrease risk factors, or surgical intervention
   b. Surgical intervention usually involves the placement of a synthetic graft within the dilated wall of the AAA; surgery is recommended for **aneurysms > 5 cm** in diameter in a good surgical candidate

10. Complications
    a. MI, renal failure (due to proximity of renal vasculature off of aorta) & colonic ischemia (AAAs usually involve the inferior mesenteric artery [IMA])
    b. Be aware of formation of **aortoduodenal fistula** in patients who have had a synthetic graft placed for AAA disease & present with GI bleeding

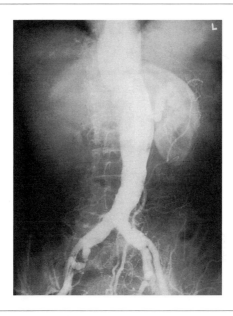

FIGURE 2-20   Suprarenal abdominal aortic aneurysm seen on angiography.

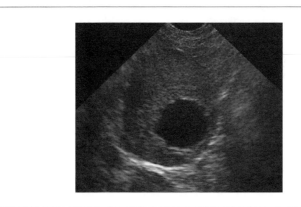

FIGURE 2-21   Transverse ultrasound of the abdomen showing the lumen (black) surrounded by thrombosis.

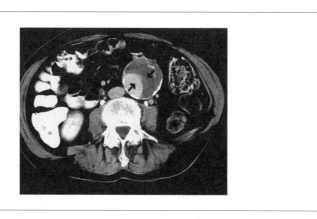

FIGURE 2-22   CT abdomen after contrast shows filling of the lumen (↑) and thrombus in an aneurysm (↓).

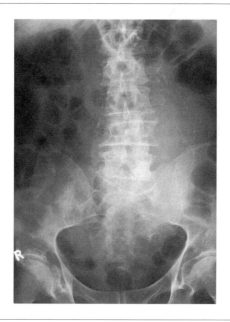

FIGURE 2-23   Plain abdomen film showing curvilinear calcification in a large abdominal aortic aneurysm.

11. **Peripheral aneurysms**
   a. Most commonly in the popliteal artery
   b. 50% of popliteal aneurysms are bilateral & 33% of patients with a popliteal aneurysm will have an AAA
   c. Si/Sx = rupture is rare, & pts usually present with thrombosis, embolization, or claudication
   d. Tx = surgical if patient is symptomatic

B. AORTIC DISSECTION

1. An intimal tear through which blood can flow, creating a plane between the intima & remainder of vessel wall
2. Usually confined to thoracic aorta (e.g., syphilis)
3. These planes can progress proximally & distally to disrupt blood supply to intestines, spinal cord, kidneys & even the coronary vessels
4. In general type A affects ascending aorta only, type B can affect both ascending & descending aorta
5. Si/Sx = **Classic severe tearing (ripping) chest pain in hypertensive patients that radiates toward the back**
6. Dx = clinical, confirm with CT or aortogram, but if pt unstable take immediately to OR
7. Tx
   a. Descending aortic dissection is usually medical (e.g., control of HTN) unless life-threatening complications arise
   b. In contrast, ascending dissection → immediate surgical intervention with graft placement

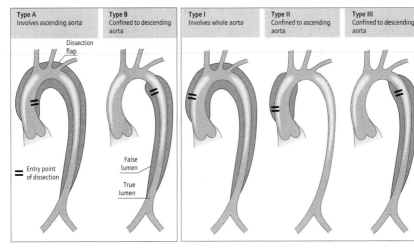

FIGURE 2-24   Aortic dissection.

C. PERIPHERAL VASCULAR DISEASE (PVD)

1. Caused by atherosclerotic dz in the lower extremities
2. Si/Sx = intermittent claudication, rest pain, ulceration, gangrene, reduced femoral, popliteal & pedal pulses, dependent rubor, muscular atrophy, trophic changes & skin blanching on foot elevation

3. Dry gangrene is the result of a chronic ischemic state & necrosis of tissue without signs of active infection
4. Wet gangrene is the superimposition of cellulitis & active infection to necrotic tissue
5. Leriche's syndrome
   a. Aortoiliac disease → claudication in hip, gluteal muscles & impotence
   b. 5% have limb loss at 5 yr with rest pain (represents more severe ischemia) & if not treated almost 50% of patients will need amputation 2° to gangrene
6. Dx
   a. Complete H&P, important to assess risk factors for atherosclerosis & limitations of lifestyle from PVD
   b. Noninvasive testing includes but is not limited to measurement of the ankle brachial index (ABI) & duplex examination
      1) ABI is the ratio of BP in the ankle to the BP in the arm
      2) Patients without disease have ABIs > 1.0 given the higher absolute pressure in the ankle
      3) Patients with severe occlusive disease (e.g., rest pain) will generally have indices < 0.4; patients with claudication generally have indices < 0.7
      4) The exercise ABI most useful diagnostically; ABI may drop with exercise in a patient with PVD
      5) Duplex (Utz) examination combines ultrasound & Doppler instruments, & can provide information regarding blood flow velocity (related to stenosis) & display blood flow as a waveform; **normal waveform is triphasic**, **moderate occlusive disease demonstrates biphasic, & severe disease shows a monophasic pattern**
      6) Preoperative angiograms are classically done to confirm the Dx & to establish distal vessel run-off, or "road-map" vessels for the surgeon
7. Tx
   a. Lifestyle modifications including smoking cessation & increasing moderate exercise
   b. Pharmacotherapy is pentoxifylline
   c. Minimally invasive therapy includes percutaneous balloon angioplasty (PTA) &/or atherectomy—best results for isolated lesions of high grade stenosis in the iliac & superior femoral arteries (SFA) vessels
   d. Treatment of iliac disease now involves PTA plus the placement of endoluminal stents
   e. Indications for surgical intervention are severe **rest pain, tissue necrosis, nonhealing infection & intractable claudication**
   f. Surgical treatment includes local endarterectomy with or without patch angioplasty & bypass procedures
   g. Results are better with autologous vein grafts; common operation for aortoiliac disease is the aortobifemoral bypass graft, while disease of the SFA is commonly treated with a femoral-popliteal bypass graft
8. Potential complication = **thrombosis**, must be addressed with either thrombolytic agents, balloon thrombectomy, or revision of graft

D. VESSEL DISEASE
1. Varicose veins
   a. Dilated, prominent tortuous superficial veins in the lower limbs
   b. Commonly seen in pregnancy (progesterone causes dilation of veins) & prolonged standing professions, may have an inherited predisposition

    c. Si/Sx = may be asymptomatic or cause itching, may also have dull aching & heaviness in legs, especially at the end of the day

    d. Dx = clinically

    e. Tx = support hose, elevate limbs, avoid prolonged standing, sclerotherapy or surgical ablation may be indicated

2. Venous ulcers

    a. 2° to venous hypertension, DVT, or varicose veins, usually located on the medial ankle & calf

    b. Si/Sx = **painless ulcers**, large, shallow & contain bleeding granulation tissue

    c. Phlegmasia alba dolens (milk leg)

        1) Venous thrombosis usually occurring in postpartum women

        2) Si/Sx = cool, pale swollen leg with impalpable pulses

        3) Tx = heparin & elevation

    d. Phlegmasia cerulea dolens (venous gangrene)

        1) Venous thrombosis with complete obstruction of arterial inflow

        2) Si/Sx = sudden intense pain, massive edema & cyanosis

        3) Tx = heparin, elevation, venous thrombectomy if unresolved

    e. Dx = clinical, Doppler studies of extremities

    f. Tx = reduction of swelling by elevation, compression stockings & Unna's boots (zinc oxide paste impregnated bandage), skin grafting is rarely indicated

3. Arterial ulcers

    a. 2° to occlusive arterial disease

    b. Si/Sx = **painful by contrast to venous ulcers**, usually found on lower leg & lateral ankle, particularly on dorsum of the foot, toes & heel, absent pulses, pallor, claudication, & may have "blue toes"

    c. Dx = clinical, work-up of PVD

    d. Tx = conservative management or bypass surgery

E. CAROTID VASCULAR DISEASE

1. Atherosclerotic plaques in carotid arteries (most commonly at carotid bifurcation)

2. DDx of carotid insufficiency = trauma, anatomic kinking, fibromuscular dysplasia & Takayasu's arteritis

3. Si/Sx = Carotid bruit, TIAs (neurologic changes that reverse in less than 24 hr), amaurosis fugax (transient monocular blindness), reversible ischemic neurologic deficits (lasting up to 3 days with no permanent changes) & CVAs that result in permanent neurologic changes

4. Dx = angiography; however, duplex scanning is noninvasive & is able to determine location, percent stenosis & assess the plaque characteristics (e.g., soft vs. calcified)

5. Tx = modification of risk factors important, anticoagulation & use of antiplatelet agents (aspirin, dipyridamole) intended to prevent thrombosis

6. Surgical therapy is carotid endarterectomy (CEA), pts are usually placed on postop aspirin therapy

7. **Surgical indications: symptomatic patient** = 1) carotid stenosis > 70%, 2) multiple TIAs (risk of stroke is 10%/year), 3) patients who have suffered a CVA & have lesion amenable to surgery (stroke recurrence is as high as 50% without surgery); **asymptomatic patient** = endarterectomy is controversial, but stenosis > 75% is an accepted indication (AHA Consensus Statement, *Stroke* 1995, 26:188–201)

8. Mortality rate of operation is very low (1%), & risk of stroke after CEA is reduced to 0.5–2%

F. SUBCLAVIAN STEAL SYNDROME

1. Caused by occlusive lesion in subclavian artery or innominate artery, causing decreased blood flow distal to the obstruction
2. This results in the "stealing" of blood from vertebral artery via retrograde flow
3. Si/Sx = arm claudication, syncope, vertigo, nausea, confusion & supraclavicular bruits
4. Dx = angiogram, Doppler, MRI
5. Tx = **carotid-subclavian bypass**

G. RENOVASCULAR HYPERTENSION

1. Caused by renal artery stenosis & subsequent activation of the renin-angiotensin pathway
2. Commonly due to atherosclerotic lesions
3. Can also be 2° to fibromuscular dysplasia, subintimal dissections & hypoplasia of renal artery
4. Si/Sx = most patients are asymptomatic, some will present with headache, abdominal bruits, or cardiac, cerebrovascular, or renal dysfunction related to hypertension; a sudden onset of hypertension is more consistent with a dysplastic process when compared to the slower evolving atherosclerosis
5. Surgically correctable HTN = **renal artery stenosis (most common)**, pheochromocytoma, unilateral renal parenchymal disease, Cushing's syndrome, primary hyperaldosteronism, hyperthyroidism, hyperparathyroidism, coarctation of the aorta, cancer & increased ICP
6. Dx = definitive Dx obtained by **angiography (string of beads appearance)**, others include IVP, renal scans & renal vein renin ratios
7. Tx = BP control & consider balloon catheter dilation of stenosis—results better with fibromuscular dysplasia vs. atherosclerotic lesions, surgical correction involves endarterectomy, bypass, or resection

H. MESENTERIC ISCHEMIA

1. **Chronic intestinal ischemia**
   a. 2° to atherosclerotic lesions of at least two of the three major vessels supplying the bowel
   b. Si/Sx = **weight loss & postprandial pain & abdominal bruit**
   c. Dx = definitive diagnosis is made with aortogram
   d. Tx = surgical intervention (endarterectomy, bypass from aorta to involved graft) is **indicated** in absence of malignancy (particularly pancreatic cancer must be ruled out)
2. **Acute intestinal ischemia**
   a. Acute thrombosis of a mesenteric vessel secondary to atherosclerotic changes or emboli from the heart
   b. Si/Sx = rapid onset of pain that is out of proportion to exam, vomiting, diarrhea & history of heart condition predisposing to emboli formation (e.g., atrial fibrillation)
   c. Dx = angiogram should be performed immediately to confirm or rule out diagnosis
   d. Tx = embolectomy/thrombectomy, resection of necrotic bowel & bypass

3. Obstetrics and Gynecology

Griselda Gutierrez

Obstetrics

I. Terminology

1. Gravidity ≡ total number of pregnancies
2. Parity ≡ number of pregnancies carried to viability—can also express parity as 4 numbers: term pregnancies, preterm, abortions & living children (TPAL)
3. Term delivery ≡ delivery of infant after 37-wk gestation
4. Premature delivery ≡ delivery of infant weighing between 500 and 2500 g & delivery between 20 and 37 wk

II. Prenatal Care

A. THE FIRST VISIT

1. Pregnancy diagnosis
   a. Si/Sx = amenorrhea, ↑ urinary frequency, breast engorgement & tenderness, nausea, fatigue, **bluish discoloration of vagina due to vascular congestion (Chadwick's sign)** & **softening of cervix (Hegar's sign)**
   b. Pregnancy test
      1) Detects human chorionic gonadotropin (hCG) or its β subunit
      2) Rapidly dividing fertilized egg produces hCG even before implantation occurs
      3) Commercial kits detect pregnancy 12–15 days after conception
      4) Home tests have low false-positive rate but high false-negative rate
   c. Ultrasound (Utz)
      1) Gestational sac identified at 5 wk, fetal image detected by 6–7 wk, cardiac activity first noted at 8 wk
      2) Utz is most accurate method to determine gestational age
2. Obstetrical Hx
   a. Duration of previous gestations
   b. Mode of delivery (e.g., normal spontaneous vaginal delivery vs. C-section vs. vacuum assisted)
   c. Duration of labor, maternal, postpartum & neonatal complications, newborn weight, newborn sex
3. Menstrual Hx including last menstrual period (LMP), regularity of cycles, age at menarche
4. Contraceptive Hx (important for risk assessment, oral contraceptive pills [OCPs] have been associated with birth defects)
5. Medical Hx
   a. Medicines, consider potential teratogens

TABLE 3-1   Teratogens

DRUG	BIRTH DEFECT
Lithium	Ebstein's anomaly (single-chambered right side of heart)
Carbamazepine & valproate	Neural tube defects
Retinoic acid	CNS defects, craniofacial defects, cardiovascular effects
ACE inhibitors	Renal failure in neonates, renal tubule dysgenesis, ↓ skull ossification
Oral hypoglycemics	Neonatal hypoglycemia
Coumadin	Skeletal & CNS defects
NSAIDs	Constriction of ductus arteriosis, necrotizing enterocolitis

    b. FHx, social Hx including tobacco ETOH, drug use, type of work, exposure to animals

    c. Diabetes & hypertension

6. Estimated date of confinement (EDC)

    a. **Nägele's rule = LMP + 7 days – 3 mo + 1 yr**: e.g., if LMP began 5/20/99, delivery due 2/27/2000

    b. This calculation depends on regular 28-day cycles (only 20–25% of women), adjustments must be made for longer or shorter cycles

7. Complete physical exam with pelvic examination including PAP smear & cultures for gonorrhea & chlamydia & estimation of uterine size

8. Labs include CBC, blood type with Rh status, urinalysis with culture, RPR test for syphilis, Rubella titer, TB skin testing, can offer HIV antibody test

9. If pt is not already immune to Rubella, do NOT vaccinate, as the vaccine is live virus

10. Genetic testing as indicated by history (e.g., hemoglobin electrophoresis in African American pt to determine sickle cell anemia likelihood)

11. Recommend 25–35 pound weight gain during pregnancy

12. Consider folate, iron & multivitamin supplements

B. FIRST TRIMESTER VISITS

1. Visit every 4 wk

2. Assess weight gain/loss, BP, pedal edema, fundal height, urine dip for glucosuria & proteinuria (**trace glucosuria is normal because of ↑ GFR, anything more than trace protein should be evaluated**)

3. Estimation of gestational age by uterine size

    a. Normal uterus is 3 × 4 × 7 cm

    b. Gravid uterus begins to enlarge & soften by 5–6 wk

TABLE 3-2   Height of Uterus by Gestational Week

12 WEEKS	16 WEEKS	20 WEEKS	20–36 WEEKS
At pubic symphysis	Midway from symphysis to umbilicus	At umbilicus	Height (cm) correlates with weeks of gestation*

*If uterine size (cm) > gestational age (wk) by more than 3 wk, consider multiple gestations, molar pregnancy, or MOST COMMONLY inaccurate dating.

C. SECOND TRIMESTER VISITS

1. Continue every 4 wk
2. After 12 wk, use Doppler Utz to evaluate fetal heartbeat at each visit
3. Offer triple marker screen (hCG, estriol, AFP) at 15–18 wk
    a. α-fetoprotein (αFP) ↓ in Down's syndrome
    b. α-fetoprotein ↑ in multiple gestation, neural tube deficit & duodenal atresia
4. At 17–19 wk (quickening) & beyond, document fetal movement
5. Amniocentesis if >35 years old or if history indicates (e.g., recurrent miscarriages, previous child with chromosomal or single gene defect, abnormal triple marker screen)
6. Glucose screening at 24 wk (1-hr Glucola)
7. Repeat hematocrit at 25–28 wk

D. THIRD TRIMESTER VISITS

1. Every 4 wk until week 32, every 2 wk from weeks 32–36, every wk until delivery
2. Inquire about preterm labor Sx: **vaginal bleeding, contractions, rupture of membranes**
3. Inquire about pregnancy-induced hypertension (PIH) (see below)
4. Screen for *Streptococcus agalactiae* (group B Strep) at 35–37 wk
5. Give RhoGAM at 28–30 wk if indicated (see below)

III. Physiologic Changes in Pregnancy

A. HEMATOLOGIC

1. Pregnancy is a **hypercoagulable** state
    a. ↑ clotting factor levels
    b. Venous stasis due to uterine pressure on lower extremity great veins
2. Anemia of pregnancy
    a. Plasma volume increases about 50% from sixth wk to week 30–34
    b. Red cell mass increases later & to a smaller degree, causing a relative anemia of about 15% due to dilution
3. Slight leukocytosis due to granulocyte demargination
4. Platelets decrease slightly, but remain within normal limits

B. CARDIAC

1. Cardiac output increases 50% (increase in both HR & stroke volume)
2. Because of ↑ flow, increased S2 split with inspiration, distended neck veins, systolic ejection murmur & S3 gallop are normal findings
3. **Diastolic murmurs are not normal findings in pregnancy**
4. ↓ peripheral vascular resistance due to progesterone-mediated smooth muscle relaxation
5. BP decreases during first 24 wk of pregnancy with gradual return to nonpregnant levels by term

C. PULMONARY

1. Nasal stuffiness & ↑ nasal secretions due to mucosal hyperemia
2. 4-cm elevation of diaphragm due to expanding uterus
3. Tidal volume & minute ventilation ↑ 30–40% (progesterone mediated)
4. Functional residual capacity & residual volume ↓ 20%

5. Hyperventilation $\rightarrow \uparrow$ PO_2, $\downarrow$ PCO_2—this allows the fetal PCO_2 to remain near 40 & still be able to give off CO_2 to maternal blood (sets up a CO_2 concentration gradient across maternal–fetal circulation & PO_2 gradient allowing maternal to fetal O_2 transfer)
6. Respiratory rate, vital capacity & inspiratory reserve do not change, total lung capacity decreases about 5%

D. GASTROINTESTINAL

1. $\downarrow$ GI motility due to progesterone
2. $\downarrow$ esophageal sphincter tone $\rightarrow$ gastric reflux also due to progesterone
3. $\uparrow$ alkaline phosphatase
4. Hemorrhoids due to constipation & $\uparrow$ venous pressure due to enlarging uterus compressing inferior vena cava

E. RENAL

1. $\downarrow$ bladder tone due to progesterone predisposes pregnant women to urinary stasis & UTIs/pyelonephritis
2. GFR increases 50%
   a. $\uparrow$ GFR $\rightarrow$ glucose excretion occurs in nearly all pregnant women
   b. Thus urine dipsticks are not useful in managing pts with diabetes
   c. **However, there should be no significant increase in protein loss**
3. Serum creatinine & blood urea nitrogen decrease

F. ENDOCRINE

1. $\downarrow$ fasting blood glucose in mother due to fetal utilization
2. $\uparrow$ postprandial glucose in mother due to $\uparrow$ insulin resistance
3. Fetus produces its own insulin starting at 9–11 wk
4. $\uparrow$ maternal thyroid bonding globulin (TBG) due to $\uparrow$ estrogen, $\uparrow$ total T3 & T4 due to $\uparrow$ TBG
5. Free T3 & T4 remain the same so pregnant women are euthyroid
6. $\uparrow$ cortisol & cortisol-binding globulin

G. SKIN

1. Normal skin changes in pregnancy mimic liver disease due to $\uparrow$ estrogen
2. Can see spider angiomas, palmar erythema
3. Hyperpigmentation occurs from $\uparrow$ estrogen & melanocyte stimulating hormone, affects umbilicus, perineum, face (chloasma) & linea (nigra)

IV. Medical Conditions in Pregnancy

A. GESTATIONAL DIABETES MELLITUS (GDM)

1. GDM = glucose intolerance or DM first recognized during pregnancy
2. **#1 medical complication of pregnancy, occurs in 2% of pregnancies**
3. GDM risk factors = previous history of GDM, maternal age ≥ 30 yr, obesity, family history of DM, previous history of infant weighing 4000 g at birth, history of repeated spontaneous abortions or unexplained stillbirths
4. GDM caused by placental-released hormone, human placental lactogen (HPL), which antagonizes insulin
5. GDM worsens as pregnancy progresses because increasing amounts of HPL are produced as placenta enlarges

6. Maternal complications = hyperglycemia, ketoacidosis, ↑ risk of UTIs, **2-fold ↑ in pregnancy induced hypertension (PIH)**, retinopathy (can occur very quickly & dramatically)
7. Fetal complications
   a. Macrosomia (≥4500 g), neonatal hypoglycemia due to abrupt separation from maternal supply of glucose, hyperbilirubinemia, polycythemia, polyhydramnios (amniotic fluid volume ≥2000 mL)
   b. **Abruption & preterm labor** due to ↑ uterine size & postpartum uterine atony, **3- to 4-fold ↑ in congenital anomalies** (often cardiac & limb deformities), spontaneous abortion & respiratory distress
8. Dx = 1-hr Glucola screening test at 24–28 wk or at onset of prenatal care in pt with known risk factors, confirm with 3-hr glucose tolerance test
9. Tx = strict glucose control, which significantly decreases complications
   a. Insulin is not required if the pt can adhere to a proper diet
   b. **Oral hypoglycemics are contraindicated** because they cross the placenta & can result in fetal & neonatal hypoglycemia
10. Delivery
    a. Route of delivery determined by estimated fetal weight
    b. If 4500 g consider C-section, if 5000 g C-section recommended
    c. Postpartum 95% of GDM patients return to normal glucose levels
    d. Glucose tolerance screening recommended 2–4 mo postpartum to pick up those few women who will remain diabetic & require Tx

B. THROMBOEMBOLIC DISEASE

1. Incidence during pregnancy is 1–2%, usually occurs postpartum (80%)
2. Si/Sx for superficial thrombophlebitis = swelling, tenderness, erythema, warmth (4 cardinal signs of inflammation), may be a palpable cord
3. Deep vein thrombosis (DVT) occurs postpartum due to spread of uterine infection to ovarian veins
4. Si/Sx of DVT = persistent fever, uterine tenderness, palpable mass, but often aSx,
5. Dx
   a. Doppler ultrasound is first line, sensitivity & specificity >90%
   b. Gold standard is venography but this is invasive
6. Tx
   a. Superficial thrombophlebitis → leg elevation, rest, heat, NSAIDs
   b. DVTs → heparin to maintain PTT 1.5–2.5x baseline
   c. **Coumadin contraindicated in pregnancy** because it crosses the placenta, is teratogenic early & causes fetal bleeding later
7. Px
   a. 25% of untreated DVTs progress to pulmonary embolism (PE)
   b. Anticoagulation decreases progression to 5%
   c. PEs in pregnancy are treated identically to DVTs

C. PREGNANCY-INDUCED HYPERTENSION (PIH)

1. Epidemiology
   a. Develops in 5–10% of pregnancies, 30% of multiple gestations
   b. Causes 15% of maternal deaths

c. Risk factors = nulliparity, age >40 years, family history of PIH, chronic hypertension, chronic renal disease, diabetes, twin gestation

2.

TABLE 3-3   Types of Pregnancy-Induced Hypertension

DISEASE	CHARACTERISTICS
Preeclampsia	• Hypertension (>140/90 or ↑ in SBP of > 30 mm Hg or DBP of >15 mm Hg compared to previous) • New onset proteinuria &/or edema • Generally occurring at ≥ 20 wk
Severe preeclampsia	• SBP > 160 mm Hg or DBP > 110 mm Hg • Marked proteinuria (>1 g/24-hr collection or > 1+ on dip), oliguria, ↑ creatinine • CNS disturbances (e.g., headaches or scotomata) • Pulmonary edema or cyanosis • Epigastric or RUQ pain, hepatic dysfunction
Eclampsia	• **Convulsions** in a woman with preeclampsia • 25% occur before labor, 50% during labor & 25% occur in first 72 hr postpartum

3. Other Si/Sx seen in preeclampsia or eclampsia
   a. Pts have rapid weight gain (2° to edema)
   b. Peripheral lower extremity edema is common in pregnancy; however, persistent edema unresponsive to rest & leg elevation, or edema involving the upper extremities or face is not normal
   c. Hyperreflexia & clonus are also noted
4. Tx
   a. The only cure for PIH is delivery of the baby, decision to do so depends on severity of preeclampsia & maturity of fetus
   b. Mild preeclampsia + immature fetus → bed rest, preferably in left lateral decubitus position to maximize blood flow to uterus, close monitoring, tell pt to return to ER if preeclampsia worsens
   c. Severe preeclampsia/eclampsia → delivery when possible, magnesium sulfate to prevent seizure, antihypertensives to maintain BP < 140/100
5. Complication of severe PIH = HELLP syndrome
   a. **HELLP** = **H**emolysis, **E**levated **L**iver enzymes, **L**ow **P**latelets
   b. Occurs in 5–10% of women with severe preeclampsia or eclampsia, more frequently in multiparous, older pts
   c. Tx = delivery (the only cure), transfuse blood, platelets, fresh frozen plasma as needed, IV fluids & pressors as needed to maintain BP

D. CARDIAC DISEASE
   1. Pts with congenital heart disease have a ↑ risk (1–5%) of having a fetus with a congenital heart disease
   2. Pts with pulmonary hypertension & ↑ right-sided pressures (e.g., Eisenmenger's complex) have poor Px with pregnancy
   3. Tx of preexisting cardiac disease = supportive, e.g., prevention &/or prompt correction of anemia, aggressive Tx of infections, ↓ physical activity/strenuous work, adherence to a low-sodium diet & proper weight gain

4. Peripartum cardiomyopathy
   a. Rare but severe pregnancy-associated condition
   b. Occurs in last month of pregnancy or first 6 mo postpartum
   c. Risk factors = African American, multiparous, age >30 yr, twin gestation, or preeclampsia
   d. Tx = bed rest, digoxin, diuretics, possible anticoagulation, consider postdelivery heart transplant especially in those whose cardiomegaly has not resolved 6 mo after Dx

E. GROUP B *STREPTOCOCCUS* (GBS = *STREPTOCOCCUS AGALACTIAE*)

1. Asymptomatic cervical colonization occurs in up to 30% of women
2. 50% of infants become colonized, clinical infection in <1%
3. Intrapartum prophylaxis with penicillin is reserved for the following situations:
   a. Preterm labor (<37 wk) or prolonged rupture of membranes (ROM) (>18 hours) or fever in labor regardless of colonization status
   b. Women identified as colonized with GBS through screening at 35–37 wk gestation
   c. Women with GBS bacteriuria or with a previous infant with GBS disease

F. HYPEREMESIS GRAVIDARUM

1. Increased nausea & vomiting that, unlike "morning sickness," persists past the sixteenth week of pregnancy
2. Causes = ↑ hCG levels, thyroid or GI hormones
3. Si/Sx = excessive vomiting, dehydration, hypochloremic metabolic alkalosis
4. Dx = clinical, rule out other cause
5. Tx = fluids, electrolyte repletion, antiemetics (IV, IM, or suppositories)
6. Some pts require feeding tubes & parenteral nutrition

V. Fetal Assessment and Intrapartum Surveillance

A. FETAL GROWTH

1. Measure by fundal height, if 2-cm deviation from expected fundal height during weeks 18–36 → repeat measurement &/or Utz
2. Utz is most reliable tool for assessing fetal growth
3. In early pregnancy measurement of gestational sac & crown-rump length correlate very well with gestational age
4. Later in pregnancy 4 measurements are done because of wide deviation in normal range = biparietal diameter of skull, abdominal circumference, femur length & cerebellar diameter

B. FETAL WELL-BEING

1. ≥4 fetal movements per hr generally indicate fetal well-being
2. Nonstress test (NST)
   a. Measures response of fetal heart rate to movement
   b. Normal (i.e., reactive) NST occurs when fetal heart rate ↑ by 15 beats/min (bpm) for 15 sec following fetal movement
   c. 2 such accelerations with 20 min are considered normal
   d. A nonreactive NST → further assessment of fetal well-being

OB/GYN

e. Test has a high false-positive rate (test suggests fetus is in trouble, but fetus is actually healthy), so it must be interpreted in the context of other tests & is often repeated within 24 hr to verify results

3. Biophysical profile (BPP)
   a. 5 measures of fetal well-being, each rated on a scale of 0–2
   b. Fetal breathing → ≥1 fetal breathing movement in 30 min lasting at least 30 sec
   c. Gross body movement → ≥3 discrete movements in 30 min
   d. Fetal tone → ≥1 episode of extension with return to flexion of fetal limbs/trunk OR opening/closing of hand
   e. Qualitative amniotic fluid volume → ≥1 pocket of amniotic fluid at least 1 cm in 2 perpendicular planes
   f. Reactive fetal heart rate → reactive NST
   g. Final score of 8–10 is normal, score of 6 is equivocal & requires further evaluation, score of 4 or less is abnormal & usually requires immediate intervention

C. TESTS OF FETAL MATURITY

1. Respiratory system is last fetal system to mature, so decisions regarding when to deliver a premature infant often depend on tests that assess the maturity of this system
2. Phospholipid production (collectively known as "surfactant") remains low until 32–33 wk of gestation, but this is highly variable
3. Lack of surfactant → neonatal respiratory distress syndrome (RDS)
4. Phospholipids enter amniotic fluid from fetal breathing & are obtained by amniocentesis & tested for maturity
5. Tests for fetal maturity
   a. Lecithin-sphingomyelin (L:S) ratio
      1) Lecithin is major phospholipid found in surfactant & increases as fetal lungs become mature
      2) Sphingomyelin production remains constant throughout pregnancy
      3) Ratio >2.0 is considered mature
   b. Phosphatidylglycerol (PG) appears late in pregnancy, its presence generally indicates maturity

D. INTRAPARTUM FETAL ASSESSMENT

1. Causes of nonreassuring fetal status
   a. Uteroplacental insufficiency
      1) Placenta impaired or unable to provide oxygen & nutrients while removing products of metabolism & waste
      2) Causes = placenta previa or abruption, placental edema from hydrops fetalis or Rh isoimmunization, postterm pregnancy, intrauterine growth retardation (IUGR), uterine hyperstimulation
      3) Fetal response to hypoxia → shunting of blood to brain, heart & adrenal glands
      4) If unrecognized can progress to metabolic acidosis with accumulation of lactic acid & damage to vital organs
   b. Umbilical cord compression due to oligohydramnios, cord prolapse or knot, anomalous cord, or abnormal cord insertion

   c. Fetal anomalies include IUGR, prematurity, postterm, sepsis, congenital anomalies
2. Fetal heart rate (FHR) monitoring
   a. Normal FHR is 120–160 bpm
   b. Tachycardia = FHR >160 bpm for 10 min or more
      1) Most common cause is maternal fever (which may signal chorioamnionitis)
      2) Other causes = fetal hypoxia, immaturity, tachyarrhythmias, anemia, infection, or maternal thyrotoxicosis or treatment with sympathomimetics
   c. Bradycardia = FHR <120 bpm for 10 min or more, caused by congenital heart block, fetal anoxia (e.g., from placental separation) & maternal treatment with β-blockers
   d. FHR variability
      1) A reliable indicator of fetal well-being, suggesting sufficient CNS oxygenation
      2) ↓ variability associated with fetal hypoxia/acidosis, depressant drugs, fetal tachycardia, CNS or cardiac anomalies, prolonged uterine contractions, prematurity & fetal sleep
3. Accelerations
   a. Types & patterns of accelerations play a role in intrapartum evaluation of the fetus
   b. Accelerations
      1) ↑ FHR of at least 15 bpm above baseline for 15–20 sec
      2) This pattern indicates a fetus unstressed by hypoxia or acidemia → reassuring & suggests fetal well-being
   c. Early decelerations (See Figure 3-1)
      1) ↓ FHR (not below 100 bpm) that mirrors a uterine contraction (i.e., begins with onset of contraction, dips at peak of contraction, returns to baseline with end of contraction)
      2) Results from pressure on fetal head → vagus nerve stimulated reflex response to release acetylcholine at fetal SA node
      3) Considered physiologic & not harmful to fetus
   d. Variable decelerations (See Figure 3-1)
      1) Do not necessarily coincide with uterine contraction
      2) Characterized by rapid dip in FHR, often <100 bpm with rapid return to baseline
      3) Also reflex-mediated, due to umbilical cord compression
      4) Can be corrected by shifting maternal position, or amnioinfusion if membranes have ruptured & cord compression is secondary to oligohydramnios
   e. Late decelerations (See Figure 3-1)
      1) Begin after contraction has already started, dip after peak of contraction, returns to baseline after contraction is over
      2) Viewed as potentially dangerous, associated with uteroplacental insufficiency
      3) Causes include placental abruption, PIH, maternal diabetes, maternal anemia, maternal sepsis, postterm pregnancy & hyperstimulated uterus
      4) Repetitive late decelerations require intervention

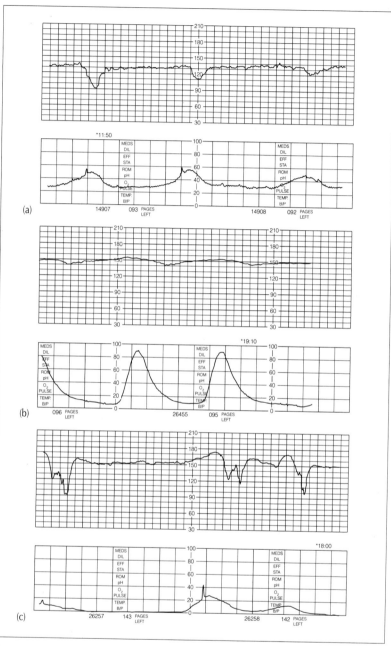

Figure 3-1 (a) An early deceleration pattern is depicted in this fetal heart rate (FHR) tracing. Note that each deceleration returns to baseline before the completion of the contraction. The remainder of the fetal heart rate tracing is reassuring. (b) Repetitive late decelerations in conjunction with decreased variability. (c) Variable decelerations are the most common periodic change of the fetal heart rate during labor. Repetitive mild-to-moderate variable decelerations are present. The baseline is normal.

E. ISOIMMUNIZATION

1. Development of maternal IgG antibodies following exposure to fetal red blood cell antigens
2. Exposure commonly occurs at delivery, but can occur during pregnancy as well
3. In subsequent pregnancies (rarely late in the same pregnancy) these antibodies can cross the placenta → attach to fetal RBC cells & hemolyze them → fetal anemia
4. Can occur with any blood group, but most often occurs when mother is Rh-negative & fetus is Rh-positive
5. Extent to which fetus is affected depends on amount of IgG antibodies crossing placenta & ability of fetus to replenish destroyed RBCs
6. Worst case scenario is hydrops fetalis
   a. Significant transfer of antibodies across placenta → fetal anemia
   b. Liver attempts to make new RBCs (fetal hematopoiesis occurs in liver & bone marrow) at the expense of other necessary proteins →↓ oncotic pressure → fetal ascites & edema
   c. High-output cardiac failure associated with severe anemia
7. Maternal IgG titer ≥ 1:16 is high enough to pose risk to the fetus
8. Tx = RhoGAM
   a. Administration of antibody to the Rh antigen (Rh immune globulin = RhoGAM) within 72 hr of delivery prevents active antibody response by the mother in most cases
   b. Risk of subsequent sensitization ↓ from 15% to 2%
   c. When RhoGAM is also given at 28 wk of gestation, risk of sensitization is further reduced to 0.2%
9. RhoGAM given to Rh-negative mothers if the father is Rh-positive
   a. At 28 wks gestation
   b. Within 72 hr of delivery of Rh-positive infant
   c. Other times maternal-fetal blood mixing can occur
      1) At time of amniocentesis
      2) After an abortion
      3) After an ectopic pregnancy
      Note: Kleinhauer-Betke test (identifies fetal RBCs in maternal blood)

F. GENETIC TESTING

1. Chromosomal abnormalities account for 50–60% of spontaneous abortion, 5% of stillbirths, 2–3% of couples with multiple miscarriages
2. 0.6% of all live births have a chromosomal abnormality
3. Indications for prenatal genetic testing
   a. Most common is advanced maternal age (AMA)
      1) Trisomy 21 (Down's syndrome) incidence ↑ 10-fold from age 35 to age 45, other polysomies ↑ similarly
      2) Amniocentesis routinely offered to all women who will be >35 yr old at estimated time of delivery
   b. Prior child with chromosome or single gene abnormality
   c. Known chromosomal abnormality such as a balanced translocation or single gene disorder in parent(s)
   d. Abnormal results from screening tests such as the triple marker screen

VI. Labor and Delivery

A. INITIAL PRESENTATION
1. Labor = progressive effacement & dilation of uterine cervix resulting from contractions of uterus
2. **Braxton Hicks contractions** (false labor) = uterine contractions without effacement & dilation of cervix
3. 85% of patients undergo spontaneous labor & delivery between 37 and 42 wk gestation
4. Pts are told to come to hospital for regular contractions q 5 min for at least 1 hr, rupture of membranes, significant bleeding, ↓ in fetal movement
5. Initial exam upon arrival
   a. Auscultation of fetal heart tones
   b. Leopold maneuvers help determine fetal lie (relation of long axis of fetus with maternal long axis), determine fetal presentation (i.e., breech vs. cephalic) & position of presenting part with respect to right or left side of maternal pelvis
   c. Vaginal examination
      1) Check for rupture of membranes, cervical effacement & cervical dilation (in cm)
      2) Fetal station (level of fetal presenting part relative to ischial spines) measured from −3 (presenting part palpable at pelvic inlet) to +3 (presenting part palpable beyond pelvic outlet)
      3) 0 station = presenting part palpable at ischial spines, significance of 0 station is that biparietal diameter (biggest diameter of fetal head) has negotiated pelvic inlet (smallest part of pelvis)

B. STAGES OF LABOR
1. Labor divided into 3 stages (See Figure 3-2)
2. Stage 1
   a. Interval between onset of labor & full cervical dilation (10 cm)
   b. Further subdivided into:
      1) Latent phase = cervical effacement & early dilation
      2) Active phase = more rapid cervical dilation occurs, usually beginning at 3–4 cm
3. Stage 2 = interval between complete cervical dilation & delivery of infant
4. Stage 3 = interval between delivery of infant & delivery of placenta
5. Stage 4 = immediate postpartum period lasting 2 hr during which pt undergoes significant physiologic changes

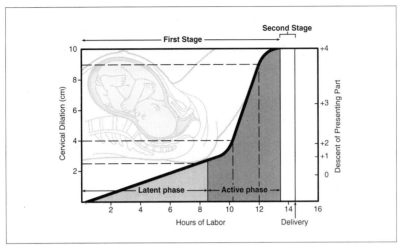

FIGURE 3-2 Schematic illustration of progress of rotation of occipitoanterior presentation in the successive stages of labor. Note relationship between changes in cervical dilation and phases of labor.

C. MANAGEMENT OF LABOR
1. First stage
    a. Continuous monitoring of fetal heart rate, either external monitoring via Doppler, or internal monitoring via fetal scalp electrode (FSE) that allows for more detailed evaluation of fetal heart rate pattern
    b. Monitoring of uterine activity
        1) External tocodynamometer measures frequency & duration of contractions, but not intensity
        2) Internal uterine pressure catheter (IUPC) measures intensity by measuring intrauterine pressure
    c. Analgesic (typically meperidine) &/or anesthetic (typically an epidural block that provides both continuous analgesia & anesthesia) can be given—agents usually not given until active stage of labor
2. Second stage
    a. Maternal effort (i.e., pushing) accelerates delivery of fetus (↑ in intra-abdominal pressure assists fetal descent down birth canal)
    b. Delivery should be well controlled with protection of the perineum
    c. If used, episiotomies are usually cut midline
    d. After head is delivered, bulb suction of nose & mouth is performed & neck is evaluated for presence of nuchal cord
    e. Shoulders are delivered by applying gentle downward pressure on head to deliver anterior shoulder followed by easy upward force to deliver posterior shoulder
    f. Delivery of body follows, cord is clamped & cut, & infant given to mother or to warmer

g. Blood from umbilical cord sent for ABO & Rh testing as well as arterial blood gases
3. Third stage
   a. 3 signs of placenta separation
      1) Uterus rises in abdomen signaling that placenta has separated
      2) Gush of blood
      3) Lengthening of umbilical cord
   b. Excessive pulling on placenta should be avoided because of risk of uterus inversion with associated profound hemorrhage & retained placenta
   c. Gentle traction should be applied at all times
   d. May take up to 30 min for placenta to be expulsed
4. Fourth stage
   a. Systemic evaluation of cervix, vagina, vulva, perineum & periurethral area for lacerations
   b. Likelihood of serious postpartum complications is greatest in first 1–2 hr postpartum

D. ABNORMAL LABOR
1. Dystocia = difficult labor
   a. Cause detected by evaluating the **3 Ps**
      1) **Power**
         a) Refers to strength, duration & frequency of contractions
         b) Measured by using tocodynamometer or IUPC
         c) For cervical dilation to occur ≥3 contractions in 10 min must be generated
         d) During active labor maternal effort comes into play, as maternal exhaustion, effects of analgesia/anesthesia, or underlying disease may prolong labor
      2) **Passenger**
         a) Refers to estimates of fetal weight + evaluation of fetal lie, presentation & position
         b) Occiput posterior presentation, face presentation & hydrocephalus are associated with dystocia
      3) **Passage**
         a) Difficult to measure pelvic diameters
         b) Adequacy of pelvis often unknown until progress (or no progress) is made during labor
         c) Distended bladder, adnexal or colon masses & uterine fibroids can all contribute to dystocia
   b. Dystocia divided into prolongation disorders
      1) Prolonged latent phase
         a) Latent phase >20 hr in primigravid or >14 hr in multigravid patient is prolonged & abnormal
         b) Causes include ineffective uterine contractions, fetopelvic disproportion & excess anesthesia
         c) Prolonged latent phase → no harm to mother or fetus
      2) Prolonged active phase

  a) Active phase >12 hr or rate of cervical dilation <1.2 cm/hr in primigravid or <1.5 cm/hr in multigravid
  b) Causes include excess anesthesia, ineffective contractions, fetopelvic disproportion, fetal malposition, rupture of membranes before onset of active labor
  c) Prolonged active phase → ↑ risk of intrauterine infection & increased risk of cesarean section
2. Arrest disorders
  a. 2° arrest occurs when cervical dilation during active phase ceases for ≥2 hr
  b. Suggests either cephalopelvic disproportion or ineffective uterine contractions
3. Management of abnormal labor
  a. Labor induction = stimulation of uterine contractions before spontaneous onset of labor
  b. Augmentation of labor = stimulation of uterine contractions that began spontaneously but have become infrequent, weak, or both
  c. Induction trial should occur only if cervix is prepared or "ripe"
  d. Bishop score used to try to quantify cervical readiness for induction

TABLE 3-4   Bishop Score

FACTOR	POINTS			
	0	**1**	**2**	**3**
Dilation	Closed	1–2 cm	3–4 cm	≥5 cm
Effacement	0–30%	40–50%	60–70%	≥80%
Station	−3	−2, −1	0	≥+1
Position		Posterior	Mid	Anterior

Score: 9–13 associated with highest likelihood of successful induction.
    0–4 associated with highest likelihood of failed induction.

4. Indications for induction = suspected fetal compromise, fetal death, PIH, premature ROM, chorioamnionitis, postdates pregnancy, maternal medical complication
5. Contraindications for induction include placenta previa, active genital herpes, abnormal fetal lie, cord presentation
6. If cervix not "ripe," prostaglandin E2 gel can be used to attempt to ripen cervix, biggest risk is uterine hyperstimulation → uteroplacental insufficiency
7. Another method is insertion of laminaria or rods inserted into the internal os that absorb moisture & expand, slowly dilating cervix, risks include failure to dilate, laceration, rupture of membranes & infection
8. Prolonged latent phase can be managed with rest, augmentation of labor with oxytocin, &/or amniotomy that may allow for fetal head to provide greater dilating force
9. During active phase of labor fetal malposition & cephalopelvic disproportion must be considered & may warrant cesarean section vs. augmentation
10. If fetus has descended far enough, forceps or vacuum can be used, if not cesarean section is carried out
11. Risks of prolonged labor include infection, exhaustion, lacerations, uterine atony with hemorrhage

12. Breech presentation occurs in 2–4% of pregnancies & risk ↑ in cases of multiple gestations, polyhydramnios, hydrocephaly, anencephaly & uterine anomalies (See Figure 3-3)

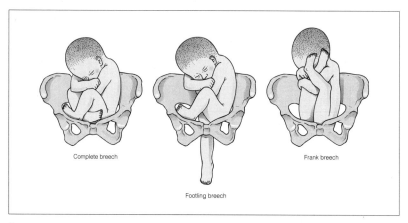

Complete breech

Frank breech

Footling breech

FIGURE 3-3   Different breech presentations.

E. POSTPARTUM HEMORRHAGE

1. Defined as blood loss >500 mL associated with delivery
2. Causes = uterine atony (most common), lacerations, retained placenta
3. Uterine atony
   a. Normally uterus quickly contracts following delivery of placenta, muscle contraction compresses down on spiral arteries & prevents excessive bleeding
   b. If contraction does not occur → postpartum hemorrhage
   c. Risk factors for uterine atony = multiple gestations, hydramnios, multiparity, macrosomia, previous history of postpartum hemorrhage, fibroids, magnesium sulfate, general anesthesia, prolonged labor, amnionitis
   d. Dx based on clinical exam of soft, "boggy" uterus
   e. Tx
      1) Start with uterine massage to stimulate contractions
      2) IV fluids & transfusions as needed, cervix & vagina visualized for lacerations
      3) Medical Tx = oxytocin, methergine (potent uterotonic always given IM—if given IV can cause severe hypertension), or prostaglandins → uterine contractions
      4) If these measures are unsuccessful, surgical interventions are used & include ligation of uterine arteries, ligation of internal iliac arteries, selective arterial embolization or hysterectomy as last resort
4. Retained placenta
   a. Occurs when separation of placenta from uterine wall or expulsion of placenta is incomplete
   b. Risk factors include previous cesarean section, fibroids & prior uterine curettage
   c. Placental tissue that abnormally implants into uterus can also result in retention
   d. Placenta accreta: placental villi abnormally adhere to superficial lining of uterine wall

e. Placenta increta: placental villi penetrate into uterine muscle layer

f. Placenta percreta: placental villi completely invade uterine muscle layer

5. Disseminated intravascular coagulation (DIC)

   a. A rare cause of postpartum hemorrhage

   b. Severe preeclampsia, amniotic fluid embolism & placental abruption are associated with DIC

   c. Tx aimed at correcting coagulopathy

VII. Postpartum Care

A. LACTATION & BREAST FEEDING

1. Engorgement occurs about 3 days postpartum

2. 3 causes of tender enlarged breasts postpartum are engorgement, mastitis & plugged duct

3. Tx engorgement with continued breast feeding, mastitis with antibiotics (nursing can be continued) & plugged duct with warm packs

4. Advantages of breast feeding = ↑ bonding between mother & child, convenience, ↓ cost, protection against infection & allergies

5. Breast milk provides all vitamins except vitamin K

B. CONTRACEPTION

1. Contraception should be discussed with all patients prior to discharge

2. About 15% of women are fertile 6 wk postpartum

3. OCPs are not contraindicated in breast-feeding & postpartum tubal ligation should be discussed as well

C. POSTPARTUM IMMUNIZATIONS

1. Rubella nonimmune women should be immunized (they can continue to breast feed)

2. Rh-negative woman who has given birth to an Rh-positive baby should receive RhoGAM

D. POSTPARTUM DEPRESSION

1. Recurrence rate for patients with previous postpartum depression is 25%

2. Postpartum depression ranges from the "blues" that affects 50% of women & typically occurs about day 2–3, resolving in 1–2 wk, to postpartum depression that affects 10% of women, to suicidal ideation that occurs more rarely

3. Especially worrisome is a mother who has estranged herself from her newborn or has become indifferent

4. Tx depends on severity of Sx & may range from simple telephone contact to psychotherapy & medication to inpatient hospitalization

E. POSTPARTUM UTERINE INFECTION

1. Incidence of infection ranges from 10–50% depending on population, mode of delivery (C-section > vaginal delivery) & risk factors

2. Risk factors = maternal obesity, immunosuppression, chronic disease, vaginal infection, amnionitis, prolonged labor, prolonged ROM, multiple pelvic examinations during labor, internal fetal monitoring or intrauterine pressure catheter, C-section

3. **Most common infection post C-section is metritis** (uterine infection)

4. Si/Sx = fever on first or second postpartum day, uterine tenderness, ↓ bowel sounds, leukocytosis (difficult to interpret because of normal leukocytosis in puerperium)
5. DDx
    a. First day postpartum: think *lungs (wind)* → atelectasis, especially if general anesthesia was used, or pneumonia
    b. Second day postpartum: think *urinary tract (water)* → UTI, pyelonephritis
    c. Third day postpartum: think *wound*
    d. Fourth day postpartum: think *extremities (walking)* → thrombophlebitis
6. Metritis usually polymicrobial with aerobic & anaerobic organisms present
7. Dx = clinical
8. Tx = first generation cephalosporin, add coverage (mezlocillin + aminoglycoside) if no response within 48–72 hr
9. Prophylactic antibiotic therapy (one-time dose) at time of C-section delivery significantly reduces incidence of postpartum infection

VIII. Obstetrical Complications

A. ABORTION
1. Termination of a pregnancy before viability, usually at 20 wk or less, occurs spontaneously in 15% of all pregnancies
2. Risk factors = ↑ parity, advanced maternal age, ↑ paternal age, conception within 3 mo of a live birth
3. Single pregnancy loss does not significantly increase risk of future loss
4. Chromosomal abnormalities cause 50% of early spontaneous abortion, mostly trisomies (the longer a pregnancy goes before undergoing spontaneous abortion, the less likely that fetus is chromosomally abnormal)
5. Other causes = endocrine dz (e.g., thyroid), structural abnormalities (e.g., fibroids, incompetent cervix), infection (e.g., *Listeria, Mycoplasma,* ToRCHS), chronic dz (e.g., DM, SLE, renal or cardiac dz), environmental factors (e.g., toxins, radiation, smoking, alcohol)
6. Vaginal bleeding in first half of any pregnancy is presumed to be a threatened abortion unless another diagnosis such as ectopic pregnancy, cervical polyps, cervicitis, or molar pregnancy can be made
7.

TABLE 3-5   Types of Abortions

Threatened	• Si/Sx = vaginal bleeding in first 20 wk of pregnancy without passage of tissue or ROM, with cervix closed
	• Occurs in 25% of pregnancies ($^1/_2$ go on to spontaneously abort)
	• ↑ risk preterm labor & delivery, low birth weight, perinatal mortality
	• Dx = Utz to confirm early pregnancy is intact
	• If no cardiac activity by 9 wk → consider D&C procedure
	• HCG levels are also used to identify viable pregnancies at various stages of development
Inevitable	• Si/Sx = threatened abortion with dilated cervical os &/or ROM, usually accompanied by cramping with expulsion of products of conception (POC)
	• Pregnancy loss is unavoidable
	• Tx = surgical evacuation of uterine contents & RhoGAM if mother is Rh-negative

TABLE 3-5   *Continued*

Completed	• Si/Sx = documented pregnancy that spontaneously aborts all POCs • POCs should be grossly examined & submitted to pathology to confirm fetal tissue &/or placental villi, if none is observed must rule out ectopic pregnancy • Pts may require curettage because of ↑ likelihood that abortion was incomplete (suspected if β-hCG levels plateau or fail to decline to zero) • RhoGAM given to Rh-negative women
Incomplete	• Si/Sx = cramping, bleeding, passage of tissue, with dilated cervix & visible tissue in vagina or endocervical canal • Curettage usually needed to remove remaining POCs & to control bleeding • Again Rh-negative patients are given RhoGAM • Hemodynamic stabilization may be required if bleeding is very heavy
Missed	• Failure to expel POC • Si/Sx = lack of uterine growth, lack of fetal heart tones & cessation of pregnancy symptoms • Evacuation of uterus required after fetal death has been confirmed, suction curettage recommended for first-trimester pregnancy, dilation & evacuation (D&E) recommended for second-trimester pregnancies • Serious but rare complication is DIC • Rh-negative patients receive RhoGAM
Recurrent	• Si/Sx = ≥2 consecutive or total of 3 spontaneous abortions • If early, often due to chromosomal abnormalities → karyotyping for both parents to determine if they carry a chromosomal abnormality • Examine mother for uterine abnormalities • Incompetent cervix is suspected by history of painless dilation of cervix with delivery of normal fetus between 18 and 32 weeks of gestation • Tx = surgical cerclage procedures to suture cervix closed until labor or rupture of membranes occurs

B. ECTOPIC PREGNANCY

1. Implantation outside of uterine cavity
2. ↑ incidence recently because of ↑ in PID, second leading cause of maternal mortality
3. Risk factors = previous ectopic pregnancy, previous history of salpingitis (scarring & adhesions impede transport of ovum down tube), age ≥35 yr old, >3 prior pregnancies, sterilization failure
4. Si/Sx = abdominal/pelvic pain, referred shoulder pain from hemoperitoneal irritation of diaphragm, amenorrhea, vaginal bleeding, cervical motion or adnexal tenderness, nausea, vomiting, orthostatic changes
5. DDx = surgical abdomen (see Surgery), abortion, salpingitis, endometriosis, ruptured ovarian cyst, ovarian torsion
6. Ectopic pregnancy should be suspected in any reproductive age woman who presents with abdominal/pelvic pain, irregular bleeding & amenorrhea—lag in treatment is a significant cause of mortality
7. Dx
    a. ⊕ pregnancy test with Utz to determine intrauterine vs. extrauterine pregnancy
    b. Very low progesterone level strongly suggests nonviable pregnancy that may be located outside the uterine cavity while higher levels suggest viable pregnancy
8. Tx

a. Surgical removal now commonly done via laparoscopy with maximum preservation of reproductive organs

b. Methotrexate can be used early, especially if pregnancy is <3.5 cm in diameter, with no cardiac activity on Utz

c. Regardless of technique used, posttreatment serial β-hCG levels must be followed to ensure proper falloff in level

d. Rh-negative women should receive RhoGAM to avoid Rh sensitization

C. THIRD-TRIMESTER BLEEDING

1. Occurs in about 5% of all pregnancies
2. Half of these are due to placenta previa or placental abruption, others due to vaginal/vulvar lacerations, cervical polyps, cervicitis, cervical cancer
3. In many cases no cause for bleeding is found
4.

TABLE 3-6 Comparison of Placenta Previa and Placental Abruption

	PLACENTA PREVIA	PLACENTAL ABRUPTION
Abnormality	Placenta implanted over internal cervical os (completely or partially)	Premature separation (complete or partial) of normally implanted placenta from decidua
Epidemiology	↑ risk grand multiparas & prior C-section	↑ risk preeclampsia, previous history of abruption, rupture of membranes in a patient with hydramnios, cocaine use, cigarette smoking & trauma
Time of onset	20–30 wk	Any time after 20 wk
Si/Sx	Sudden, **painless** bleeding	**Painful** bleeding, can be heavy, painful & frequent uterine contractions
Dx	Utz → placenta abnormal location	Clinical, based on presentation of painful vaginal bleeding, frequent contractions & fetal distress. **Utz not useful**
Tx	Hemodynamic support, expectant management, deliver by C-section when fetus mature enough	Hemodynamic support, urgent C-section or vaginal induction if pt is stable & fetus is not in distress
Complications	Associated with 2-fold ↑ in congenital malformations so evaluation for fetal anomalies should be undertaken at Dx	↑ risk of fetal hypoxia/death, DIC may occur as a result of intravascular & retroplacental coagulation

D. PRETERM LABOR (PTL)

1. Regular uterine contractions at ≤10 min intervals, lasting ≥30 sec, between 20 and 36 wk gestation & accompanied by cervical effacement, dilation &/or descent of fetus into the pelvis

2. It is a major cause of preterm birth → significant perinatal morbidity & mortality

3. Risk factors = premature rupture of membranes (PROM), infection (UTI, vaginal, amniotic), dehydration, incompetent cervix, smoking, fibroids, placenta previa, placental abruption, many cases are idiopathic

4. Si/Sx = cramps, dull low back pain, abdominal/pelvic pressure, vaginal discharge (mucous, water, or bloody) & contractions (often painless)

5. Dx = external fetal monitoring to quantify frequency & duration of contractions, vaginal exam → extent of cervical dilation/effacement

6. Utz to confirm gestational age, amniotic fluid volume (helps to determine if rupture of membranes has occurred), fetal presentation & placental location

7. Tx focused on delaying delivery if possible until fetus is mature
   a. 50% of patients have spontaneous resolution of preterm uterine contractions
   b. IV hydration important because dehydration is well known to cause uterine irritability
   c. Empiric antibiotic therapy is given for suspected chorioamnionitis or vaginal infection
   d. Tocolytic regimens
      1) Magnesium sulfate, β-2 agonists like terbutaline & ritodrine, Ca^{2+}-blockers like nifedipine, or indomethacin may be instituted although they have never been shown to substantially prolong delivery more than several days
      2) Contraindications to tocolysis = advanced labor (cervical dilation >3 cm), mature fetus, chorioamnionitis, significant vaginal bleeding, anomalous fetus, acute fetal distress, severe preeclampsia or eclampsia
   e. From 24 to 34 wk steroids such as betamethasone are generally used to enhance pulmonary maturity
   f. Management of infants at 34–37 wk is individualized; survival rates for infants born at 34 wk is within 1% of the survival rate for infants born at 37 wk & beyond; assessment of fetal lung maturity may help decide who to deliver between 34 and 37 wk

8. Common complications include death, respiratory distress syndrome & subsequent bronchopulmonary dysplasia, sepsis, intraventricular hemorrhage, necrotizing entero-colitis, developmental delays & seizures

E. PREMATURE RUPTURE OF MEMBRANES (PROM)

1. Rupture of chorioamniotic membrane before onset of labor, occurs in 10–15% of all pregnancies

2. Labor usually follows PROM; 90% of patients & 50% of preterm patients go into labor within 24 hr after rupture

3. Biggest risk is labor & delivery of preterm infant with associated morbidities/mortality, second biggest complication is infection (chorioamnionitis)

4. PROM at 26 wk of gestation or less is associated with pulmonary hypoplasia

5. Dx = vaginal exam with testing of nonbloody fluid from the vagina
   a. Nitrazine test: uses pH to distinguish alkaline amniotic fluid (pH > 7.0) with more acidic urine & vaginal secretions (note false-positive seen with semen, cervical mucus, *Trichomonas* infection, blood, unusually basic urine)
   b. Fern test: amniotic fluid placed on slide that is allowed to dry in room (up to 30 min); the branching fern leaf pattern that results when the slide is completely dry is caused from sodium chloride precipitates from amniotic fluid

OB/GYN

    c. Utz confirms Dx by noting oligohydramnios, labor is less likely to occur if sufficient fluid remains

  6. Tx

    a. If intrauterine infection is suspected, empiric broad spectrum antibiotics are started

    b. Otherwise treat as for preterm labor above

F. MULTIPLE GESTATIONS

  1. 1 in 90 incidence in US (slightly higher in black women, slightly lower in white women)

  2. **Dizygotic twins occur when 2 separate ova are fertilized by 2 separate sperm, incidence ↑ with ↑ age & parity**

  3. Monozygotic twins represent division of the fertilized ovum at various times after conception

  4. Multiple gestations are considered high-risk pregnancies because of the disproportionate increase in perinatal morbidity & mortality as compared with a singleton gestation

    a. **Spontaneous abortions & congenital anomalies occur more frequently in multiple pregnancies as compared with singleton pregnancies**

    b. Maternal complications = anemia, hydramnios, eclampsia, PTL, postpartum uterine atony & hemorrhage, increased risk for C-section

    c. Fetal complications: congenital anomalies, spontaneous abortion, IUGR, prematurity, PROM, umbilical cord prolapse, placental abruption, placenta previa & malpresentation

  5. Average duration of gestation ↓ with ↑ number of fetuses (twins deliver at 37 wk, triplets deliver at 33 wk, quadruplets deliver at 29 wk)

  6. Twin-twin transfusion syndrome

    a. Occurs in 10% of twins sharing a chorionic membrane

    b. Occurs when blood flow is interrupted by a vascular anastomoses such that one twin becomes the donor twin & can have impaired growth, anemia, hypovolemia, & the other twin (recipient twin) can develop hypervolemia, hypertension, polycythemia & congestive heart failure as a result of the increased blood flow from one twin to the other

  7. Dx of twins usually suspected when uterine size exceeds calculated gestational age & can be confirmed with ultrasound

  8. DDx = incorrect dates, fibroids, polyhydramnios & molar pregnancy

  9. Delivery method largely depends on presentation of twins; usually if first fetus is in vertex presentation, vaginal delivery is attempted; if not C-section is often performed

  10. Important to watch for uterine atony & postpartum hemorrhage because overdistended uterus may not clamp down normally

Gynecology

I. Benign Gynecology

A. MENSTRUAL CYCLE (See Figure 3-4)

1. Due to hypothalamic pulses of gonadotropin releasing hormone (GnRH), pituitary release of follicle stimulating hormone (FSH) & luteinizing hormone (LH), & ovarian sex steroids estradiol & progesterone
2. ↑ or ↓ of any of these hormones → irregular menses or amenorrhea
3. At birth, the human ovary contains approximately 1 million primordial follicles each with an oocyte arrested in the prophase stage of meiosis
4. Process of ovulation begins in puberty = follicular maturation
   a. After ovulation the dominant follicle released becomes the corpus luteum, which secretes progesterone to prepare the endometrium for possible implantation
   b. If the ovum is not fertilized the corpus luteum undergoes involution, menstruation begins & cycle repeats
5. Phases of the menstrual cycle
   a. First day of menstrual bleeding is day 1 of the cycle
   b.

TABLE 3-7   Phases of the Menstrual Cycle (See Figure 3-4)

FOLLICULAR PHASE (PROLIFERATIVE PHASE)	OVULATORY PHASE	LUTEAL PHASE (SECRETORY PHASE)
Day 1–13 of cycle: estradiol-induced negative feedback on FSH & ⊕ feedback on LH in anterior pituitary leads to LH surge on day 11–13	**Day 13–17 of cycle:** dominant follicle secretion of estradiol → ⊕ feedback to anterior pituitary FSH & LH, ovulation occurs 30–36 hr after the LH surge, small FSH surge also occurs at time of LH surge	**Day 15 to first day of menses:** marked by change from estradiol to progesterone predominance, corpus luteal progesterone acts on hypothalamus, causing negative feedback on FSH & LH, resulting in ↓ to basal levels prior to next cycle, if fertilization & implantation do not occur → rapid ↓ in progesterone

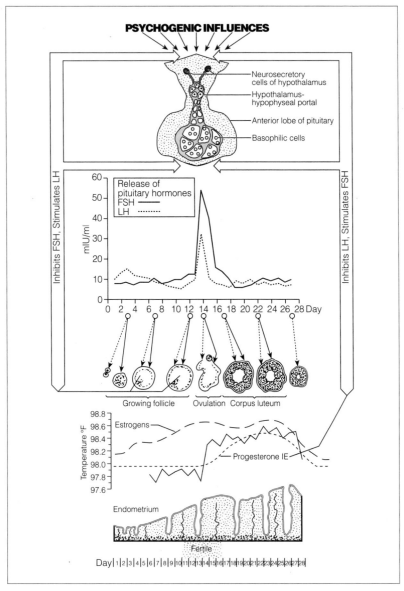

FIGURE 3-4 Normal menstrual cycle. Note the suprahypothalamic (cerebral, pineal), hypothalamic, pituitary, ovarian, and endometrial interrelations.

B. CONTRACEPTION

1. Oral contraceptive pills (OCPs) = combination estrogen & progestin

   a. Progestin is major contraceptive by suppressing LH & thus ovulation, also thickens cervical mucus so it is less favorable to semen

   b. Estrogen participates by suppressing FSH thereby preventing selection & maturation of a dominant follicle

   c. Estrogen & progesterone together inhibit implantation by thinning endometrial lining, also resulting in light or missed menses

   d. Monophasic pills deliver a constant dose of estrogen & progestin

   e. Phasic OCPs alter this ratio (usually by varying the dose of progestin) that slightly ↓ the total dose of hormone per month, but also has slightly ↑ rate of breakthrough bleeding between periods

   f. Pts usually resume fertility once OCPs are discontinued; however, **3% may have prolonged postpill amenorrhea**

   g.

TABLE 3-8   Risks and Benefits of OCPs

ADVANTAGES	DISADVANTAGES

• Highly reliable, failure rate <1% (failure usually related to missing pills)
• Protect against endometrial & ovarian CA
• ↓ incidence of pelvic infections & ectopic pregnancies
• Menses are more predictable, lighter, less painful
	• Require daily compliance
	• Does not protect against STDs
	• 10–30% have breakthrough bleeding
	• Side effects:
	  ◊ Estrogen → bloating, weight gain, breast tenderness, nausea, headaches
	  ◊ Progestin → depression, acne, HTN*

*Try lower progesterone pill, if hypertension doesn't resolve, D/C OCPs—pts with preexisting hypertension can try OCPs if they are ≤35 yr old & in good medical control.

   h. Absolute contraindications to use of OCPs = pregnancy, DVT or thromboembolic dz, endometrial CA, cerebrovascular or coronary artery dz, breast CA, cigarette smoking in women > 35 yr old, hepatic dz/neoplasm, abnormal vaginal bleeding, hyperlipidemia

TABLE 3-9   Alternatives to OCPs

METHOD	INDICATION	ADVANTAGE	DISADVANTAGE
Progestin only pills ("Mini-pills")	• **Lactating women**	• Can start immediately postpartum • No impact on milk production or the baby	• ↑ failure rate than OCP (ovulation continues in 40%) • Requires strict compliance—low dose of progesterone requires that pill be taken at same time each day
Depo-Provera (Medroxy-progesterone)	• Contraception for ≥1 yr • Noncompliance with daily OCPs • Breast feeding	• **IM injection** maintained for 14 wk	• Irregular vaginal bleed[a] • 50% pts infertile for 10 mo after last injection • Risk of abortion[b]

TABLE 3-9   *Continued*

METHOD	INDICATION	ADVANTAGE	DISADVANTAGE
Norplant	• Long-term contraception	• Subcutaneous implants provide **contraception for 5 yr** • Prompt fertility when DC'd	• 30% of breakthrough pregnancies are ectopic
Intrauterine device	• For those at low risk for STDs	• Inserted into endometrial cavity, left in place for several years	• Contraindicated in cervical or vaginal infxn, Hx of PID or infertility • Spontaneous expulsion, menstrual pain, ↑ rate of ectopic pregnancy, septic abortion & pelvic infxns
Postcoital	• Emergency contraception	• **Progestin/estrogen taken within 72 hr of intercourse**, repeat in 12 hr • Allows for early termination of unwanted pregnancy	• Follow pt to ensure withdrawal bleeding occurs within 5 days • Nausea

[a] Oral estrogen or NSAIDs can ↓ bleeding, bleeding ↓ with each use, 50% pts are amenorrheic in 1 yr.
[b] Injection given within first 5 days of menses (ensuring pt not pregnant).

C. PAP SMEAR

1. First Pap smear should be done when woman becomes sexually active or by age 18, then yearly thereafter
2. In pts with 1 sexual partner, 3 consecutive normal Pap smears & onset of sexual activity after age 25, may be able to screen less frequently
3. Reliability depends on presence/absence of cervical inflammation, adequacy of specimen & prompt fixation of specimen to avoid artifact
4. If Pap → mild- or low-grade atypia → repeat Pap—atypia may spontaneously regress
5. Recurrent mild atypia or high-grade atypia → more intensive evaluation
   a. Colposcopy
      1) Allows for magnification of cervix allowing subtle areas of dysplastic change to be visualized, optimizing selection of biopsy sites
      2) Cervix washed with acetic acid solution, white areas, abnormally vascularized areas & punctate lesions are selected for biopsy
   b. Endocervical curettage (ECC) → sample of endocervix obtained at same time of colposcopy so that disease further up in endocervical canal may be detected
   c. Cone biopsy
      1) Cone-shaped specimen encompassing squamocolumnar junction (SCJ) & any lesions on ectocervix removed from cervix by knife, laser, or wire loop
      2) Allows for more complete ascertainment of extent of disease & in many cases is therapeutic as well as diagnostic
      3) Indications = ⊕ ECC, unsatisfactory colposcopy meaning that entire squamocolumnar junction was not visualized, & discrepancy between Pap smear & colposcopy biopsy
6. Tx = excision of premalignant or malignant lesions—if cancer, see Section VIII below for appropriate adjunctive modalities

D. VAGINITIS

1. 50% of cases due to *Gardnerella* ("bacterial vaginosis"), 25% due to *Trichomonas*, 25% due to *Candida* (↑ frequency in diabetics, in pregnancy & in HIV)
2. Most common presenting symptom in vaginitis is discharge
3. Rule out noninfectious causes, including chemical or allergic sources
4. Dx by pelvic examination with microscopic examination of discharge
5. DDx of vaginitis

TABLE 3-10   Differential Diagnosis of Vaginitis

	CANDIDA	*TRICHOMONAS*	*GARDNERELLA*
Vaginal pH	4–5	>6	>5
Odor	None	Rancid	"Fishy" on KOH prep
Discharge	Cheesy white	Green, frothy	Variable
Si/Sx	Itchy, burning erythema	Severe itching	Variable to none
Microscopy	Pseudohyphae, more pronounced on 10% KOH prep (See Figure 3-5)	Motile organisms (See Figures 3-6 and 3-7)	Clue cells (large epithelial cells covered with dozens of small dots)
Treatment	Fluconazole	Metronidazole— treat partner also	Metronidazole

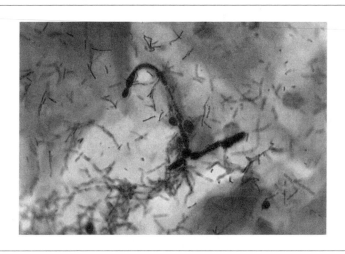

FIGURE 3-5   Gram's-stain appearance of candidal pseudohyphae and cells.

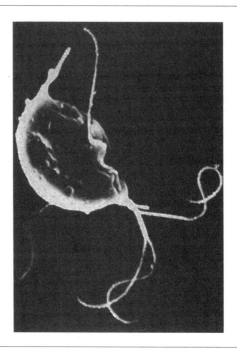

Figure 3-6   Scanning electronmicrograph of *Trichomonas vaginalis.* The undulating membrane and flagellae of *Trichomonas* are its characteristic features.

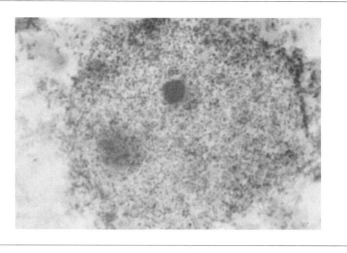

Figure 3-7   Gram's-stain appearance of a "clue cell"—a vaginal epithelial cell covered with bacteria. No lactobacilli are present.

E. ENDOMETRIOSIS

1. Affects 1–2% of women (up to 50% in infertile women), peak age = 20s–30s
2. Endometrial tissue in extrauterine locations, most commonly ovaries (60%), but can be anywhere in the peritoneum & rarely extraperitoneal
3. Adenomyosis = endometrial implants within the uterine wall
4. Endometrioma = endometriosis involving an ovary with implants large enough to be considered a tumor, filled with chocolate-appearing fluid (old blood) that gives them their name of "chocolate cysts"
5. Si/Sx = **the 3 D's = dysmenorrhea, dyspareunia, dyschezia** (painful defecation), pelvic pain, infertility, uterosacral nodularity palpable on rectovaginal exam, severity of Sx often do not correlate with extent of dz
6. Dx requires direct visualization via laparoscopy or laparotomy with histologic confirmation
7. Tx
   a. Start with NSAIDs, can add combined estrogen & progestin pills, allowing maintenance without withdrawal bleeding & dysmenorrhea
   b. Can use progestin-only pills, drawback is breakthrough bleeding
   c. GnRH agonists inhibit ovarian function → hypoestrogen state
   d. Danazol inhibits LH & FSH midcycle surges, side effects include hypoestrogenic & androgenic (hirsutism, acne) states
   e. Conservative surgery involves excision, cauterization, or ablation of endometrial implants with preservation of ovaries & uterus
   f. Recurrence after cessation of medical Tx is common, definitive Tx requires hysterectomy, ⊕ oophorectomy (TAH/BSO), lysis of adhesions & removal of endometrial implants
   g. Pts can take estrogen replacement therapy following definitive surgery, risk of reactivation of endometriosis is very small compared to risk of prolonged estrogen deficiency

II. Reproductive Endocrinology and Infertility

A. AMENORRHEA

1. Amenorrhea ≡ absence of menstruation, primary amenorrhea = a woman who has never menstruated, secondary amenorrhea = a menstrual-aged woman who has not menstruated in 6 mo
2. Causes of amenorrhea
   a. **Pregnancy = most common cause**, thus every evaluation should begin with an exclusion of pregnancy before any further work-up
   b. Asherman's syndrome
      1) Scarring of the uterine cavity after a D&C procedure
      2) **The most common anatomic cause of 2° amenorrhea**
   c. Hypothalamic deficiency due to weight loss, excessive exercise (e.g., marathon runner), obesity, drug induced (e.g., marijuana, tranquilizers), malignancy (prolactinoma, craniopharyngioma), psychogenic (chronic anxiety, anorexia)
   d. Pituitary dysfunction results from either ↓ hypothalamic pulsatile release of GnRH or ↓ pituitary release of FSH or LH
   e. Ovarian dysfunction

1) Ovarian follicles are either exhausted or resistant to stimulation by FSH & LH
2) Si/Sx = those of estrogen deficiency = hot flashes, mood swings, vaginal dryness, dyspareunia, sleep disturbances, skin thinning
3) **Note that estrogen deficiency 2° to hypothalamic-pituitary failure does not cause hot flashes, while ovarian failure does**
4) Causes = inherited (e.g., Turner's syndrome), premature natural menopause, autoimmune ovarian failure (Blizzard's syndrome), alkylating chemotherapies

  f. Genital outflow tract alteration, usually the result of congenital abnormalities (e.g., imperforate hymen or agenesis of uterus/vagina)

3. Tx
  a. Hypothalamic → reversal of underlying cause & induction of ovulation with gonadotropins
  b. Tumors → excision or bromocriptine for prolactinoma
  c. Genital tract obstruction → surgery if possible
  d. Ovarian dysfunction → exogenous estrogen replacement

B. DYSFUNCTIONAL UTERINE BLEEDING

1. Irregular menstruation without anatomic lesions of the uterus
2. **Usually due to chronic estrogen stimulation** (vs. amenorrhea, an estrogen deficient state), more rarely to genital outflow tract obstruction
3. Abnormal bleeding = bleeding at intervals <21 days or >36 days, lasting longer than 7 days, or blood loss > 80 mL
4. Menorrhagia (excessive bleeding) is usually due to anovulation
5. Dx
  a. Rule out anatomic causes of bleeding including uterine fibroids, cervical or vaginal lesions or infection, cervical & endometrial cancer
  b. Evaluate stress, exercise, weight changes, systemic disease such as thyroid, renal or hepatic disease & coagulopathies, & pregnancy
6. Tx
  a. Convert proliferative endometrium into secretory endometrium by administration of a progestational agent for 10 days
  b. Alternative is to give OCPs that suppress the endometrium & establish regular, predictable cycles
  c. NSAIDs ⊕ iron used in pts who want to preserve fertility
  d. **Postmenopausal bleeding is cancer until proven otherwise**

C. HIRSUTISM & VIRILIZATION (See Figure 3-8)

1. Hirsutism ≡ excess body hair, usually associated with acne, most commonly due to polycystic ovarian dz or adrenal hyperplasia
2. Virilization ≡ masculinization of a woman, associated with marked ↑ testosterone, clitoromegaly, temporal balding, voice deepening, breast involution, limb-shoulder girdle remodeling

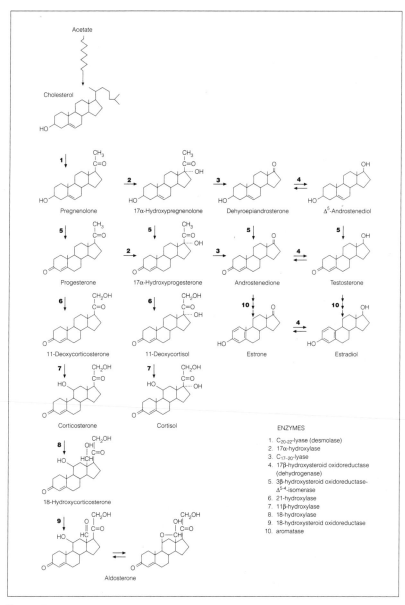

ENZYMES

1. C₂₀₋₂₂-lyase (desmolase)
2. 17α-hydroxylase
3. C₁₇₋₂₀-lyase
4. 17β-hydroxysteroid oxidoreductase (dehydrogenase)
5. 3β-hydroxysteroid oxidoreductase-Δ⁵⁻⁴-isomerase
6. 21-hydroxylase
7. 11β-hydroxylase
8. 18-hydroxylase
9. 18-hydroxysteroid oxidoreductase
10. aromatase

FIGURE 3-8 Biosynthesis of androgens, estrogens, and corticosteroids.

TABLE 3-11   Differential Diagnosis of Hirsutism and Virilization

DISEASE	CHARACTERISTICS	TREATMENT
Polycystic ovarian disease	• **#1 cause of androgen excess & hirsutism** • Etiology likely related to LH overproduction • Si/Sx = oligo- or amenorrhea, anovulation, infertility, hirsutism, acne • Labs → ↑ **LH/FSH**, ↑ **testosterone**	• Break feedback cycle with OCPs → ↓ LH production • Weight loss may allow ovulation, sparing fertility • Refractory pts may require clomiphene to ⊕ ovulation
Sertoli-Leydig cell tumors	• Ovarian tumors secreting testosterone, usually in women aged 20–40 • Si/Sx = **rapid onset** of hirsutism, acne, amenorrhea, virilization • Labs → ↓ **LH/FSH**, ↑↑↑ **testosterone**	• Removal of involved ovary (tumors usually unilateral) • 10-yr survival = 90–95%
Congenital adrenal hyperplasia	• Usually due to 21-α-hydroxylase defect • Autosomal recessive, variable penetrance • When severe → virilized newborn, milder forms can present at puberty or later • Labs → ↑ **LH/FSH**, ↑**DHEA**	• Glucocorticoids to suppress adrenal androgen production

D. MENOPAUSE

1. Defined as the cessation of menses, **average age in US is 51 yr**
2. Suspect when menstrual cycles are not regular & predictable & when cycles are not associated with any premenstrual symptoms
3. Si/Sx = rapid onset hot flashes & sweating with resolution in 3 min, mood changes, sleep disturbances, vaginal dryness/atrophy, dyspareunia (painful intercourse) & osteoporosis
4. Dx = irregular menstrual cycles, hot flashes & ↑ FSH level (> 30 mIU/mL)
5. Depending on clinical scenario other laboratory tests should be conducted to exclude other diagnoses that can cause amenorrhea such as thyroid disease, hyperprolactinemia, pregnancy
6. Tx
   a. **First line is estrogen hormone replacement therapy (HRT)**
   b. HRT can be via continuous estrogen with cyclic progestin to allow controlled withdrawal bleeding or via daily administration of both estrogen & progestin, which does not cause withdrawal bleeding
   c. There are risks & benefits of HRT

TABLE 3-12   Risks and Benefits of Hormone Replacement Therapy

RISKS	BENEFITS
Endometrial CA ↑ risk with HRT, but risk significantly ↓ by addition of ≥10 days of progesterone to induce uterine wall sloughing	Relief of menopause Sx
Breast CA • Very controversial, studies equivocal, some show that prolonged HRT (≥5–10yr) → ↑ relative risk of breast CA • Regardless, breast CA or heavy risk factors for its development are contraindications to HRT	↓ risk of heart dz or stroke, ↑ HDL, ↓ LDL
DVT/PE Only seen with oral estrogen (not transdermal)	↓ osteoporosis
Breast pain Due to constant estrogen stimulation	↓ risk of dementia

OB/GYN

    d. Raloxifene

        1) Second-generation tamoxifen-like drug = mixed estrogen agonist/antagonist, FDA approved to prevent osteoporosis

        2) So far raloxifene shown to act like estrogen in bones (good), ↓ serum LDL (good) but does not stimulate endometrial growth (good) (unlike tamoxifen & estrogen alone), effects on breast are not yet known

    e. **Calcium supplements are not a substitute for estrogen replacement**

E. INFERTILITY

    1. Defined as failure to conceive after 1yr of unprotected sex

    2. Affects 10–15% of reproductive-age couples in the US

    3. Causes = abnormal spermatogenesis (40%), anovulation (30%), anatomic defects of the female reproductive tract (20%), unknown (10%)

    4. Dx

        a. **Start work-up with male partner not only because it is the most common cause**, but because the work-up is simpler, noninvasive & more cost-effective than work-up of infertility in the female

        b. **Normal semen excludes male cause in > 90% of couples**

        c. Work-up of female partner should include measurement of basal body temperature, which is an excellent screening test for ovulation

           1) Temperature drops at time of menses, then rises 2 days after LH surge at the time of progesterone rise

           2) Ovulation probably occurs 1 day before first temperature elevation & temperature remains elevated for 13–14 days

           3) A temperature elevation of > 16 days suggests pregnancy

    d. Anovulation
        1) Hx of regular menses with premenstrual Sx (breast fullness, ↓ vaginal secretions, abdominal bloating, mood changes) strongly suggests ovulation
        2) Sx such as irregular menses, amenorrhea episodes, hirsutism, acne, galactorrhea, suggest anovulation
        3) FSH measured at day 2–3 is best predictor of fertility potential in women, FSH > 25 IU/L correlated with a poor prognosis
        4) Dx confirm with basal body temperature, serum progesterone (↑ postovulation, >10 ng/mL → ovulation), endometrial Bx
    e. Anatomic disorder
        1) **Most commonly results from an acquired disorder, especially acute salpingitis 2° to *N. gonorrhoeae* & *C. trachomatis***
        2) Endometriosis, scarring, adhesions from pelvic inflammation or previous surgeries, tumors & trauma can also disrupt normal reproductive tract anatomy
        3) Less commonly a congenital anomaly such as septate uterus or reduplication of the uterus, cervix, or vagina is responsible
        4) **Dx with hysterosalpingogram**
  5. Tx
    a. Anovulation → restore ovulation with use of ovulation-inducing drugs
        1) First line = clomiphene, an estrogen antagonist that relieves negative feedback on FSH, allowing follicle development
        2) Anovulatory women who bleed in response to progesterone are candidates for clomiphene, as are women with irregular menses or midluteal progesterone levels <10 ng/mL
        3) 40% get pregnant, 8–10% ↑ rate of multiple births, mostly twins
        4) If no response, FSH can be given directly → pregnancy rates of 60–80%, multiple births occur at an ↑ rate of 20%
    b. Anatomic abnormalities → surgical lysis of pelvic adhesions
    c. If endosalpinx is not intact & transport of the ovum is not possible, an assisted fertilization technique, such as in vitro fertilization, may be used with 15–25% success

III. Urogynecology

A. PELVIC RELAXATION & URINARY INCONTINENCE
  1. ↑ incidence with age, also with birth trauma, obesity, chronic cough

2. Si/Sx = prolapse of urethra (urethrocele), uterus, bladder (cystocele), or rectum (rectocele), pelvic pressure & pain, dyspareunia, bowel & bladder dysfunction, & urinary incontinence
3. Types of urinary incontinence (See Figure 3-9)
   a. Stress incontinence = bladder pressure exceeds urethral pressure briefly at times of strain or stress such as coughing or laughing
   b. Urge incontinence & overflow incontinence result from ↓ innervation & control of bladder function resulting in involuntary bladder contraction (urge) or bladder atony (overflow)
4. Dx = urodynamic testing, assess for underlying medical conditions such as diabetes, neurologic dz, genitourinary surgery, pelvic irradiation, trauma & medications that may account for Sx
5. Tx = correct underlying cause
   a. Kegel exercises to tone pelvic floor
   b. Insertion of pessary devices to add structural support
   c. Useful drugs = anticholinergics, Ditropan/Detrol, β-agonists
   d. Surgical repair aimed at restoring structures to original anatomic position

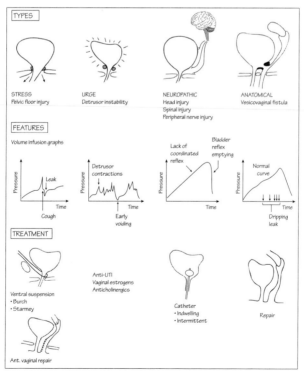

FIGURE 3-9 Urinary incontinence.

IV. Gynecology Oncology

A. ENDOMETRIAL CANCER

1. Most common reproductive tract cancer with approximately 35,000 new cases per year
2. "Estrogen-dependent" cancer
   a. Estrogen source can be glandular from the ovary
   b. Extraglandular from peripheral conversion of androstenedione to estrone or from a granulosa cell tumor
   c. Exogenous from oral estrogen, cutaneous patches, vaginal creams & now tamoxifen (reduces risk of breast cancer by 50%, but associated with 3x ↑ incidence of endometrial cancer)
3. Risk factors
   a. Unopposed postmenopausal estrogen replacement therapy
   b. Menopause after 52 yr
   c. Obesity, nulliparity, feminizing ovarian tumors (e.g., ovarian granulosa cell tumors), chronic anovulation, polycystic ovarian syndrome, postmenopausal (75% of patients), diabetes
4. Si/Sx = abnormal uterine bleeding, especially postmenopausal—any woman over age 35 yr with abnormal uterine bleeding should have a sample of endometrium taken for histologic evaluation
5. DDx = endometrial hyperplasia
   a. Abnormal proliferation of both glandular & stromal elements, can be simple or complex
   b. Atypical hyperplasia
      1) Significant numbers of glandular elements that exhibit cytological atypia & disordered maturation
      2) Analogous to carcinoma in situ → 20–30% risk for malignancy
6. Dx
   a. **Pap smear IS NOT reliable in Dx of endometrial cancer; however, if atypical glandular cells of undetermined significance (AGCUS) are found on the smear then endometrial evaluation is mandatory**
   b. Bimanual exam for masses, nodularity, induration & immobility
   c. Endometrial biopsy by endocervical curettage, D&C, hysteroscopy with directed biopsies
7. Tx
   a. Simple or complex hyperplasia → progesterone to reverse hyperplastic process promoted by estrogen (e.g., Provera × 10 d)
   b. Atypical hyperplasia → hysterectomy because of likelihood that it will become invasive endometrial carcinoma
   c. Endometrial carcinoma
      1) Total abdominal hysterectomy with bilateral salpingo-oophorectomy (TAH/BSO), lymph node dissection
      2) Adjuvant Tx may include external-beam radiation
      3) Tx for recurrence is high-dose progestins (e.g., Depo-Provera)
8. Px
   a. **Most important prognostic factor is histological grade**

PLATE 1 Café au lait patch (polyostotic fibrous dysplasia, neurofibromatosis can appear similarly).

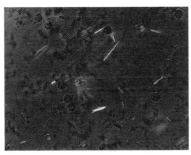

PLATE 2 Gout. Synovial fluid microscopy under compensated polarized light showing the slender needle-shaped and negatively birefringent urate crystals. The axis of slow vibration is from bottom left to top right.

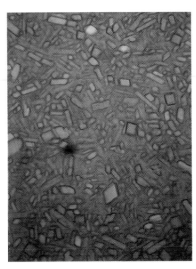

PLATE 3 CPPD dihydrate crystals (extracted from synovial fluid). These are pleomorphic, rectangular, and weakly positively birefringent. The axis of slow vibration is from bottom left to top right.

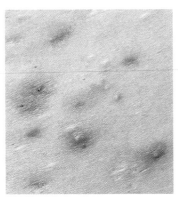

PLATE 4 Comedones, pustules, and scars (acne vulgaris).

PLATE 5 Impetigo

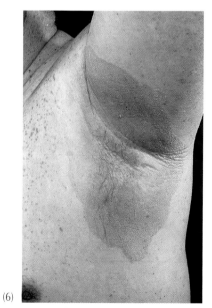

(6)

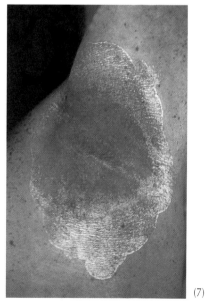

(7)

PLATES 6 & 7 Erythrasma: (6) normal light; (7) coral-red axillary fluorescent, due to proporphyria III elaborated by *Corynebacterium minutissimum* in erythrasma, under Wood's lamp.

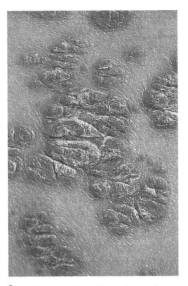

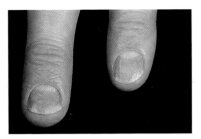

PLATE 9 Nail involvement in psoriasis. Note dystrophy, pits, and irregular yellowing onychylosis.

PLATE 8 Hyperkeratotic (scaly), erythematous plaques (psoriasis).

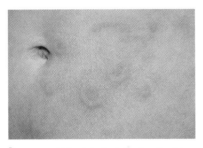

PLATE 11 Urticarial wheals (acute urticaria).

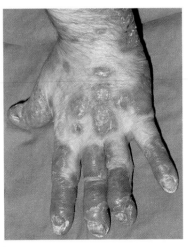

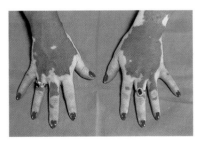

PLATE 10 Psoriatic arthropathy (arthritis mutilans); severe nail dystrophy.

PLATE 12 Macules and patches of hypopigmentation (vitiligo).

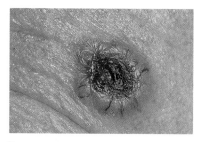

PLATE 13   Classic crateriform basal cell carcinoma. Ulcerating nodule.

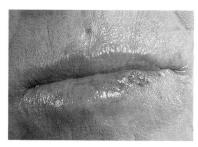

PLATE 14   Squamous cell carcinoma of the lip (early ulcer).

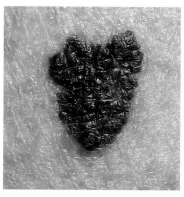

PLATE 15   Superficial spreading melanoma.

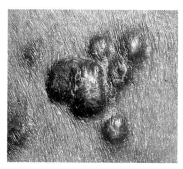

PLATE 16   Papules and nodules (Kaposis sarcoma–AIDS).

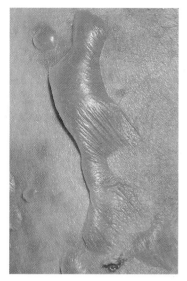

PLATE 17 Vesicles and bulla (bullous pemphigoid).

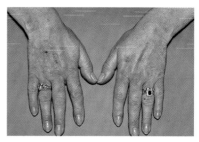

PLATE 18 Porphyria cutanea tarda.

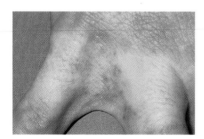

PLATE 19 Scabies.

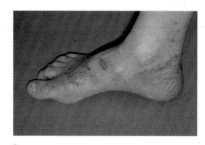

PLATE 20 Tinea pedis. Well-marginated erythematous scaly eruption (moccasin pattern).

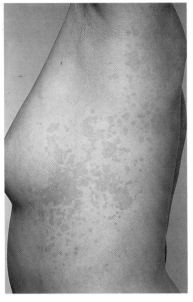

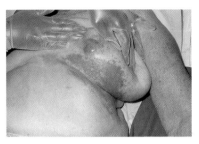

PLATE 22   Candidiasis. Erythematous, almost eroded intertrigo.

PLATE 21   Pityriasis versicolor. Petaloid, scaly macules.

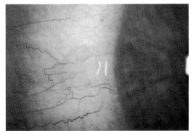

(23)

(24)

PLATES 23 & 24   The clinical apearance of (23) a pingueculum; (24) a pterygium.

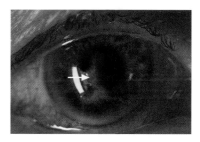

PLATE 25 A dendritic ulcer seen in herpes simplex infection.

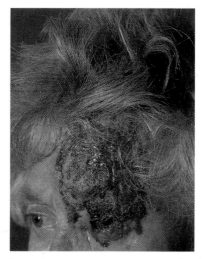

PLATE 26 The clinical appearance of herpes zoster ophthalmicus.

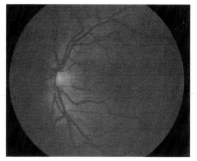

PLATE 27 A normal left fundus. note the optic disc with retinal veins and arteries passing from it to branch over the retina. The large temporal vessels are termed *arcades*. The macula lies temporal to the disc with the fovea at its center.

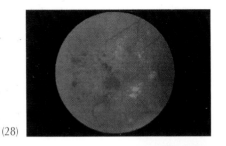
(28)

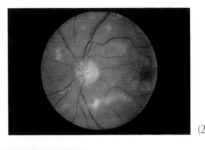
(29)

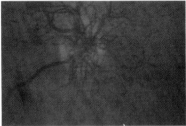
(30)

PLATES 28, 29 & 30   The signs of retinal vascular disease: (28) hemorrage and exudate; (29) cotton wool spots; (30) new vessels, here particularly florid arising at the disc. Note the yellowish nature and distinct margin to the exudates compared to the less distinct and white appearance of the cottom wool spot.

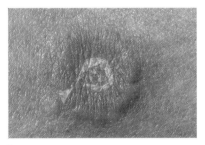

PLATE 31   Sweet's syndrome.

b. G1 is highly differentiated, G2 is moderately differentiated, G3 is predominantly solid or entirely undifferentiated carcinoma

c. **Depth of myometrial invasion is second most important Px factor**

d. Pt with G1 tumor that does not invade the myometrium has a 95% 5-yr survival, pt with G3 tumor with deep myometrial invasion has 5-yr survival rate closer to 20%

B. UTERINE LEIOMYOMAS = FIBROIDS

1. Benign tumors, growth related to estrogen production, usually most rapid growth occurs perimenopausally

2. Most common indication for hysterectomy (30% of cases)

3. Si/Sx = bleeding (usually menorrhagia or ↑ amount & duration of flow), pelvic pressure, pelvic pain often manifested as dysmenorrhea

4. Dx = Utz, confirm with tissue sample by either D&C or biopsy (especially in post-menopausal pts)

5. Tx

   a. If Sx are mild → reassurance & observation

   b. Medical Tx → estrogen inhibitors such as GnRH agonists shrink uterus, resulting in a simpler surgical procedure or can be used as a temporizing measure until natural menopause occurs

   c. Surgery → myomectomy indicated in young pts who want to preserve fertility (risk of intraoperative & postoperative hemorrhage ↑ compared to hysterectomy); hysterectomy is considered definitive treatment, but should be reserved for symptomatic women who have completed childbearing

C. LEIOMYOSARCOMA

1. Rare malignancy accounting for only 3% of cancers involving uterine corpus

2. ↑ suspicion for postmenopausal uterine enlargement

3. Si/Sx suggestive of sarcoma = postmenopausal bleeding, pelvic pain & ↑ vaginal discharge

4. Tx = hysterectomy with intraoperative lymph node biopsies

5. Surgical staging same as that for endometrial adenocarcinoma

6. Survival rate is much lower than that for endometrial cancer, only 50% of patients survive 5 yr

7. Adjunctive therapies are of minimal benefit

D. CERVICAL CANCER

1. Annual Pap smear is most important screening tool available to detect disease

2. Risk factors = early sexual intercourse, multiple sexual partners, HPV infection (especially types 16, 18), cigarette smoking, early childbearing & immunocompromised patients

3. Average age of Dx = 50 yr, but can occur much earlier

4. 85% are of squamous cell origin, 15% are adenocarcinomas arising from endocervical glands

5. Si/Sx = postcoital bleeding, but there is no classic presentation for cervical cancer

6. Dx = Pap screening, any visible cervical lesion should be biopsied

7. Tx

   a. Local dz → hysterectomy + lymph node dissection—ovaries may remain → survival >70% at 5 yr

   b. Extensive or metastatic dz → pelvic irradiation → survival <40% at 5 yr

E. OVARIAN NEOPLASMS

TABLE 3-13   Ovarian Neoplasms

NEOPLASM	CHARACTERISTICS	TX
Benign cysts	• Functional growth resulting from failure of normal follicle to rupture • Si/Sx = pelvic pain or pressure, rupture of cyst → acute, severe pain & hemorrhage mimicking acute abdomen • Confirm cyst with Utz	• Typically self-limiting • Rupture may require laparotomy to stop bleeding
Benign Tumors: more common than malignant, but risk of malignancy ↑ with age		
Epithelial	• Serous cystadenocarcinoma most common type, almost always benign unless bilateral → ↑ risk of malignancy • Other types = mucinous, endometrioid, Brenner tumors, all rarely malignant • Dx = clinical, can see on CT/MRI	• Surgical excision
Germ cell	• Teratoma is most common (also called "dermoid cyst") • Very rarely malignant, contain differentiated tissue from all 3 embryologic germ layers • Si/Sx = unilateral cystic, mobile, nontender adnexal mass, often aSx • Dx confirmed with Utz	• Excision to prevent ovarian torsion or rupture
Stromal cell	• Functional tumors secreting hormones • Granulosa tumor makes estrogens → gynecomastia, loss of body hair, etc. • Sertoli-Leydig cells make androgens, virilize females	• Excision

Malignant Tumors
• Usually occur in women >50 yr old
• Risk factors = low parity, ↓ fertility, delayed childbearing—**OCP use is a protective factor**
• Most lethal gynecologic cancer due to lack of early detection → ↑ rate of metastasis (60% at Dx)
• Dz are typically asymptomatic until extensive metastasis has occurred
• Can follow dz with Ca-125 marker, not specific enough for screening
• Yearly pelvic exams remain most effective screening tool
• Si/Sx = vague abdominal/pelvic complaints, e.g., distension, early satiety, constipation, pelvic pain, urinary frequency—shortness of breath due to pleural effusion may be only presenting Sx
• Tx = debulking surgery with chemo- & radiotherapy

SUBTYPES	CHARACTERISTICS	TREATMENT
Epithelial cell	• Cause 90% of all ovarian malignancies • Serous cystadenocarcinoma is most common, often originate from benign precursors • Others = endometrioma & mucinous cystadenocarcinoma	• Excision
Germ cell	• Most common ovarian cancers in women <20 years old • Can produce HCG or α-fetoprotein, useful as tumor markers • Subtypes = dysgerminoma, which is very radiosensitive, & immature teratoma	• Radiation first line • Chemotherapy second line • 5-yr survival >80% for both
Stromal	• Granulosa cell makes estrogen, can result in 2° endometriosis or endometrial carcinoma • Sertoli-Leydig tumor makes androgens	• Total hysterectomy with oophorectomy

F. VULVAR & VAGINAL CANCER
1. Vulvar intraepithelial neoplasia (VIN)
   a. VIN I & II = mild & moderate dysplasia, ↑ risk progressing to advanced stages & then carcinoma
   b. VIN III = carcinoma in situ
   c. Si/Sx = pruritus, irritation, presence of raised lesion
   d. Dx = biopsy for definitive diagnosis
   e. DDx includes Paget's disease, malignant melanoma
   f. Tx = excision, local for VIN I & II & wide for VIN III
2. Vulvar cancer
   a. 90% are squamous
   b. Usually presents postmenopausally
   c. Si/Sx = pruritus, with or without presence of ulcerative lesion
   d. Tx = excision
   e. 5-yr survival rate is 70–90% depending on nodal status, if deep pelvic nodes are involved survival is a dismal 20%
3. Vaginal CIS & carcinoma are very rare
   a. 70% of patients with vaginal CIS have either previous or coexistent genital tract neoplasm
   b. Tx = radiation, surgery reserved for women with extensive dz

G. GESTATIONAL TROPHOBLASTIC NEOPLASIA (GTN) = HYDATIDIFORM MOLE OR MOLAR PREGNANCY
1. Rare variation of pregnancy in which a neoplasm is derived from abnormal placental tissue (trophoblastic) proliferation
2. Usually a benign disease called a "molar pregnancy" that is further subdivided into complete mole (90%) in which there is no fetus & incomplete mole in which there is a fetus & molar degeneration
3. Persistent or malignant disease develops in 20% of pts (mostly in complete moles)
4. Complete moles are 46 XX, do not form fetus
5. Partial moles are 69 XXY triploids, often form partial fetus
6. Si/Sx = exaggerated pregnancy Sx, with missing fetal heart tones & enlarged uterus (size > dates), painless bleeding commonly occurs in early second trimester
7. Pts can also present with PIH
8. Utz → characteristic "snowstorm" pattern
9. Dx = Utz + ↑↑↑ hCG levels (See Figures 3-10 and 3-11)
10. Tx = removal of uterine contents by D&C & suction curettage
11. Nonmetastatic persistent GTN is treated with methotrexate
12. Follow-up = check that hCG levels are appropriately dropping
13. Contraception is recommended during first yr of follow-up

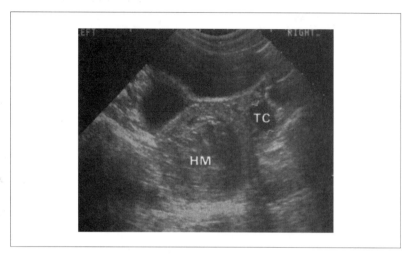

FIGURE 3-10   Ultrasound scan of a hydatidiform mole (HM) with a theca-luteal cyst (TC) in the ovary.

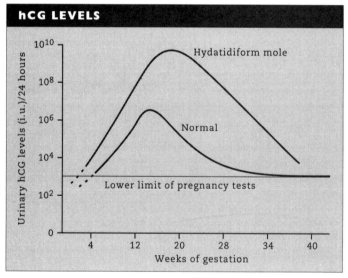

FIGURE 3-11   Means of levels of hCG in women with normal pregnancies and hydatidiform moles.

4. Pediatrics

Beatriz Mares

I. Development

A.

TABLE 4-1   Development Milestones

AGE	GROSS MOTOR	FINE MOTOR	LANGUAGE	SOCIAL/ COGNITION
Newborn	Head side to side, **Moro & grasp reflex**			
2 mos	Holds head up	Swipes at object	Coos	Social smile
4 mos	Rolls front to back	**Grasps object**	Orients to voice	Laughs
6 mos	Rolls back to front, **sits upright**	Transfers object	Babbles	**Stranger anxiety, sleeps all night**
9 mos	Crawl, pull to stand	**Pincer grasp,** eats with fingers	**Mama-dada (nonspecific)**	Waves bye-bye, responds to name
12 mos	**Stands**	**Mature pincer**	**Mama-dada (specific)**	Picture book
15 mos	**Walks**	Uses cup	4–6 words	**Temper tantrum**
18 mos	Throws ball, walks upstairs	Uses spoon for solids	Names common objects	**Toilet training may begin**
24 mos	Runs, up/down stairs	Uses spoon for semisolids	**2-word sentence** (2 word at 2 yr)	Follows 2-step command
36 mos	Rides tricycle	Eats neatly with utensils	**3-word sentence** (3 word at 3 yr)	Knows first & last name

B. PUBERTY

TABLE 4-2   Tanner Stages

BOYS	GIRLS
Testicular enlargement at 11.5 yr*	Breast buds at 10.5 yr*
Increase in genital size	Pubic hair
Pubic hair	Linear growth spurt at 12 yr
Peak growth spurt at 13.5 yr*	Menarche at 12.5 yr*

*Years represent population averages.

II. Infections

A. ToRCHS

TABLE 4-3   The ToRCHS

DISEASE	CHARACTERISTICS
Toxoplasmosis	• Acquired in mothers via ingestion of poorly cooked meat or through contact with cat feces • Carriers common (10–30%) in population, only causes neonatal dz if acquired during pregnancy (1%) • 1/3 of women who acquire during pregnancy transmit infection to fetus, & 1/3 of fetuses are clinically affected • Sequelae = intracerebral calcifications, hydrocephalus, chorioretinitis, microcephaly, severe mental retardation, epilepsy, intrauterine growth retardation (IUGR), hepatosplenomegaly • Screening is useless since acquisition prior to infection is common & clinically irrelevant • Pregnant women should be told to avoid undercooked meat, wash hands after handling cat, do not change litter box • If fetal infection established → Utz to determine major anomalies & provide counseling regarding termination if indicated
Rubella	• First trimester maternal Rubella infxn → 80% chance of fetal transmission • Second trimester → 50% chance of transmission to fetus, third trimester → 5% • Si/Sx of fetus = intrauterine growth retardation, cataracts, glaucoma, chorioretinitis, patent ductus arteriosus, pulmonary stenosis, atrial or ventricular septal defect, myocarditis, microcephaly, **hearing loss, "blueberry muffin rash,"** mental retardation • Dx confirmed with IgM Rubella Ab in neonate's serum, or viral culture • Tx = prevention by universal immunization of all children against Rubella, there is no effective therapy for active infection
Cytomegalovirus (CMV)	• # 1 congenital infection, affecting 1% of births • Transmitted through bodily fluids/secretions, infection often asymptomatic • 1° seroconversion during pregnancy → ↑ risk of severely affected infant, but congenital infection can occur if mother reinfected during pregnancy • About 1% risk of transplacental transmission of infection, about 10% of infected infants manifest congenital defects of varying severity • Congenital defects = microcephaly, intracranial calcifications, severe mental retardation, chorioretinitis, IUGR • 10–15% of asymptomatic but exposed infants will develop later neurologic sequelae
Herpes simplex virus	• **C-section delivery for pregnant women with active herpes** • Vaginal → 50% chance that the baby will acquire the infection & is associated with significant morbidity & mortality • Si/Sx = vesicles, seizures, respiratory distress, can cause pneumonia, meningitis, encephalitis → impaired neurologic development after resolution • Tx = acyclovir (markedly decreases mortality)
Syphilis	• Transmission from infected mother to infant during pregnancy nearly 100%, **occurs after the first trimester in the vast majority of cases** • Fetal/perinatal deaths in 40% of affected infants • Early manifestations in first 2 years, later manifestations in next 2 decades • Si/Sx of early dz = jaundice, ↑ liver function tests, hepatosplenomegaly, hemolytic anemia, rash followed by desquamation of hands & feet, wart-like lesions of mucous membranes, **blood-tinged nasal secretions (snuffles), diffuse osteochondritis, saddle nose** (2° to syphilitic rhinitis) • Si/Sx of late dz = **Hutchinson teeth** (notching of permanent upper 2 incisors), mulberry molars (both at 6 yr), bone thickening (frontal bossing), **anterior bowing of tibia (saber shins)** • Dx = RPR/VDRL & FTA serologies in mother with clinical findings in infant • Tx = procaine penicillin G for 10–14 days

B. INFANT BOTULISM

1. Acute, flaccid paralysis caused by *Clostridium botulinum* neurotoxin that irreversibly blocks acetylcholine release from peripheral neurons
2. Dz acquired via **ingestion of spores in honey** or via inhalation of spores
3. 95% cases in infants 3 wk to 6 mo old, peak 2–4 mo
4. Si/Sx = constipation, lethargy, poor feeding, weak cry, ↓ spontaneous movement, hypotonia, drooling, ↓ gag & suck reflexes, as dz progresses → **loss of head control & respiratory arrest**
5. Dx = clinical, **based on acute onset of flaccid descending paralysis with clear sensorium, without fever or paresthesias**, can confirm by demonstrating botulinum toxin in serum or toxin/organism in feces
6. Tx = intubate, supportive care, no antibiotics or antitoxin needed in infants

C. EXANTHEMS

TABLE 4-4   Viral Exanthems

DISEASE/VIRUS	SI/SX
Measles (Rubeola) Paramyxovirus	• Erythematous maculopapular rash, **erupts 5 days after onset of prodromal Sx, begins on head & spreads to body, lasting 4–5 days**, resolving from head downward • **Koplik spots (white spots on buccal mucosa) are pathognomonic**, but leave before rash starts so often not found when pt presents • Dx = fever & Hx of the 3 C's: **cough, coryza, conjunctivitis**
Rubella (German measles) Togavirus	• **Suboccipital lymphadenopathy** (very few dzs do this) • Maculopapular rash begins on face then generalizes • Rash lasts 5 days, fever may accompany rash on first day only • May find reddish spots of various sizes on soft palate
Hand, foot & mouth disease Coxsackie A virus	• Vesicular rash on hands & feet with ulcerations in mouth • Rash clears in about 1 wk • Contagious by contact
Roseola infantum (Exanthem subitum) (HHV6)*	• **Abrupt high fever persisting for 1–5 days even though child has no physical Sx to account for fever & does not feel ill** • When fever drops, macular or maculopapular rash appears on trunk & then spreads peripherally over entire body, lasts 24 hr
Erythema infectiosum (Fifth disease) Parvovirus B-19	• **Classic sign = "slapped cheeks,"** erythema of the cheeks • Subsequently an erythematous maculopapular rash spreads from arms to trunk & legs forming a reticular pattern • **Dz is dangerous in sickle cell pts (& other anemias) due to parvovirus B-19's tendency to cause aplastic crises**
Varicella (Chicken pox) Varicella Zoster Virus (VZV)	• Highly contagious, pruritic "tear drop" vesicles that break & crust over, start on face or trunk (centripetal) & spread to extremities • New lesions appear for 3–5 days & typically take 3 days to crust over, so rash persists for about 1 wk • **Lesions are contagious until they crust over** • Zoster (shingles) = reactivation of old varicella infxn, painful skin eruptions are seen along the distribution of dermatomes that correspond to the affected dorsal root ganglia

Dx = clinical for all, Tx = supportive for all.
*HHV6 = human herpes virus 6.

D. VACCINATIONS

TABLE 4-5   Recommended Childhood Immunization Schedule[a]

AGE	VACCINE			
Newborn	Hepatitis B (1)			
2 mo	Hepatitis B (2)	DTaP (rotavirus[b])	Hib	Polio[c]
4 mo		DTaP (rotavirus[b])	Hib	Polio[c]
6 mo	Hepatitis B (3)	DTaP (rotavirus[b])	Hib	
12 mo	MMR	Varicella	Hib	Polio[c]
15 mo		DTaP (may combine with Hib at 12 mo)		
4–6 yr	MMR	DTaP		Polio[c]
11–12 yr	MMR (if second dose not yet given)	Varicella	Td	

[a] The immunization schedule above is one example of a schedule that is frequently revised as new immunization findings are released. Always refer to the appropriate current, updated guidelines for pediatrics immunization schedules.
[b] New vaccine, standard guidelines not yet available.
[c] First 3 doses IM; others can be oral.

III. Respiratory Disorders

A. OTITIS MEDIA

1. Usually in children, precipitated by a viral URI
2. Congenital disorders (e.g., Down's syndrome, cleft palate) that prevent eustachian tube drainage ↑ risk of infection
3. Si/Sx = ear pressure, ↓ hearing, fever, **erythema & ↓ mobility of tympanic membrane** (TM), TM bulging & a meniscus of fluid behind the TM (effusion)
4. Caused by *S. pneumoniae, H. influenzae, Moraxella,* or viral infection such as respiratory syncytial virus (RSV)
5. Tx = amoxicillin (first line), Augmentin (second line)
6. Surgical tube placement may be required for chronic effusions to prevent developmental delay secondary to hearing loss

B. BRONCHIOLITIS (See Figure 4–1)

1. Commonly seen in children under 2 yr, peak incidence at 6 mo
2. **>50% due to RSV**, others include parainfluenzae & adenovirus
3. Si/Sx = mild rhinorrhea & fever progress to cough, wheezing with crackles, tachypnea, nasal flaring, decreased appetite
4. Dx by culture or antigen detection of nasopharyngeal secretions
5. Tx = bronchodilators, oxygen as needed

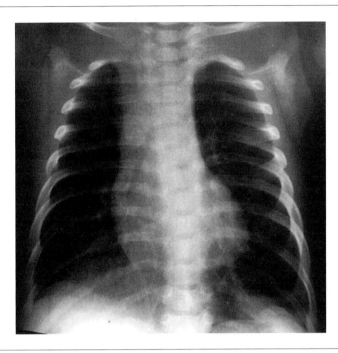

FIGURE 4-1   Chest x-ray of an 8-week-old baby with bronchiolitis. The x-ray shows gross overinflation of the lungs clearly seen by the level of the diaphragm and the intercostal spaces. There is also some bronchial wall thickening.

C. UPPER RESPIRATORY DISEASES

TABLE 4-6   Pediatric Upper Respiratory Disorders

DISEASE	CAUSE	SI/SX	LABS	TX
Croup (Laryngotrach-eobronchitis)	Parainfluenza, influenza, RSV, *Mycoplasma*	**Presents in fall & winter, 3mo—3 yr old, with barking cough, inspiratory stridor, Sx worse at night,** hoarse voice, preceded by URI	Neck x-ray → "steeple sign"	O₂, cool mist, racemic Epi & steroids if severe, ribavirin may be used for immunocompromised
Epiglottitis	*H. influenzae* type B	**Medical emergency!!! Fulminant inspiratory stridor, drooling, sits leaning forward,** dysphagia, "hot potato" voice	"Thumb print" sign on lateral neck film, cherry-red epiglottitis on endoscopy	**Examine pt in OR,** Intubate as needed, ceftriaxone
Bacterial tracheitis	*Staph.* & *Strep.* spp.	Inspiratory stridor, high fever, toxic appearing	Leukocytosis	Nafcillin or ceftriaxone

TABLE 4-6 *Continued*

DISEASE	CAUSE	SI/SX	LABS	TX
Foreign body aspiration		**Usually presents after 6 mo old** (need to grasp object to inhale it) with **inspiratory stridor** (chronic), wheeze, ↓ breath sounds, dysphagia & unresolved pneumonia	CXR → hyperinflation on affected side, ENT consult (See Figure 4-2)	Endoscopic or surgical removal

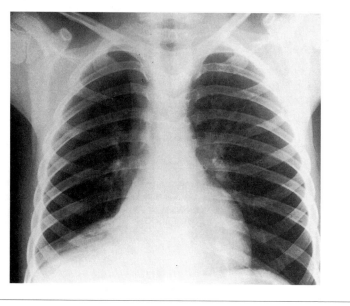

FIGURE 4-2 X-ray of a child admitted with fever and cough that failed to respond to treatment. At bronchoscopy a toy car steering wheel was found in the right intermediate bronchus. The chest x-ray shows collapse of the right middle and lower lobe with loss of definition of the right hemidiaphragm and right heart border.

D. PNEUMONIA

1. Common etiologies vary with age
   a. Newborns get *S. agalactiae* (group B *Strep*), gram-negative rod, *Chlamydia trachomatis*
   b. Infants get *S. pneumoniae, H. influenzae, Chlamydia, S. aureus, Listeria monocytogenes* & viral
   c. Preschoolers get RSV, other viruses & *Mycoplasma*
   d. Adolescents get *S. pneumoniae, Mycoplasma* & *Chlamydia*

2. Si/Sx = cough (productive in older children), fevers, nausea/vomiting, diarrhea, tachypnea, grunting, retractions, crackles
3. Pertussis presents with 3 stages
   a. Catarrhal stage = 1–2 weeks of cough, rhinorrhea, wheezing
   b. Paroxysmal stage = 2–4 weeks of paroxysmal cough with "whoops"
   c. Convalescent stage = 1–2 weeks of persistent chronic cough
4. *Chlamydia* causes classic "staccato cough" & conjunctivitis, pts afebrile
5. RSV causes wet cough, often with audible wheezes
6. *Staphylococcus* infections may be associated with skin lesions as well
7. Dx = rapid antigen detection or culture of secretions, CXR → infiltrates
8. Tx = infants get hospitalized, bronchodilators & O_2 for RSV, erythromycin for atypical dz (e.g., *Chlamydia*, *Mycoplasma*), cefuroxime for bacteria

IV. Musculoskeletal

A. LIMP

1. Painful limp is usually acute onset, may be associated with fever & irritability, toddlers may refuse to walk
2. DDx painful limp

TABLE 4-7 Pediatric Painful Limp

DISEASE	CHARACTERISTICS	TX
Septic arthritis	• **#1 cause of painful limp in 1–3-yr-old** • Usually monoarticular → hip, knee, or ankle • Causes = *S. aureus* **(most common)**, *H. influenzae*, *N. gonorrhoeae* • Si/Sx = **acute onset pain**, arthritis, fever, ↓ range of motion, child may lie still & refuse to walk or crawl, ↑ **WBC**, ↑ **ESR** • X-ray → joint space widening, soft tissue swelling • Dx = joint aspiration → turbid gray, **WBC ≥ 10,000 with neutrophil predominance**, low glucose	Tx = drainage, antibiotics appropriate to Gram's stain or cultures
Toxic synovitis	• Most common in males 5–10 yr old, may precede viral URI • Si/Sx = **insidious onset pain**, low grade fever, **WBC & ESR normal** • **Typically no tenderness, warmth, or joint swelling** • X-ray → usually normal • Dx → technetium scan → ↑ **uptake of epiphysis**	Rest & analgesics for 3–5 days
Aseptic avascular necrosis	• Legg-Calve-Perthes dz = head of femur, Osgood-Schlatter = tibial tubercle, Kohler's bone dz = navicular bone • Legg-Calve-Perthes → usually 4–9 yr old (boys-girls = 5:1), bilateral in 10–20% of cases, ↑ incidence with delayed growth & ↓ birth weight • Si/Sx = **afebrile, insidious onset** hip pain, inner thigh, or knee, ↑ pain with movement, ↓ with rest, antalgic gait, **normal WBC & ESR** • X-ray → **femoral head sclerosis** & ↑ width of femoral neck (See Figure 4-3) • Dx → technetium scan → ↓ **uptake in epiphysis**	↓ weight bearing on affected side over long time

TABLE 4-7   *Continued*

DISEASE	CHARACTERISTICS	TX
Slipped capital femoral epiphysis	• Often in **obese male adolescents** (8–17 yr old), 20–30% bilateral • 80% → slow, progressive, 20% → acute, associated with trauma • Si/Sx → **dull, aching pain** in hip or knee, ↑ pain with activity • X-ray → lateral movement of femur shaft in relation to femoral head, looks like **"ice-cream scoop falling off cone"** • Dx = clinical	Surgical pinning
Osteomyelitis	• Neonates → *S. aureus* (50%), *S. agalactiae, E. coli* • Children → *Staph. & Strep., Salmonella* (sickle cell), *P. aeruginosa* • Si/Sx young infants → fever may be only symptom • Si/Sx older children → fever, malaise, ↓ extremity movement, edema • X-ray lags changes by 3–4 weeks • Dx → neutrophilic leukocytosis, ↑ ESR (50%), blood cultures, bone scan (90% sensitive), **MRI is the gold standard**	IV antibiotics for 4–6 wk

3. Painless limp usually has insidious onset, may be due to weakness or deformity of limb 2° to developmental hip dysplasia, cerebral palsy, or leg length discrepancy

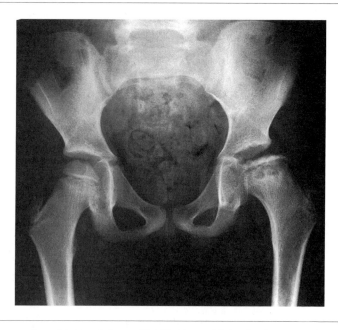

FIGURE 4-3   X-ray of the hips of a 5-year-old child with Legg-Calvé-Perthes disease. Note the increased density, flattening, and fragmentation of the left capital femoral epiphysis.

B. COLLAGEN VASCULAR DISEASES

1. Juvenile rheumatoid arthritis
   a. Chronic inflammation of ≥1 joints in pt ≤ 16 yr old
   b. Most commonly in children 1–4 yr old, females > males
   c. 3 categories = systemic, pauciarticular, polyarticular

TABLE 4-8   Types of Juvenile Rheumatoid Arthritis

Systemic (10–20%)	• High, **spiking fevers** with return to normal daily, generalized lymphadenopathy • **Rash of small, pale pink macules with central pallor on trunk & proximal extremities with possible involvement of palms & soles** • Joint involvement may not occur for weeks to months after fever • 1/3 have disabling chronic arthritis
Pauciarticular (40–60%)	• Involves ≤ 4 joints, large joints primarily affected (knees, ankles, elbows, asymmetric) • Other Si/Sx = fever, malaise, anemia, lymphadenopathy, **chronic joint dz is unusual** • Divided into 2 types ◊ *Type 1* (most common) → females < 4 yr, ↑ risk for chronic iridocyclitis, 90% ANA+ ◊ *Type 2* → males > 8 yr, ANA −, 75% HLA-B27+, ↑ risk of ankylosing spondylitis or Reiter's later in life
Polyarticular	• ≥5 joints involved, small & large, insidious onset, fever, lethargy, anemia • 2 types depending on if rheumatoid factor is present or not • Rheumatoid factor ⊕ → 80% females, late onset, more severe, rheumatoid nodules present, 75% ANA+ • Rheumatoid factor − → occurs any time during childhood, mild, rarely associated with rheumatoid nodules, 25% ANA+

   d. Dx = Sx persists for 3 consecutive mo with exclusion of other causes of acute/chronic arthritis or collagen vascular diseases
   e. Tx = NSAIDs, low-dose methotrexate, prednisone only in acute febrile onset
2. Kawasaki's disease (mucocutaneous lymph node syndrome)
   a. Large & medium vessel vasculitis in children < 5 yr old, predilection for Japanese children
   b. Dx = fever > 104° for > 5 days, unresponsive to antibiotics ⊕ 4 out of 5 of the following criteria (**mnemonic: CRASH**)
      1) **C**onjunctivitis
      2) **R**ash, primarily truncal, protean
      3) **A**neurysms of coronary arteries
      4) **S**trawberry tongue, crusting of lips, fissuring of mouth & oropharyngeal erythema
      5) **H**ands & feet show induration, erythema of palms & soles, desquamation of fingers & toes
   c. Complications = cardiac involvement, 10–40% of untreated cases show evidence of coronary vasculitis (dilation/aneurysm) within first weeks of illness
   d. Tx = immediate IVIG to prevent coronary vasculitis, **high-dose aspirin—prednisone is contraindicated & will exacerbate the dz!**
   e. Px
      1) Response to IVIG & aspirin is rapid, 2/3 pts afebrile within 24 hr

2) Evaluate pts one week after discharge, repeat echocardiography 3–6 wk after onset of fever, if baseline & repeat echo do not detect any coronary abnormalities, further imaging is unnecessary

3. Henoch-Schönlein purpura
   a. IgA small vessel vasculitis, related to IgA nephropathy (Berger's disease)
   b. Si/Sx = **pathognomonic palpable purpura** on legs & buttocks (in children), abdominal pain, may cause intussusception
   c. Tx = self-limited, rarely progresses to glomerulonephritis

C. Histiocytosis X
1. Proliferation of histiocytic cells resembling Langerhans' skin cells
2. 3 common variants
   a. Letterer-Siwe disease
      1) Acute, aggressive, disseminated variant, usually fatal in infants
      2) Si/Sx = hepatosplenomegaly, lymphadenopathy, pancytopenia, lung involvement, recurrent infections
   b. Hand-Schuller-Christian
      1) Chronic progressive variant, presents prior to 5 yr old
      2) **Classic triad = skull lesions, diabetes insipidus, exophthalmus**
   c. Eosinophilic granuloma
      1) Extraskeletal involvement generally limited to lung
      2) Has the best Px, rarely fatal, sometimes spontaneously regresses

V. Metabolic

A. Congenital Hypothyroidism
1. Due to 2° agenesis of thyroid or defect in enzymes
2. **T4 is crucial during first 2 yr of life for normal brain development**
3. Birth Hx → normal Apgars, prolonged jaundice (↑ indirect bilirubin)
4. Si/Sx = presents at 6–12 wk old with poor feeding, lethargy, **hypotonia, coarse facial features, large protruding tongue**, hoarse cry, constipation, developmental delay
5. Dx = ↓ T4, ↑ TSH
6. Tx = levothyroxine replacement
7. **If Dx delayed beyond 6 wk, child will be mentally retarded**
8. Newborn screening is mandatory by law

B. Newborn Jaundice
1. Physiologic jaundice is clinically benign, occurs 24–48 hr after birth
   a. Characterized by unconjugated hyperbilirubinemia
   b. 50% of neonates have jaundice during first wk of life
   c. Results from increased bilirubin production & relative deficiency in glucuronyl transferase in the immature liver
   d. Requires no Tx
2. **Jaundice present AT birth is ALWAYS pathologic**
3. Unconjugated hyperbilirubinemia
   a. Caused by hemolytic anemia or congenital deficiency of glucuronyl transferase (e.g., Crigler-Najjar & Gilbert's syndromes)
   b. Hemolytic anemia can be congenital or acquired
      1) Congenital due to spherocytosis, G6PD, pyruvate kinase deficiency

2) Acquired due to ABO/Rh isoimmunization, infection, drugs, twin-twin transfusion, chronic fetal hypoxia, delayed cord clamping, maternal diabetes

4. Conjugated hyperbilirubinemia
    a. Infectious causes = sepsis, the ToRCH group, syphilis, *Listeria monocytogenes*, hepatitis
    b. Metabolic causes = galactosemia, α-1-antitrypsin deficiency
    c. Congenital causes = extrahepatic biliary atresia, Dubin-Johnson & Rotor syndromes

TABLE 4-9   Differential Diagnosis of Neonatal Jaundice by Time of Onset

Within 24 hr of birth	• Hemolysis (ABO/Rh isoimmunization, hereditary spherocytosis) • Sepsis
Within 48 hr of birth	• Hemolysis • Infection • Physiologic
After 48 hr	• Infection • Hemolysis • Breast milk (liver not mature to handle lipids of breast milk) • Congenital malformation (biliary atresia) • Hepatitis

5. Tx = UV light to break down bilirubin pigments & Tx underlying cause
6. Complications of UV light = retinal damage, dehydration, dermatitis, diarrhea
7. Tx urgently to prevent mental retardation 2° to kernicterus (biliary precipitation in basal ganglia)

C. REYE SYNDROME
    1. Acute encephalopathy & fatty degeneration of the liver associated with **use of salicylates in children with varicella or influenza-like illness**
    2. Most cases in children 4–12 yr old
    3. Si/Sx = biphasic course with prodromal fever → aSx interval → abrupt onset vomiting, delirium, stupor, hepatomegaly with abnormal liver function tests, may rapidly progress to seizures, coma & death
    4. Dx = clinical ⊕ ↑↑ liver enzymes, normal CSF
    5. Tx = control of ↑ intracranial pressure due to cerebral edema (major cause of death) with mannitol, fluid restriction, give glucose because glycogen stores are commonly depleted
    6. Px = ↑ chance to progress into coma if ≥3-fold ↑ in serum ammonia level, ↓ prothrombin not responsive to vitamin K
    7. Recovery rapid in mild dz, severe dz may → neuropsychologic defects

D. FEBRILE SEIZURES
    1. Usually occurs between 3 mo & 5 yr, associated with a fever without evidence of infection (intracranial) or defined cause
    2. It is the most common convulsive order in young children, rarely develops into epilepsy
    3. Risk = very high fever (≥39°C) & family history, seizure occurs during rise in temperature, not at the peak of temperature

4. Si/Sx = commonly tonic-clonic seizure with most lasting < 10 min with a drowsy postictal period
5. **Note:** if seizure lasts > 15 min, most likely due to infection or toxic process and careful work-up should follow
6. Dx = clinical, routine lab tests should only be performed to evaluate fever source, EEG not indicated unless febrile seizure is atypical (complex febrile seizure)
7. Consider lumbar puncture to rule out meningitis
8. Tx = careful evaluation for source of fever, control of fever with antipyretics, parental counseling & reassurance to decrease anxiety
9. Px = 33–50% of children experience recurrence of seizure

VI. Genetic and Congenital Disorders

A. FAILURE TO THRIVE (FTT)
1. Failure of children to grow & develop at an appropriate rate
2. Due to inadequate calorie intake or inadequate calorie absorption
3. Can be idiopathic or due to gastroesophageal reflux, urinary tract infections, cardiac disease, cystic fibrosis, hypothyroidism, congenital syndromes, lead poisoning, malignancy
4. Additional factors include poverty, family discord, neonatal problems, maternal depression
5. Dx requires 3 criteria
   a. Child < 2 yr old with weight < third to fifth percentile for age on more than one occasion
   b. Child < 2 yr old whose weight is < 80% of ideal weight for age
   c. Child < 2 yr old whose weight crosses 2 major percentiles downward on a standardized growth chart
   d. Exceptions = children of genetically short stature, small-for-gestational-age infants, preterm infants, normally lean infants, "overweight" infants whose rate of height gain increases while rate of weight gain decreases
6. Tx
   a. Organic causes → treat underlying condition & provide sufficient caloric supplementation
   b. Idiopathic → observe the parent feeding the infant & educate parents on appropriate formulas, foods & liquids that are appropriate for the infant
   c. In older infants & children it is important to offer solid foods before liquids, decrease distractions during meal times, & child should eat with others & not be force-fed
   d. Monitor closely for progressive weight gain in response to adequate calorie feeding
7. Px poor in first year of life due to maximal postnatal brain growth during the first 6 mo of life—1/3 of children with nonorganic FTT are developmentally delayed

B. CRANIOFACIAL ABNORMALITIES
1. Mildest form is bifid uvula, no clinical significance
2. Cleft lip
   a. Can occur unilaterally or bilaterally, due to failure of fusion of maxillary prominences

  b. **Unilateral cleft lip is the most common malformation of the head & neck**

  c. Does not interfere with feeding

  d. Tx = surgical repair

3. Cleft palate

  a. Can be anterior or posterior (determined by position relative to incisive foramen)

  b. Anterior cleft palate due to failure of palatine shelves to fuse with primary palate

  c. Posterior cleft palate due to failure of palatine shelves to fuse with nasal septum

  d. **Interferes with feeding, requiring a special nipple for the baby to feed**

  e. Tx = surgical repair

4. Macroglossia

  a. Congenitally enlarged tongue seen in Down's syndrome, gigantism, hypothyroidism

  b. Can also be acquired in amyloidosis & acromegaly

  c. This is different from glossitis (redness & swelling, with burning sensation) that is seen in vitamin B deficiencies

  d. Tx is directed at underlying cause

C. DOWN'S SYNDROME

1. **Invariably caused by trisomy 21, ↑ risk if maternal age > 35 yr**

2. Si/Sx → cardiac septal defects, psychomotor retardation, classic Down's facies, ↑ risk of leukemia, premature Alzheimer's dz

3. Down's facies = flattened occiput (brachycephaly), **epicanthal folds, up-slanted palpebral fissures, speckled irises (Brushfield spots)**, protruding tongue, small ears, redundant skin at posterior neck, **hypotonia, simian crease in palms (50%)**

4. Px = typically death in 30s–40s

D. TURNER'S SYNDROME

1. **#1 cause of 1° amenorrhea**, due to XO genotype

2. Si/Sx = newborns have ↑ skin at dorsum of neck (**neck webbing**), lymphedema in hands & feet, as develop → short stature, ptosis, **coarctation of aorta, amenorrhea but uterus is present**, juvenile external genitalia, bleeding due to GI telangiectasias, no mental retardation

3. Tx = hormone replacement to allow 2° sex characteristics to develop

E. FRAGILE X SYNDROME

1. X-linked dominant trinucleotide repeat expansion disorder

2. **#1 cause of mental retardation in boys**

3. Si/Sx = long face, prominent jaw, large ears, enlarged testes (postpubertal), developmental delay, mental retardation

4. Tx = none

F. ARNOLD-CHIARI MALFORMATION

1. Congenital disorder

2. Si/Sx = caudally displaced cerebellum, elongated medulla passing into foramen magnum, flat skull base, hydrocephalus, meningomyelocele & aqueductal stenosis

3. Px = death as neonate or toddler

G. NEURAL TUBE DEFECTS

1. Associated with ↑ α-fetoprotein levels in maternal serum

2. **Preventable by folic acid supplements during pregnancy**

3. Si/Sx = spina bifida (posterior vertebral arches don't close) & meningocele (no vertebrae cover lumbar cord)
4. Tx = prevention, neurologic deficits often remain after surgical correction

H. FETAL ALCOHOL SYNDROME

1. Seen in children born to alcoholic mothers
2. Si/Sx = characterized by facial abnormalities & developmental defects (mental & growth retardation), **smooth filtrum of lip,** microcephaly, atrial septal defect
3. Tx = prevention

I. CONGENITAL PYLORIC STENOSIS

1. Causes projectile vomiting in first **2 wk–2 mo of life**
2. More common in males & in first-born children
3. **Pathognomonic physical finding is palpable "olive" nodule in midepigastrium,** representing hypertrophied pyloric sphincter
4. If olive is not present, diagnosis made by ultrasound
5. Tx = longitudinal surgical incision in hypertrophied muscle

J. CONGENITAL HEART DISEASE

1. Atrial septal defect (ASD)
   a. Usually aSx, often found on routine preschool physicals
   b. Predispose to CHF in second & third decades, also predispose to stroke due to embolus bypass tract (Eisenmenger's complex)
   c. Si/Sx = loud S_1, **wide fixed-split S_2,** midsystolic ejection murmur
   d. Dx = echocardiography
   e. Tx = surgical patching of bypass, more important for females due to eventual increased cardiovascular stress of pregnancy
2. Ventricular septal defect (VSD)
   a. **Most common congenital heart defect**, 30% of small to medium defects close spontaneously by age 2
   b. Si/Sx = small defects may be completely aSx throughout entire life, large defects → CHF, ↓ development/growth, frequent pulmonary infections, holosystolic murmur over entire precordium, maximally at fourth LICS
   c. Eisenmenger's complex = R → L shunt 2° to pulmonary HTN
      1) RV hypertrophy → flow reversal through the shunt, so that an R → L shunt develops
      2) Causes cyanosis 2° to lack of blood flow to lung
      3) Allows venous thrombi (e.g., DVT) to bypass lung, causing systemic paradoxical embolization
   d. Dx = echocardiography
   e. Tx = complete closure for simple defects
3. Tetralogy of Fallot
   a. 4 physical defects comprising the tetralogy are
      1) Ventricular septal defect
      2) Pulmonary outflow obstruction
      3) Right ventricular hypertrophy
      4) Overriding aorta (aorta inlet spans both ventricles)

b. Si/Sx = acyanotic at birth, ↑ cyanosis over first 6 mo, **"Tet spell"** = acute cyanosis & panic in child, child adopts a squatting posture to improve blood flow to lungs, **CXR shows classic boot-shaped contour** due to RV enlargement

c. Dx = echocardiography

d. Tx = surgical repair of VSD, repair of pulmonary outflow tracts

4. Transposition of the great arteries

a. Aorta comes off right ventricle, pulmonary artery off left ventricle

b. Must have persistent arteriovenous communication or dz is incompatible with life (can be via patent ductus arteriosus or persistent foramen ovale)

c. Si/Sx = marked cyanosis at birth, early digital clubbing, often no murmur, **CXR →** **enlarged egg-shaped heart** & ↑ pulmonary vasculature

d. Dx = echocardiography

e. Tx = surgical switching of arterial roots to normal positions with repair of communication defect

f. Px = invariably fatal within several months of birth without Tx

5. Coarctation of the aorta

a. Congenital aortic narrowing, often aSx in young child

b. Si/Sx = ↓ BP in legs with normal BP in arms, **continuous murmur over collateral vessels in back, classic CXR sign = rib notching**

c. Dx confirmed with aortogram or CT

d. Tx = surgical resection of coarctation & reanastomosis

6. Patent ductus arteriosus (PDA)

a. ↑ incidence with premature births, predisposes pt to endocarditis & pulmonary vascular disease

b. Si/Sx = **continuous machinery murmur heard best at second left interspace, wide pulse pressure**, hypoxia

c. Dx = echocardiography or heart catheterization

d. Tx = indomethacin (block prostaglandins, induces closure) for infants, surgical repair for older children

VII. Trauma and Intoxication

A. Child Abuse

1. Can be physical trauma, emotional, sexual, or neglect

2. Nutritional neglect is the most common etiology for underweight infants

3. Most common perpetrator of sexual abuse is family member or family friends, 97% of reported offenders are males

4. **Physicians are required by law to report suspected child abuse or neglect (law provides protection to mandated reporters who report in good faith), clinical & lab evaluations are allowed without parental/guardian permission**

5. Epidemiology

a. 85% of children reported to children's protective services (CPS) are < 5 yr old, 45% are < 1 yr old

b. 10% of injuries to children < 5 yr old seen in the ER are due to abuse, & 10% of abuse cases involve burns

c. **High-risk children** = premature infants, children with chronic medical problems, colicky babies, those with behavioral problems, children living in poverty, children of teenage parents, single parents, or substance abusers

6. Si/Sx = injury is unexplainable or not consistent with Hx, bruises are the most common manifestation
   a. Accidental injuries seen on shins, forearms, hips
   b. Less likely to be accidental are bilateral & symmetric, seen on buttocks, genitalia, back, back of hands, different color bruises (repeat injuries over time)
   c. Highly suspicious for abuse are fractures due to pulling or wrenching, causing damage to the metaphysis
7. **Classic findings**
   a. Chip fracture, where the corner of metaphysis of long bone is torn off with damage to epiphysis
   b. Periosteum spiral fracture before infant can walk
   c. Rib fractures
8. Dating fracture can be done by callus formation (callus appears in 10–12 days)
9. Burns
   a. Shape/pattern of burn may be diagnostic
   b. **Cigarette** → circular, punched out lesions of similar size, hands & feet common
   c. **Immersion** → most common in infants, affecting buttocks & perineum (hold thighs against abdomen), or with scalded line clearly demarcated on thighs or waist without splash marks
   d. Stocking-glove burn on hands or feet
10. Injury to head is the most common cause of death from physical abuse, infants can present with convulsions, apnea, increased intracranial pressure, subdural hemorrhages, retinal hemorrhages (marker for acceleration/deceleration injuries), or in a coma
11. Sexual abuse
    a. Child may talk to mother or teacher, friend, relative about situation
    b. Si/Sx = vaginal, penile, or rectal pain, erythema, discharge, bleeding, chronic dysuria, enuresis, constipation, encopresis
    c. Behaviors = sexualized activity with peers or objects, seductive behavior
12. Dx
    a. Labs → PT/PTT & platelets to screen for bleeding diathesis
    b. Consider bone survey in children < 2 yr old, plain films or MRI for severe injuries or refusal/inability to communicate
    c. For sexual abuse collect specimens of offender's sperm, blood & hair, collect victim's nail clipping & clothing, obtain *Chlamydia* & gonorrhea cultures from mouth, anus & genitalia
    d. Dx is tentatively based on H&P, record all information, photograph when appropriate
13. Tx
    a. Medical, surgical, psychiatric treatment for injuries
    b. Report immediately, do not discharge before talking to CPS
    c. Admit pt if injuries are severe enough, if Dx unclear, or if no other safe placement available

B. POISONINGS

1. Accidental seen in younger children left unsupervised momentarily, usually a single agent ingested or inhaled (plants, household products, medications)

2. Intentional seen in adolescents/adults, toxic substances for recreational purposes or overdose taken with intent to produce self-harm
3. Epidemiology
   a. Nearly 50% of cases occur in children < 6 yr old, as a result of an accidental event or as abuse
   b. 92% occur at home, 60% with nonpharmacologic agent, 40% with pharmacologic agent
   c. Ingestion occurs in 75% of cases, 8% dermal, 6% ophthalmic, 6% inhalation
4. Hx is crucial during initial contact with patient or guardian
   a. Evaluation of severity (asymptomatic, symptomatic)
   b. Age & weight
   c. Time, type, amount & route of exposure
   d. Past medical history
5. Si/Sx

TABLE 4-10   Pediatric Toxicology

SI/SX	POSSIBLE TOXIN
Lethargy/Coma	Ethanol, sedative-hypnotics, narcotics, antihistamines, antidepressants, neuroleptic
Seizures	Theophylline, cocaine, amphetamines, antidepressants, antipsychotics, pesticides
Hypotension (with bradycardia)	Organophosphate pesticides, beta blockers
Arrhythmia	Tricyclic antidepressants, cocaine, digitalis, quinidine
Hyperthermia	Salicylates, anticholinergics

6. Tx
   a. Syrup of ipecac followed by clear liquid (water) induces vomiting, should not use in children < 6 mo, those with depressed sensorium, those with seizures or who ingested strong acids or bases
   b. Lavage usually unnecessary in children, may be useful with drugs that decrease gastric motility
   c. Charcoal may be most effective & safest procedure to prevent absorption, repeat doses every 2–6 hr with cathartic for first dose, ineffective in heavy metal or volatile hydrocarbon poisoning

VIII. Adolescence

A. EPIDEMIOLOGY
1. Injuries
   a. 50% of all deaths in adolescents attributed to injuries
   b. Many occur under the influence of alcohol & other drugs
   c. Older adolescents more likely to be killed in motor vehicle accidents while younger adolescents are at risk for drowning & fatal injuries with weapons
   d. Homicide rate is 5x higher for black males than white males
2. Suicide
   a. Second leading cause of adolescent death

b. Females more likely to attempt than males but males are 5x more likely to succeed than females

c. Pts with preexisting psychiatric problems or those who abuse alcohol & drugs more likely to attempt suicide

3. Substance abuse
   a. A major cause of morbidity in adolescents
   b. Average age of first use is 12–14 yr old
   c. 1 of every 2 adolescents have tried an illicit drug by their high school graduation
   d. Survey of high school seniors (1994–1995) noted that 90% had experience with alcohol & ≥40% had tried marijuana

4. Sex
   a. 61% of all male & 47% of all female high school students have had sex
   b. Health risks of early sexual activity are unwanted pregnancies, sexually transmitted diseases (STDs) such as gonorrhea, *Chlamydia* & HIV
   c. 86% of all STDs occur among adolescents & young adults 15–29 yr old
   d. More than 1 million adolescent females become pregnant yearly, 33% are < 15 yr old—this is a second major cause of morbidity in adolescents

5. Eating disorders
   a. Anorexia nervosa occurs in 0.5% of adolescent females & bulimia in 1–3%
   b. Si/Sx = cardiovascular symptoms, fluid & electrolyte abnormalities, amenorrhea, decreased bone density, anemia, parotid gland enlargement, tooth decay, constipation (hallmark of anorexia)
   c. Adolescents with anorexia lose 15% of ideal body weight & appear sick, but those with bulimia may look well nourished
   d. Anorexia nervosa is seen at 2 peak ages, one at 14.5 yr, the next at 18 yr, but 25% of females with anorexia may be < 13 yr old

B. CONFIDENTIALITY

1. Most issues revealed by adolescents to physicians in an interview are confidential
2. **Exceptions** include suicidal or homicidal behavior, sexual or physical abuse
3. It is strongly encouraged for physicians to inform adolescents about confidentiality at the beginning of the interview to help develop a trusting relationship between adolescent & physician

C. SCREENING

1. Annual risk behavior screening in every adolescent is strongly recommended
2. **HEADSSS** assessment allows physicians to evaluate critical areas in each adolescent's life that may be detrimental to growth & development
   a. **H**ome environment → who does adolescent live with?, any recent changes?, quality of parental interaction (if applicable)?, has he/she ever run away from home?
   b. **E**mployment & **E**ducation → is child in school?, favorite subjects?, academic performance?, are friends in school?, any recent changes?, does child have a job?, future plans?
   c. **A**ctivities → what does child like to do in spare time?, who does child spend time with?, involved in any sports/exercise?, hobbies?, attends parties or clubs?

d. **D**rugs → has child ever used tobacco?, alcohol?, marijuana?, other illicit drugs? if so, when was the child's last use?, how often?, do friends or family members use drugs?, who does the child use these substances with?

e. **S**exual activity → sexual orientation?, is child sexually active?, number of sexual partners?, does the child use condoms or other forms of contraception?, any history of STDs or pregnancy?

f. **S**uicide → does the child ever feel sad, tired, or unmotivated?, has the child ever felt that life was not worth living?, any feelings of wanting to harm self?, if so, does the child have a plan?, has the child ever tried to harm self in the past?, does the child know anyone who has attempted suicide?

g. **S**afety → does the child use a seat belt or bike helmet?, does the child enter into high-risk situations?, does the child have access to a firearm?

PEDIATRICS

5. Outpatient Medicine

Pedro Cheung

I. Headache

A. Signs/Symptoms & Differential Diagnosis

Table 5-1   Summary of Headaches

Type	Epidemiology	Characteristics
Tension	Usually after age 20 (rarely > age 50)	• Most common headache type • **Bilateral, band-like, dull in quality** • Worse with stress; not aggravated by activity • Chronic HA associated with depression
Cluster	**Male**-female = 6:1 Mean age 30 yr	• **Unilateral**, stabbing peri/retro-orbital pain, lasting 15 min to 3 hr • Seasonal attacks occur in series (6x/day) lasting weeks, followed by months of remission • **Associated with ipsilateral lacrimation (85%), ptosis, nasal congestion & rhinorrhea** • Often occurs within 90 min of onset of sleep
Migraine	80% have positive FHx **Female**-male = 3:1	• Classically, HA is **unilateral (60%)** with **aura (only 15%)**; pt looks for quiet place to rest • Visual aura: **scotoma** (blind spots), **teichopsia** (jagged zigzag lines), **photopsias** (shimmering lights), or **rhodopsins** (colors) • Accompanied by **nausea & photophobia** • Triggered by stress, odors, certain foods, alcohol, menstruation, or sleep deprivation
Temporal arteritis (Giant cell)	**Female**-male = 2:1 Age > 50	• **Unilateral temporal** headache • **Associated with jaw claudication, temporal artery tenderness with palpation, ESR ≥ 50** • 50% also have polymyalgia rheumatica • If not treated leads to optic neuritis & **blindness** • Screen by ESR; Dx with temporal artery Bx
Trigeminal neuralgia	Peak age at 60	• Episodic, severe pain shooting from side of mouth to ipsilateral ear, eye, or nose
Withdrawal headache		• Common cause of frequent headaches • Can be withdrawal from various drugs
SAH*		• Head trauma is most common cause • Spontaneous: usually berry aneurysm rupture • Classically the "worst headache of my life"

*Subarachnoid hemorrhage.

B. Dx Is Made by Clinical History & Physical Except:

1. **Temporal arteritis Dx requires temporal artery biopsy**
2. **Trigeminal neuralgia Dx requires head CT or MRI** to rule out sinusitis, cerebellopontine angle neoplasm, multiple sclerosis, herpes zoster
3. **Subarachnoid hemorrhage requires** confirmation by CT scan or lumbar puncture to detect CSF xanthochromia (can be detected 6 hr after onset of HA)

4. Suspect intracranial lesion causing headache in **pts > 50 or pts with headaches immediately upon waking up**
5. **Suspect ↑ ICP in pts awakened in middle of night by headache, who have projectile vomiting, or focal neural deficits; obtain head CT**

C. TREATMENT

TABLE 5-2   Treatment of Headache

HEADACHE	TREATMENT
Tension	• Acutely NSAIDs or Midrin® • Prophylaxis with antidepressants or β-blockers
Cluster	• Acutely 100% O_2, sumatriptan* or dihydroergotamine • Prophylaxis with verapamil, lithium, methysergide, or ergotamine
Migraine	• Acutely sumatriptan,* dihydroergotamine, NSAIDs, antiemetics • Prophylaxis with β-blockers (first line) or calcium blockers
Temporal arteritis	• High-dose prednisone or cytotoxic drug to prevent blindness
Trigeminal neuralgia	• Carbamazepine (first line) or phenytoin, clonazepam, valproic acid
Withdrawal	• NSAIDs
SAH	• Immediate neurosurgical evaluation & nimodipine to reduce incidence of postrupture vasospasm & ischemia

*Sumatriptan contraindicated with known coronary dz or ergot drugs taken within 24 hr.

II. Ears, Nose, and Throat

A. OTITIS EXTERNA
   1. Si/Sx = **pulling on pinna or pushing on tragus causes pain**
   2. *Pseudomonas* is usual cause in patients with diabetes, can be chronic in pts with seborrhea
   3. Tx = antibiotic ear drops
   4. DDx = Ramsay Hunt syndrome (herpes zoster otiticus)
      a. Herpes infection of geniculate ganglia (CN VII)
      b. Si/Sx = painful vesicles in external auditory meatus
      c. Tx = urgent acyclovir to prevent extension to meningitis
   5. In diabetics, get CT/MRI of temporal bone to rule out osteomyelitis (**malignant otitis externa**), which requires surgical débridement

B. INNER EAR DISEASE
   1. Tinnitus (ringing in the ears)
      a. Objective (heard by observer) or subjective (heard only by patient)
      b. Causes = foreign body in external canal, pulsating vascular tumors, or medications (aspirin), hearing loss
   2. Vertigo
      a. Feel as though surroundings are spinning when eyes are open, whereas in dizziness pt feels as if he/she is spinning, not the surroundings

TABLE 5-3   Causes of Vertigo

DISEASE	CHARACTERISTICS	TX
Benign positional vertigo	• Sudden, episodic vertigo with head movement lasting for seconds	Hallpike maneuver
Ménière's disease	• Dilation of membranous labyrinth due to excess endolymph • **Classic triad = hearing loss, tinnitus & episodic vertigo lasting several hours**	Medical (thiazide, anticholinergics, antihistamines) or surgery (labyrinthectomy)
Viral labyrinthitis	• Preceded by viral respiratory illness • Vertigo lasting days to weeks	Meclizine
Acoustic neuroma	• CN VIII schwannoma, commonly affects vestibular portion but can also affect cochlea • Si/Sx = vertigo, sudden deafness, tinnitus • Dx = MRI of cerebellopontine angle	Tx = local radiation or surgical excision

C. EPISTAXIS

1. 90% of bleeds occur at Kiesselbach's plexus (anterior nasal septum)
2. **#1 cause of epistaxis in children is trauma (induced by exploring digits)**
3. Also precipitated by rhinitis, nasal mucosa dryness, septal deviation & bone spurs, alcohol, antiplatelet medication, bleeding diathesis
4. Tx = direct pressure, topical nasal vasoconstrictors (Neo-Synephrine), consider anterior nasal packing if unable to stop, 5% originate in posterior nasal cavity requiring packing to occlude choana

D. SINUSITIS

1. Maxillary sinuses most commonly involved
2. DDx

TABLE 5-4   Sinusitis

	ORGANISMS	SI/SX	TX
Acute bacterial (<4 wk)	S. pneumoniae, H. influenzae, Moraxella catarrhalis	**Purulent rhinorrhea**, headache, **pain on sinus palpation**, fever, **halitosis**, anosmia, **tooth pain**	Bactrim, amoxicillin, decongestants
Chronic bacterial (>3 mo)	Bacteroides, Staph. aureus, Pseudomonas, Streptococcus spp.	Same as for acute but lasts longer, also otitis media in children	Surgical correction of obstruction, nasal steroids
Fungal	Aspergillus—**diabetics get** mucormycosis!	Usually seen in the immunocompromised	Surgery & amphotericin

3. Dx = CT scan showing inflammatory changes or bone destruction (See Figure 5-1)
4. Potential complications of sinusitis include meningitis, abscess formation, orbital infection, osteomyelitis

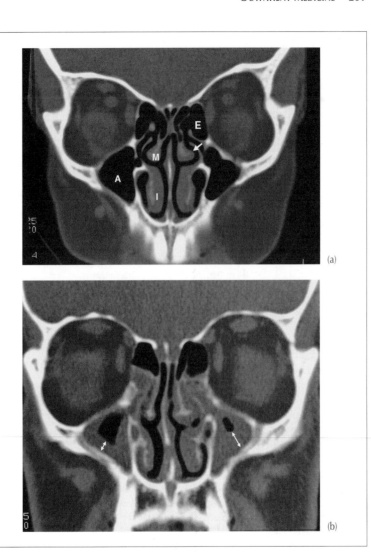

(a)

(b)

FIGURE 5-1   Coronal CT scan. (a) Normal sinuses. Note the excellent demonstration of the bony margins. The arrow points to the middle meatus into which the maxillary antrum, frontal, anterior, and middle ethmoid sinuses drain. A = maxillary antrum; E = ethmoid sinus; I = inferior turbinate; M = middle turbinate. (b) Sinusitis. Mucosal thickening prevents drainage of the sinuses. Both antra are almost opaque. The arrows indicate mucosal thickening in the antra.

E.

TABLE 5-5   Pharyngitis

DISEASE	SI/SX	DX	TX
Group A Strep throat	High fever, **severe throat pain without cough**, edematous tonsils with white or yellow **exudate, cervical adenopathy**	• H&P 50% accurate • Antigen agglutination kit for screening • Throat swab culture is gold standard	Penicillin to prevent acute rheumatic fever
Membranous (diphtheria)	High fever, dysphagia, drooling, **can cause respiratory failure** (airway occlusion)	**Pathognomonic gray membrane on tonsils extending into throat**	**STAT antitoxin**
Fungal (*Candida*)	Dysphagia, sore throat with white, cheesy patches in oropharynx (oral thrush), **seen in AIDS & small children**	Clinical or endoscopy	Nystatin liquid, swish & swallow
Adenovirus	**Pharyngoconjunctival fever (fever, red eye, sore throat)**	Clinical	Supportive
Mononucleosis (EBV)	Generalized lymphadenopathy, exudative tonsillitis, palatal petechiae & splenomegaly	• ⊕ **heterophile antibody** • **skin rash** occurs in pts given ampicillin	Supportive
Herpangina (coxsackie A)	Fever, pharyngitis, body ache, tender vesicles along tonsils, uvula & soft palate	Clinical	Supportive

III. Outpatient Gastrointestinal Complaints

A. DYSPEPSIA

1. Si/Sx = upper abdominal pain, early satiety, postprandial abdominal bloating or distention, nausea, vomiting, often exacerbated by eating
2. DDx = peptic ulcer, gastroesophageal reflux disease (GERD), cancer, gastroparesis, malabsorption, intestinal parasite, drugs (e.g., NSAIDs), etc.
3. Dx = clinical
4. Tx = empiric for 4 wk, if Sx not relieved → endoscopy
   a. Avoid caffeine, alcohol, cigarettes, NSAIDs, eat frequent small meals, stress reduction, maintain ideal body weight, elevate head of bed
   b. H_2 blockers & antacids, or proton pump inhibitor
   c. **Antibiotics for *H. pylori* are NOT indicated for nonulcer dyspepsia**

B. GASTROESOPHAGEAL REFLUX DISEASE (GERD)

1. Causes = obesity, relaxed lower esophageal sphincter, esophageal dysmotility, hiatal hernia
2. Si/Sx = heartburn occurring 30–60 min postprandial & upon reclining, usually relieved by antacid self-administration, dyspepsia, postprandial burning sensation in esophagus, also regurgitation of gastric contents into the mouth, cough, hoarseness, and globus sensation
3. Atypical Si/Sx sometimes seen = asthma, chronic cough/laryngitis, atypical chest pain
4. Upper endoscopy → tissue damage but may be normal in 50% of cases
5. Dx = clinical, can confirm with ambulatory pH monitoring
6. Tx
   a. First line = lifestyle modifications: avoid lying down postprandial, avoid spicy foods & foods that delay gastric emptying, reduction of meal size, weight loss

b. Second line = H2-receptor antagonists—aim to discontinue in 8–12 wk

c. Promotility agents may be comparable to H2-antagonists

d. Third line = proton pump inhibitors, reserve for refractory dz, often will require maintenance Tx since Sx return upon discontinuation

e. Fourth line = surgical fundoplication, relieves Sx in 90% of pts, may be more cost-effective in younger pts or those with severe dz

7. Sequelae

a. Barrett's esophagus

1) Chronic GERD → metaplasia from squamous to columnar epithelia in lower esophagus

2) Requires close surveillance with endoscopy & aggressive Tx as 10% progress to adenocarcinoma

b. Peptic stricture

1) Results in gradual solid food dysphagia often with concurrent improvement of heartburn symptoms

2) Endoscopy establishes diagnosis

3) Requires aggressive proton pump inhibitor Tx & surgical opening if unresponsive

C. DIARRHEA

1. Diarrhea ≡ stool weight > 300 g/day (normal = 100–300 g/day)

2. Small bowel dz → stools typically voluminous, watery & fatty

3. Large bowel dz → stools smaller in volume but more frequent

4. Prominent vomiting suggests viral enteritis or *Staph. aureus* food poisoning

5. Malabsorption diarrhea characterized by high fat content

a. Lose fat soluble vitamins, iron, calcium & B vitamins

b. Can cause iron deficiency, megaloblastic anemia (B_{12} loss) & hypocalcemia

6. General Tx = oral rehydration, IV fluids & electrolytes (supportive)

7. Specific diarrheas

TABLE 5-6   Diarrheas

TYPE	CHARACTERISTICS	DX	TX
Infectious	• **#1 cause of acute diarrhea** • Si/Sx = vomiting, pain; blood/mucus & fevers/chills suggest invasive dz	• Stool leukocytes, Gram's stain & culture, O & P for parasitic • *C. difficile* toxin test	• Ciprofloxacin • Metronidazole for *C. difficile*[a]
Osmotic	• Causes = lactose intolerance, oral Mg, sorbitol/mannitol	• ↑ osmotic gap • Check fecal fat	• Withdraw inciting agent
Secretory	• Causes = toxins (cholera), enteric viruses, ↑ dietary fat	• Normal osmotic gap • Fasting → no change	• Supportive
Exudative	• Mucosal inflammation → plasma & serum leakage • Causes = enteritis, TB, colon CA, inflammatory bowel dz	• ↑ ESR & CRP[b] • Radiologic imaging or colonoscopy to visualize intestine	• Varies by cause—see appropriate section of text
Rapid transit	• Causes = laxatives, surgical excision of intestinal tissue	• Hx of surgery or laxative use	• Supportive
Encopresis	• Oozing around fecal impaction in children or sick elderly	• History of constipation	• Fiber rich diet & laxatives

TABLE 5-6   *Continued*

TYPE	CHARACTERISTICS	DX	TX
Malabsorption			
Celiac sprue	• Gluten allergy (wheat, barley, rye, oats contain gluten) • Sx/Si = weakness, failure to thrive, growth retardation • Classic rash = **dermatitis herpetiformis** = pruritic, red papulovesicular lesions on shoulders, elbows & knees • 10–15% of pts develop intestinal lymphoma	**Dx by small bowel biopsy → pathognomonic blunting of intestinal villi**	Avoid dietary gluten
Tropical sprue	• Diarrhea probably caused by a tropical infection • Si/Sx = glossitis, diarrhea, weight loss, steatorrhea	Dx = clinical	Tetracycline ⊕ folate
Whipple's disease	• GI infection by *Tropheryma whippelii* • Si/Sx = diarrhea, arthritis, rash, anemia	Dx = biopsy → PAS ⊕ macrophages in intestines	Penicillin or tetracycline
Lactase deficiency	• Most of world is lactase deficient as adults, people lose as they emerge from adolescence • Si/Sx = abdominal pain, diarrhea, flatulence after ingestion of any lactose-containing product	Dx = clinical	Avoid lactose or take exogenous lactase
Intestinal lymphangiectasia	• Seen in children, congenital or acquired dilation of intestinal lymphatics leads to marked GI protein loss • Si/Sx = diarrhea, hypoproteinemia, edema	Dx = jejunal biopsy	Supportive
Pancreas dz	• Typically seen in pancreatitis & cystic fibrosis due to deficiency of pancreatic digestive enzymes • Si/Sx = foul smelling steatorrhea, megaloblastic anemia (folate deficiency), weight loss	Hx of prior pancreatic disease	Pancrease supplementation

[a] Vancomycin reserved for resistance.
[b] CRP = C-reactive protein.

8. Common infectious pathogens for diarrhea

TABLE 5-7   Infectious Causes of Diarrhea

	BACTERIAL	VIRAL	PARASITIC
Etiology	*E. coli, Shigella, Salmonella, Campylobacter jejuni, Vibrio parahaemolyticus, Vibrio cholera, Yersinia enterocolitica*	Rotavirus Norwalk virus	*Giardia lamblia, Cryptosporidium, Entamoeba histolytica*
Tx	Ciprofloxacin, Bactrim	Supportive	Metronidazole

IV. Urogenital Complaints

A. URINARY TRACT INFECTION (UTI)

1. Epidemiology
   a. 40% of females have ≥ 1 UTI, 8% have bacteriuria at a given time
   b. Most common in sexually active young women, elderly, posturethral catheter or instrumentation—rare in males (↑ risk with prostate dz)
   c. Due to *E. coli* (80%), *S. saprophyticus* (15%), other gram-negative rods
2. Si/Sx = **burning during urination**, urgency, sense of incomplete bladder emptying, hematuria, lower abdominal pain, nocturia
3. Systemic Sx = fever, chills, **back pain suggest pyelonephritis**
4. Dx = **UA → pyuria**; ⊕ bacteria on Gram's stain; positive culture results
5. Tx
   a. Lower UTI → Bactrim (first line), fluoroquinolone for refractory dz
   b. Uncomplicated pyelonephritis → same antibiotics given IV or PO depending on severity of pt's illness
   c. Men cured within 7 days of Tx do not warrant further work-up, but **adolescents & men with pyelonephritis or recurrent infxn require renal Utz & intravenous pyelogram to rule out anatomic etiology**
   d. UTI 2° to bacterial prostatitis requires 6–12 wk of antibiotics
   e. Asymptomatic bacteriuria
      1) Defined as urine culture > 100,000 CFU/mL but no Sx
      2) Only Tx in 1) pregnancy (use penicillins or nitrofurantoin), or pts with 2) renal transplant, 3) about to undergo GU procedure, 4) severe vesicular-ureteral reflux & 5) struvite calculi

B. SEXUALLY TRANSMITTED DISEASES (STDs)—SEE SECTION C FOR AIDS

TABLE 5-8   Sexually Transmitted Diseases

DISEASE	CHARACTERISTICS	TX
Herpes simplex virus (HSV)	• Most common cause of genital ulcers (causes 60–70% of cases) • Si/Sx = **painful vesicular & ulcerated** lesions 1–3 mm diameter, onsets 3–7 days after exposure • Lesions generally resolve over 7 days • Primary infection also characterized by malaise, low grade fever & inguinal adenopathy in 40% of patients • Recurrent lesions are similar appearing, but milder in severity & shorter in duration, lasting about 2–5 days • Dx confirmed with direct fluorescent antigen (DFA) staining, Tzanck prep, serology, HSV PCR, or culture	• Tx = acyclovir, famciclovir, or valacyclovir to ↓ duration of viral shedding & shorten initial course

TABLE 5-8 *Continued*

DISEASE	CHARACTERISTICS	TX
Pelvic inflammatory disease	• *Chlamydia trachomatis* & *Neisseria gonorrhoeae* are primary pathogens, but PID is polymicrobial involving both aerobic & anaerobic bacteria • PID includes endometritis, salpingitis, tuboovarian abscess (TOA) & pelvic peritonitis • Infertility occurs in 15% of pts after 1 episode of salpingitis, ↑ to 75% after ≥ 3 episodes • Risk of ectopic pregnancy ↑ 7–10 times in women with history of salpingitis • Dx = abdominal, adnexal & cervical motion tenderness + at least 1 of the following: ⊕ Gram's stain, temp > 38°C, WBC > 10,000, pus on culdocentesis or laparoscopy, tuboovarian abscess on bimanual or Utz	• Toxic pts, ↓ immunity & noncompliant should be Tx as inpatients with IV antibiotics • Use fluoroquinolone + metronidazole or cephalosporin + doxycycline • Start antibiotic as soon as PID is suspected, even before culture results are available
Human papillomavirus (HPV)	• Serotypes 16, 18 most commonly associated with cervical cancer • Incubation period varies from 6 wk to 3 mo, spread by direct skin-to-skin contact • Infection after single contact with an infected individual results in 65% transmission rate • Si/Sx = condyloma acuminata (genital warts) = soft, fleshy growths on vulva, vagina, cervix, perineum & anus • Dx = clinical, confirmed with biopsy	• Topical podophyllin or trichloracetic acid, if refractory → cryosurgery or excision • If pregnant, C-section recommended to avoid vaginal lacerations
Syphilis (*Treponema pallidum*)	• Si/Sx = **painless ulcer** with bilateral inguinal adenopathy, chancre heals in 3–9 wk • Because of lack of Sx, Dx of primary syphilis is often missed • 4–8 wk after appearance of chancre, 2° dz → fever, lymphadenopathy, maculopapular rash affecting palms & soles, condyloma lata in intertriginous areas • Dx = serologies, VDRL & RPR for screening, FTA-ABS to confirm	• Benzathine penicillin G

C. ACQUIRED IMMUNODEFICIENCY SYNDROME (AIDS)

1. Epidemiology
   a. AIDS is a global pandemic (currently the fastest spread is in SE Asia & central Europe)
   b. **Heterosexual transmission is the most common mode worldwide**
   c. In the US, IV drug users & their sex partners are the fastest growing population of HIV⊕ patients
   d. Homosexual transmission is slowing dramatically [see *N Engl J Med* 1999, 341:1046-1050]

2. HIV biology
   a. Retrovirus with the usual *gag, pol* & *env* genes
   b. p24 is a core protein encoded by *gag* gene, can be used clinically to follow disease progression
   c. gp120 & gp41 are envelope glycoproteins that are produced on cleavage of gp160, coded by *env*

d. Reverse transcriptase (coded by *pol*) converts viral RNA to DNA so it can integrate into the host's DNA

e. Cellular entry is by binding to both CD4 & an additional ligand (can be CCR4, CCR5, others) that typically is a cytokine receptor

f. HIV can infect CD4⊕ T cells, macrophages, thymic cells, astrocytes, dendritic cells & others

g. The mechanisms of T-cell destruction are not well understood but probably include direct cell lysis, induction of CTL responses against infected CD4⊕ cells & exhaustion of bone marrow production (suppression of production of T cells)

h. In addition, the virus induces alterations in host cytokine patterns rendering surviving lymphocytes ineffective

3. Disease course

a. In most patients AIDS is relentlessly progressive & death occurs within 10–15 yr of HIV infection

b. Long-term survivors

1) Up to 5% of patients are "long-term survivors," meaning the disease does not progress even after 15–20 yr without Tx

2) This may be due to infection with defective virus, a potent host immune response, or genetic resistance of the host

3) People with homozygous deletions of CCR5 or other viral coreceptors are highly resistant to infection with HIV, while heterozygotes are less resistant

c. Although patients can have no clinical evidence of disease for many years, **HIV has no latent phase in its life cycle**; clinical silence in those patients who eventually progress is due to daily, temporarily successful host repopulation of T cells

d. Death is usually caused by opportunistic infections (OIs)

1) OIs typically onset after CD4 counts fall below 200

2) Below 200 CD4 cells, all pts should be on permanent Bactrim prophylaxis against *P. carinii* pneumonia (PCP) & *Toxoplasma encephalitis*

3) Below 50 CD4 cells, all patients should receive azithromycin prophylaxis against *M. avium-intracellulare* complex (MAC)

4) Kaposi's sarcoma = common skin cancer found in homosexual HIV patients, thought to be caused by cotransmission of human herpes virus 8 (HHV 8)

5) Other diseases found in AIDS patients include generalized wasting & dementia

4. Treatment

a. Triple combination therapy is now the cornerstone

1) Cocktail includes 2 nucleoside analogues (e.g., AZT, ddl, d4T) ⊕ a protease inhibitor

2) Protease inhibitors block the splicing of the large *gag* precursor protein into its final components, p24 & p7

3) Newest addition to arsenal is hydroxyurea

a) Inhibits host ribonucleotide reductase → decreased concentration of purines

b) ddl is a purine analogue (competitor), so hydroxyurea ↑ efficacy of ddl

c) In theory, virus should not be able to become resistant to hydroxyurea, since it acts on a host enzyme & not on the virus

b. **No patient should ever be on any single drug regimen for HIV—resistance is invariable in monotherapy**

c. Current Tx is able to suppress viral replication to below detectable limits in the majority of patients, but **up to 50% of patients end up "failing" therapy (viral loads rebound)**

d. **Failure of the regimen is associated with poor compliance** (missed doses lead to resistance) & **prior exposure to one or more drugs in the regimen** (the virus is already resistant to the agent)

e. The long-term significance of viral suppression is unclear, but **it is known that the virus is NOT cleared from the body at up to 2 yr after it ceases to be detectable in the blood** (it can be found latent in lymph nodes)

D. HEMATURIA

1. Red/brown urine discoloration 2° to RBCs, correlates with presence of >5 RBCs/high-powered field on microanalysis
2. Can be painful or painless
   a. Painless = 1° renal dz (tumor, glomerulonephritis), TB infection, vesicular dz (bladder tumor), prostatic dz
   b. Painful = nephrolithiasis, renal infarction, UTI
3. DDx = myoglobinuria or hemoglobinuria, where hemoglobin dipstick is positive but no RBCs are seen on microanalysis
4. Dx = finding of RBCs in urinary sediment
   a. Urinalysis → WBCs (infection) or RBC casts (glomerulonephritis)
   b. CBC → anemia (renal failure), polycythemia (renal cell CA)
   c. Urogram will show nephrolithiasis & tumors (Utz → cystic vs. solid)
   d. Cystoscopy only after UA & IVP; best for lower urinary tract
5. Tx varies by cause

E. PROSTATE

1. Benign prostatic hyperplasia
   a. Hyperplasia of the periurethral prostate causing bladder outlet obstruction
   b. Common after age 45 (autopsy shows that 90% of men over 70 have BPH)
   c. Does not predispose to prostate cancer
   d. Si/Sx urinary frequency, urgency, nocturia, ↓ size & force of urinary stream leading to hesitancy & intermittency, sensation of incomplete emptying worsening to continuous overflow incontinence or urinary retention, rectal exam → enlarged prostate (classically a rubbery vs. firm, hard gland that may suggest prostate cancer) with loss of median furrow
   e. Labs → PSA elevated in up to 50% of pts, not specific—not useful marker for BPH
   f. Dx based on symptomatic scoring system, i.e., prostate size >30 mL (determined by Utz or exam), maximum urinary flow rate (<10 mL/sec) & postvoid residual urine volume (>50 mL) (see *J Urology* 1992, 148:1549)
   g. Tx = α-blocker (e.g., terazosin), 5-α-reductase inhibitor (e.g., Finasteride); avoid anticholinergics, antihistaminergics, or narcotics
   h. Refractory dz requires surgery = transurethral resection of prostate (TURP); open prostatectomy recommended for larger glands (>75 g)
2. Prostatitis
   a. Si/Sx = fever, chills, low back pain, urinary frequency & urgency, tender, possible fluctuant & swollen prostate

b. Labs → leukocytosis, pyuria, bacteriuria

c. Dx = clinical

d. Tx = systemic antibiotics

F. IMPOTENCE

1. Affects 30 million men in US, strongly associated with age (about 40% among 40-yr-olds & 70% among 70-yr-olds)

2. Causes

  a. 1° erectile dysfunction = never been able to sustain erections

    1) Psychological (sexual guilt, fear of intimacy, depression, anxiety)

    2) ↓ testosterone 2° to hypothalamic-pituitary-gonadal disorder

    3) Hypo- or hyperthyroidism, Cushing's syndrome, ↑ prolactin

  b. 2° erectile dysfunction = acquired, **>90% due to organic cause**

    1) Vascular dz = atherosclerosis of penile arteries &/or venous leaks causing inadequate impedance of venous outflow

    2) Drugs = diuretics, clonidine, CNS depressants, tricyclic antidepressants, high-dose anticholinergics, antipsychotics

    3) Neurologic dz = stroke, temporal lobe seizures, multiple sclerosis, spinal cord injury, autonomic dysfunction 2° to diabetes, post-TURP or open prostatic surgery

3. Dx

  a. Clinical, rule out above organic causes

  b. **Nocturnal penile tumescence** testing differentiates psychogenic from organic—nocturnal tumescence is involuntary, ⊕ in psychogenic but not in organic dz

4. Tx

  a. Sildenafil (Viagra)

    1) Selective inhibitor of cGMP specific phosphodiesterase type 5a → improves relaxation of smooth muscles in corpora cavernosa

    2) Side effects = transient headache, flushing, dyspepsia & rhinitis, transient visual disturbances (blue hue) is very rare, drug may lower blood pressure → **use of nitrates is an absolute contraindication**, deaths have resulted from combo

  b. Vacuum-constriction devices use negative pressure to draw blood into penis with band placed at base of penis to retain erection

  c. Intracavernosal prostaglandin injection has mean duration about 60 min; risks = penile bruising/bleeding & priapism

  d. Surgery = penile prostheses implantation; venous or arterial surgery

  e. Testosterone therapy for hypogonadism

  f. Behavioral therapy & counseling for depression & anxiety

V. Common Sports Medicine Complaints

A. LOW BACK PAIN

1. 80% of people experience low back pain—second most common complaint in 1° care (next to common cold)

2. **50% of cases will recur within the subsequent 3 yr**

3. **Majority cases attributed to muscle strains**, but always consider disk herniation

4. Si/Sx of disk herniation = shooting pain down leg (sciatica), pain on **straight leg raise (>90% sensitive)** & pain on **crossed straight leg raise (>90% specific, not sensitive)**

OUTPATIENT MEDICINE

5. Dx

    a. **Always rule out RED FLAGS** (see below) with Hx & physical exam

    b. If no red flags detected, presume Dx is muscle strain & not serious—**no radiologic testing is warranted**

    c. Dz not remitting after 4 wk of conservative Tx should be further evaluated with repeat Hx & physical; consider radiologic studies

    d. Red Flags

TABLE 5-9   Low Back Pain Red Flags

DIAGNOSIS	SI/SX	DX
Fracture	• Hx of trauma (fall, car accident) • Minor trauma in elderly (e.g., strenuous lifting)	• Spine x-rays
Tumor	• **Pt > 50 yr old** (accounts for >80% of cancer cases) or <20 yr old • Prior Hx of CA • **Constitutional Sx** (fever/chills, weight loss) • Pain worse when supine or at night	• Spinal MRI is gold standard, can get CT also
Infection	• Immunosuppressed pts • Constitutional Sx • Recent bacterial infection or IV drug abuse	• Blood cultures, spinal MRI to rule out abscess
Cauda equina syndrome	• Acute urinary retention, **saddle anesthesia**, lower extremity weakness or paresthesias & ↓ reflexes, ↓ anal sphincter tone	• Spinal MRI
Spinal stenosis	• Si/Sx = **pseudoclaudication** (neurogenic) with pain ↑ with walking **& standing**; relieved by sitting or leaning forward	• Spinal MRI
Radiculopathy (herniation compressing spinal nerves)*	• Sensory loss: (L5 → **L**arge toe/ medial foot, S1→ **S**mall toe/ lateral foot) • Weakness: (L1–L4 → quadriceps, L5 → foot dorsiflexion, S1 → plantar flexion) • ↓ reflexes (L4 → patellar, S1 → achilles)	• **Clinical**—MRI may confirm clinical Dx but false-positive are common (clinically insignificant disk herniation) (See Figure 5-2)

*Radiculopathy ≠ herniation; radiculopathy indicates evolving spinal nerve impingement & is a more serious Dx than simple herniation indicated by straight leg testing & sciatica.

6. Tx

    a. No red flags → conservative with acetaminophen (safer) or NSAIDs, **muscle relaxants have not been shown to help**; avoid narcotics

    b. **Strict bed rest is NOT warranted** (extended rest shown to be debilitating, especially in older patients)—encourage return to normal activity, low-stress aerobic & back exercises

    c. **90% of cases resolve within 4 wk with conservative Tx**

    d. Red flags:

        1) Fracture → surgical consult

        2) Tumor → urgent radiation/steroid (↓ compression), then excise

        3) Infection → abscess drainage & antibiotics per pathogen

        4) Cauda equina syndrome → emergent surgical decompression

        5) Spinal stenosis → complete laminectomy

6) Radiculopathy → anti-inflammatories, nerve root decompression with laminectomy or microdiscectomy only if (1) sciatica is severe & disabling, (2) Sx persist for 4 wk or worsening progression & (3) strong evidence of specific nerve root damage with MRI correlation of level of disk herniation

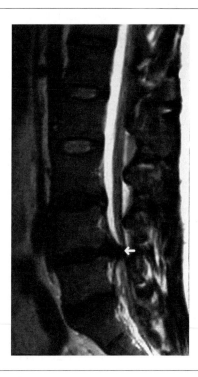

FIGURE 5-2   MRI scan demonstrating a prolapsed disk at L4/L5 with posterior deviation of the theca (arrow).

B. SHOULDER DISLOCATION

1. Subluxation = symptomatic translation of humeral head relative to glenoid articular surface
2. Dislocation = complete displacement out of the glenoid
3. Anterior instability (about 95% of cases) usually due to subcoracoid dislocation is the most common form of shoulder dislocation
4. Si/Sx = pain, joint immobility, arm "goes dead" with overhead motion
5. Dx = clinical, assess axillary nerve function in neuro exam, look for signs of rotator cuff injury, confirm with x-rays if necessary
6. Tx = initial reduction of dislocation by various traction-countertraction techniques, 2–6 wk period of immobilization (longer for younger patients), intense rehabilitation; rarely is surgery required

C. Clavicle Fracture
1. Occurs primarily due to contact sports in adults
2. Si/Sx = pain & deformity at clavicle
3. Dx = clinical, confirm fracture with standard AP view x-ray
4. Must rule out subclavian artery injury by checking pulses, brachial plexus injury with neuro examination & pneumothorax by checking breath sounds
5. Tx = sling until range of motion is painless (usually 2–4 wk)

D. Elbow Injuries
1. Epicondylitis (tendinitis)
   a. Lateral epicondylitis **(tennis elbow)**
      1) Usually in tennis player (>50%), or racquetball, squash, fencing
      2) Si/Sx = pain 2–5 cm distal & anterior to lateral epicondyle reproduced with wrist extension while elbow is extended
   b. Medial epicondylitis **(golfer's elbow)**
      1) Commonly in golf, racquet sports, bowling, baseball, swimming
      2) Si/Sx = acute onset of medial elbow pain & swelling localized 1 or 2 cm area distal to medial epicondyle, pain usually reproduced with wrist flexion & pronation against resistance
   c. Tx for both = ice, rest, NSAIDs, counterforce bracing, rehabilitation
   d. Px for both varies, can become chronic condition; surgery sometimes indicated (débridement & tendon reapproximation)
2. Olecranon fracture
   a. Usually direct blow to elbow with triceps contraction after fall on flexed upper extremity
   b. Tx = long arm cast or splint in 45–90° flexion for ≥ 3 wk
   c. Displaced fracture requires open reduction & internal fixation
3. Dislocation
   a. Elbow joint most commonly dislocated joint in children, second most in adults (next to shoulder)
   b. Fall onto outstretched hand with fully extended elbow (posterolateral dislocation) or direct blow to posterior elbow (anterior dislocation)
   c. May also be seen after jerking child's arm by hurried parent or guardian (**nursemaid's elbow**) (See Figure 5-3)
   d. Key is associated nerve injury (ulnar, median, radial or anterior interosseous nerve), vascular injury (brachial artery) or other structural injury (associated coronoid process fracture common)
   e. Tx = reduce elbow by gently flexing supinated arm, long arm splint or bivalved cast applied at 90° flexion

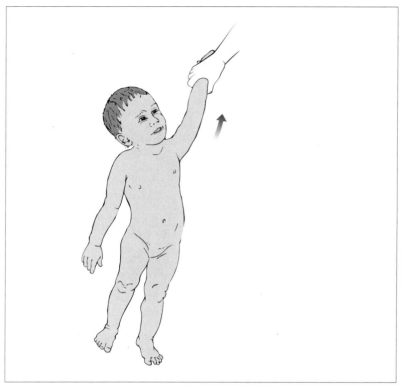

FIGURE 5-3 Nursemaid's elbow. Sudden forceful traction dislocates the elbow joint.

4. Olecranon bursitis
   a. Inflammation of bursa under olecranon process
   b. Seen with direct blow to elbow by collision or fall on artificial turf
   c. Si/Sx = swollen & painful posterior elbow with restricted motion
   d. Dx = clinical, confirm with bursa aspiration to rule out septic bursitis
   e. Tx = bursa aspiration, compression dressing & pad

E. ANKLE INJURIES
   1. Achilles tendonitis
      a. 2° to overuse, commonly seen in runners, gymnasts, cyclists & volleyball players
      b. Si/Sx = swelling or erythema along area of Achilles tendon with tenderness 2–5 cm proximal to calcaneus
      c. Evaluate for rupture = Thompson test (squeezing leg with passive plantar flexion) positive only with complete tear
      d. Tx = rest, ice, NSAIDs, taping or splinting to ↓ stress & ↑ support
      e. Rupture requires long leg casting × 4 wk, short leg walking cast × 4 wk, then wear heel lift × 4 wk
      f. Open repair speeds recovery & is recommended with complete tears in younger patients

2. Ankle sprains
   a. Lateral sprain occurs when ankle is plantar-flexed (90% of sprains)
   b. Anterior drawer sign is done with foot in 10–15° plantar flexion
   c. Medial sprain is rare (10%) because ligament is stronger
   d. Dx = multiple view x-rays both free & weight bearing
   e. Tx = **RICE** = **R**est (limit activity +/– crutches), **I**ce, **C**ompression (ACE bandage), **E**levation above level of heart to decrease swelling
   f. Severe sprains may benefit from casting, open repair rarely indicated

VI. Preventive Medicine

A. Cancer Screening

TABLE 5-10   Cancer Screening

DISEASE	INTERVENTION
Cervical CA	• Annual PS in women ≥ 18 yr or sexually active (ACS) • Perform less often if ≥3 consecutive Paps are nl & pt is monogamous
Breast CA	• Exam & mammogram every 1–2 yr women 50–69 yr (AAFP, USPTF) • Self exams; annual exam & mammogram in women >40 yr (ACS)
Colorectal CA	• Hemoccult annually >50 yr (screen earlier with positive family Hx) • Pt > 50 yr → sigmoidoscopy q 5 yr or colonoscopy q 10 yr (ACS)
Prostate CA	• Annual digital exam & PSA should be offered to all men >50 yr (ACS)
Endometrial CA	• High-risk patients should have biopsy shortly after menopause (ACS)
Other CA	• Annual physical exam for signs of thyroid, skin, oral, testicular or ovarian CA (ACS)

B. Adult Immunization

TABLE 5-11   Adult Immunization

Tetanus	All require primary series & periodic boosters q 10 yr (A)
MMR	All require vaccination if born after 1956 without immunity (A)
Hepatitis B	Recommended for all young adults & ↑ risk pts (A)
Pneumococcal	Give once in immunocompetent pts ≥ 65 yr or to any pt with ↑ risk (B)
Influenza	Annually for all pts ≥ 50 yr or high-risk pts (B)
Hepatitis A	Only for high-risk patients like travelers (B)
Varicella	Adults without Hx of disease or previous vaccination (B)
In HIV pts avoid live preparations, but MMR should be given if CD4 count >500	
In pregnant pts live vaccinations are not recommended (MMR, OPV, VZV)	

A = proven benefit, B = probably benefit.

C. TRAVEL PROPHYLAXIS

TABLE 5-12   Travel Prophylaxis

Traveler's diarrhea	Prevent w/ Pepto-Bismol; Tx w/ ciprofloxacin & loperamide
Malaria	Chloroquine; mefloquine (endemic chloroquine-resistant areas)
Hepatitis A	Most travelers; vaccine requires 4 wk; give IVIG for short-term
Typhoid	Endemic in India, Pakistan, Peru, Chile, Mexico; oral or inject
Yellow fever	Endemic in parts of South America & Africa
Meningococcus	Endemic in meningococcal belt (sub-Saharan Africa)
	Ensure all other routine immunizations are up to date (MMR, polio, Hep B)

Note: current cholera & plague vaccines are not very effective.

D. SMOKING CESSATION

1. 20–50 million US smokers attempt to quit; 6% long-term success rate
2. **Nicotine replacement (gum or patch) increases success about twofold**
3. Support from weekly counseling session, telephone calls, family & other support groups shown ↑ success
4. For best success, set a precise quit date to begin complete abstinence
5. Pts with negative affect (e.g., depression) have more difficulty quitting
6. **Bupropion +/– nicotine replacement** has 12 mo abstinence rate of >30%, **2x better than nicotine replacement alone** [*N Engl J Med* 1999, 340:9, 655]
7. On average, pts who quit successfully will gain weight (mean = 5 lb)

E. OTHER PERIODIC HEALTH EXAMINATION CONCERNS

1. Adolescence (11–24 yr)
   a. Leading cause of death are MVA & injuries & homicide/suicide
   b. BP check, Pap smears, rubella status, drug & STD education, safety
2. HTN: check BP every 2 yr in normotensive pts 21+ yr (USPTF)
3. Hyperlipidemia: check cholesterol & lipids in normal population about every 5 yr in men 35–65 yr & women 45–65 yr (USPTF)
4. Endocarditis: antibiotic prophylaxis (amoxicillin or erythromycin) given before & after dental procedures & certain surgeries; consider prophylaxis for (1) prosthetic values, (2) mitral or aortic valvular dz, (3) congenital heart dz & (4) prior Hx of infectious endocarditis

VII. Biostatistics

A. TABLE OF DEFINITIONS

TABLE 5-13   Biostatistics

TERM	DEFINITION
Sensitivity	Probability that test results will be positive in pts with disease
Specificity	Probability that test results will be negative in pts without disease
False-positive	Pt without disease who has a positive test result
False-negative	Pt with disease who has a negative test result
PPV	Positive predictive value: probability pt with positive test actually has disease

TABLE 5-13   *Continued*

TERM	DEFINITION
NPV	Negative predictive value: probability pt with negative test actually has no disease
Incidence	# of newly reported cases of disease divided by total population
Prevalence	# existing cases of disease divided by total population at a given time
Relative risk	From cohort study (prospective)—risk of developing dz for people with known exposure compared to risk of developing dz without exposure
Odds ratio	From case control study (retrospective)—approximates relative risk by comparing odds of developing dz in exposed pts to odds of developing dz in unexposed pts (if dz is rare, odds ratio approaches true relative risk)
Variance	An estimate of the variability of each individual data point from the mean
Std deviation	Square root of the variance
Type I error (α error)	Null hypothesis is rejected even though it is true—e.g., the study says the intervention works but it only appears to work because of random chance
Type II error (β error)	Null hypothesis is not rejected even though it is false—e.g., the study fails to detect a true effect of the intervention
Power ($1 - \beta$)	An estimate of the probability a study will be able to detect a true effect of the intervention—e.g., power of 80% means that if the intervention works, the study has an 80% chance of detecting this but a 20% chance of randomly missing it

B. STUDY TYPES
Prospective is more powerful than retrospective
Interventional is more powerful than observational

1. Clinical trial: **Prospective interventional trial** in which pts are randomized into an intervention group & a control group. **Randomization blunts effect of confounding factors. Blinding both clinician & patient (double-blind) further decreases bias.**
2. Cohort study: Population is divided by exposure status. Requires large population (cannot study rare disease). Can study multiple effects by exposure. Gives **relative risk if prospective**. Can be prospective or retrospective.
3. Case control study: Pts divided by those with dz (cases) & those without dz (controls). Fewer patients are needed (good for rare disease). Can study correlation of multiple exposures. Gives **odds ratio**. **Always retrospective**.

C. CALCULATION OF STATISTICAL VALUES

TABLE 5-14   Sample Calculation of Statistical Values

	PT HAS DZ	PT DOES NOT HAVE DZ
Positive test	a = true-positive	b = false-positive
Negative test	c = false-negative	d = true-negative

PPV = a/a + b
NPV = d/c + d
Sensitivity = a/a + c
Specificity = d/b + d

Sensitivity & specificity are inherent characteristics of the test—they must be given in the question. **Predictive values vary with the prevalence of the disease.** They are NOT inherent characteristics of the test, but rather reflect an interaction of sensitivity & specificity with the frequency of the disease in the population.

EXAMPLE 1: For disease X, a theoretical screening test is **90% sensitive** & **80% specific**. In Africa, where the disease has a **prevalence of 50%**, the test's **PPV = 82%** (a / a + b = 45 / 55), & the **NPV is 89%** (d / c + d = 40 / 45).

	PT HAS DZ	PT DOES NOT HAVE DZ
POSITIVE TEST	45	10
NEGATIVE TEST	5	40

Always fill the table in assuming 100 patients—it's easier to do the math this way. The prevalence of the disease (50%) tells you that 50 patients should be in the first column, because 50% of 100 patients have the disease. Therefore, 50 patients should also be in the second column (if 50 of 100 patients have the disease, 50 patients also do NOT have the disease). The sensitivity tells you that 45 of the patients in the first column should be in the top row because the test will find 90% of the 50 patients who have the disease. The specificity tells you that 40 of the patients in the second column should be in the bottom row because the test will correctly describe 80% of the 50 people who truly don't have the disease (& incorrectly claim that 20% of the 50 patients who truly don't have the disease do have the disease).

EXAMPLE 2: Now study the **same test for the same disease (X)** in America, where the **prevalence of the disease is 10%**. The test characteristics remain the same: **90% sensitive** & **80% specific**. The test's **PPV = 33%** (a / a + b = 9 / 27) & the **NPV = 99%** (d / c + d = 72 / 73). **The same test has drastically different predictive values depending on the disease prevalence!!!**

	PT HAS DZ	PT DOES NOT HAVE DZ
POSITIVE TEST	9	18
NEGATIVE TEST	1	72

Now the disease prevalence tells you that 10 patients should be in the first column (10% of 100 patients have the disease). Therefore, 90 patients should be in the second column (if 10 of 100 patients have the disease, 90 patients do NOT have the disease). The sensitivity tells you that 9 of the patients in the first column should be in the top row because the test will find 90% of the 10 patients who have the disease. The specificity tells you that 72 of the patients in the second column should be in the bottom row because the test will correctly describe 80% of the 90 people who truly don't have the disease (& incorrectly claim that 20% of the 90 patients who don't have the disease do have the disease).

OUTPATIENT MEDICINE

6. Psychiatry

Charles Lee

I. Introduction

A. DSM-IV (DIAGNOSTIC & STATISTICAL MANUAL)
1. The DSM-IV lists current US diagnostic criteria for psychiatric conditions
2. **The USMLE will rely on DSM-IV diagnostic criteria**
3. **Do not try memorizing all the possible Sx mentioned by the DSM** to define a given condition. It is impossible and not a good use of time. This review will focus on the Sx you are **most likely to see on the exam.**

B. PRINCIPLES OF PSYCHIATRY FOR THE USMLE (MORE COMPLEX IN REAL LIFE)
1. Major psychiatric Dx requires **significant impairment in the pt's life**
2. **Always rule out drug abuse** (frequent comorbidity in psychiatric dz)
3. **Combination Tx** (pharmacology & psychotherapy) **is superior** to either alone but **pharmacologic Tx is first line for severe dz in acute setting**
4. **Criteria for hospitalization (any single criterion is acceptable)**
   a. Danger to self (suicide)
   b. Danger to others
   c. Unable to provide food, clothing, shelter (grave disability)
5. Psychiatric dz is chronic—if asked about dz course, **"cures" are rare**
6. Prognosis depends on symptom onset, insight & premorbid function

TABLE 6-1   Prognosis of Psychiatric Disorders

PROGNOSIS	SYMPTOM ONSET	INSIGHT*	PREMORBID FUNCTION
Favorable	Acute	Good	High
Unfavorable	Subacute/Chronic	Poor	Low

*Insight = pt recognizes symptoms as abnormalities & is distressed by them.

II. Mood Disorders

A. MAJOR DEPRESSIVE DISORDER (MDD)
1. A syndrome of **repeated major depressive episodes**
2. One of the most common psychiatric disorders, with lifetime prevalence of 15–25%, with a greater incidence in women & elderly (often overlooked)
3. Si/Sx for depression in general
   a. Major Si/Sx = ↓ **mood** &/or **anhedonia** (inability to experience pleasure)
   b. Others = insomnia (less commonly hypersomnia), ↓ appetite/weight loss (less commonly ↑ appetite/weight gain), fatigue, ↓ concentration, guilt or feeling worthless, recurrent thoughts of death & suicide
   c. **Commonly presents with various somatic complaints & ↓ energy level rather than complaints of depression**—beware of clinical scenarios in which pts have multiple unrelated physical complaints

218

4. DDx = dysthymic disorder, bipolar disorder, medical dz (**classically hypothyroidism**), bereavement
5. Dx requires depressive episode to continue for ≥2 wk, with ≥2 episodes separated by ≥2 mo (**2 episodes of 2 wk, 2 mo apart**)
6. Tx
    a.

TABLE 6-2   Pharmacologic Therapy for Depression[a]

DRUG	EXAMPLES	SIDE EFFECTS
SSRIs[b]	Fluoxetine, paroxetine	Favorable profile: rare impotence
TCAs[b]	Amitriptyline, desipramine, imipramine, nortriptyline	More severe: confusion, sedation, **orthostatic hypotension, prolonged QRS duration** (think autonomic/cholinergic)
MAO[b] Inhibitors	Phenelzine, tranylcypromine	Very severe: classic syndromes • *Serotonin syndrome* = caused by **MAO inhibitor interaction with SSRIs, demerol, or pseudoephedrine** & others, presents with hyperthermia, muscle rigidity, altered mental status • *Hypertensive crisis* = malignant hypertension when ingested with foods rich in **tyramine** (wine & cheese)

[a] Takes 2–6 wk for effect.
[b] SSRIs (selective serotonin reuptake inhibitors) are first line; TCAs (tricyclic antidepressants) are second line; MAO inhibitors (monoamine oxidase inhibitors) are third line.

b. Psychotherapy = **psychodynamic** (understanding self/inner conflicts), **cognitive-behavioral** (recognizing negative thought or behavior & altering thinking/behavior accordingly), **interpersonal** (examines relation of Sx to negative/absent relationships with others)
c. **Electroconvulsive therapy (ECT)** is effective for refractory cases, main side effect is short-term memory loss

B. Dysthymic Disorder

1. Si/Sx as per major depressive episodes but is continuous
2. Dx = **steady Sx duration for minimum of 2 yr**—dysthymic disorder is longer but less acute than MDD
3. If major depressive episode takes place during the 2 yr of dysthymia, then by definition the Dx is MDD rather than dysthymic disorder
4. Tx as per MDD

C. Bereavement

1. **Bereavement** is a commonly asked test question!
2. Si/Sx = an older adult whose partner has died & who has been feeling sad, losing weight & sleeping poorly (depression symptoms)
3. Dx: key is **how much time** has elapsed since the partner died—**if Sx persist for >2 mo, Dx is MDD rather than normal bereavement**
4. Although bereavement is normal behavior, grief management may be helpful.

D. Bipolar Disorder (Manic-Depression)

1. Seen in 1% of population, genders equally affected but **often presents in young people** while **major depression is a dz of middle age (40s)**
2. Si/Sx = abrupt onset of ↑ **energy**, ↓ **need to sleep, pressured speech** (speaks quickly

to the point of making no sense), ↓ attention span, **hypersexuality, spending large amounts of money,** engaging in outrageous activities (e.g., directing traffic at an intersection while naked)

3. DDx = cocaine & amphetamine use, personality disorders (cluster B, see below, Section V.B), schizophrenia (see below, Section III), hypomania
4. Dx
   a. **Manic episode causes significant disability,** whereas hypomania presents with identical Sx but no significant disability
   b. Episodes **must last ≥1 wk & should be abrupt, not continuous,** which would suggest personality disorder or schizophrenia
   c. **Bipolar I** = manic episode with or without depressive episodes (pts often have depressive episodes before experiencing mania)
   d. **Bipolar II** = depressive episodes **with hypomanic episodes** but, by definition, **the absence of manic episodes**
   e. **Rapid cycling** = 4 episodes (depressive, manic, or mixed) in 12 mo; can be precipitated by antidepressants
5. Tx
   a. Hospitalization, often involuntary since manic pts rarely see the need
   b. **Valproate** or **carbamazepine** are first line, **lithium** second line
   c. Valproate & carbamazepine cause **blood dyscrasias**
   d. Lithium blood levels must be checked due to frequent toxicity, including **tremor** & polyuria due to **nephrogenic diabetes insipidus**
6. Px worse than major depression, episodes more frequent with age

E. DRUG-INDUCED MANIA
1. Cocaine & amphetamines are major culprits
2. Si/Sx = mania as above, also tachycardia, hypertension, dilated pupils, **EKG arrhythmia or ischemia in young people is highly suggestive**
3. Dx = urine or serum toxicology screen
4. Tx = calcium-channel blockers for acute autonomic Sx, drug Tx programs longer term

III. Psychosis

A. SI/SX
1. **Hallucinations & delusions** are hallmark
   a. Hallucination ≡ false sensory perception not based on real stimulus
   b. Delusion ≡ false interpretation of external reality
   c. Can be paranoid, grandiose (thinking one possesses special powers), religious (God is talking to the pt), or ideas of reference (every event in the world somehow involves the pt)

B. DDX

TABLE 6-3   Diagnosis of Psychotic Disorders

DISEASE	CHARACTERISTICS
Schizophrenia	• **Presents in late teens–20s (slightly later in women), very strong genetic predisposition** • Often accompanied by **premorbid** sign, including poor school performance, poor emotional expression & lack of friends • Positive Sx = hallucinations (**more often auditory than visual**) & delusions • Negative Sx = lack of affect, alogia • Other Sx = disorganized behavior &/or speech • **Schizophrenia lasts ≥6 continuous mo** • **Schizophreniform disorder lasts 1–6 mo** • **Brief psychotic disorder lasts 1 day–1 mo**, with full recovery of baseline functioning—look for acute stressor, e.g., the death of a loved one
Other psychoses	• Schizoaffective disorder = meets criteria for mood disorders & schizophrenia • Delusional disorder = **nonbizarre delusions** (they could happen, e.g., pt's spouse is unfaithful, a person who is trying to kill the pt, etc.), without hallucinations, disorganized speech or disorganized behavior
Mood disorders	• Major depression & bipolar disorder can cause delusions & in extreme cases, hallucinations—can be difficult to differentiate from schizophrenia
Delirium	• Seen in pts with underlying illnesses, often in ICU (ICU psychosis) • **Patients are not orientated to person, place, time** • **Severity waxes & wanes even during the course of 1 day** • Resolves with treatment of underlying dz
Drugs	• LSD & PCP → predominantly visual, taste, touch, or olfactory hallucination • Cocaine & amphetamines → paranoid delusions & **classic sensation of bugs crawling on the skin (formication)** • Anabolic steroids → body-builder with bad temper, acne, shrunken testicles • Corticosteroids → psychosis/mood disturbances early in course of therapy
Medical	• Metabolic, endocrine, neoplastic & seizure dz can all cause psychosis • **Look for associated Si/Sx not explained by psychosis**, including focal neurologic findings, seizure, sensory/motor deficits, abnormal lab values

C. Tx

1. Hospitalization if voices tell pts to hurt themselves or others, or if condition is disabling to the point that pts cannot care for themselves
2. Pharmacologic therapy
   a. All antipsychotics act as dopamine-blockers
   b. Differences among agents relate to side-effect profile

TABLE 6-4   Antipsychotic Drugs

DRUG		ADVERSE EFFECTS[a]
Typical Antipsychotics[b]		
Chlorpromazine	Low potency	↑ anticholinergic effects, ↓ movement disorders
Haloperidol	High potency	↓ anticholinergic effects, ↑ movement disorders
Atypical Antipsychotics[b]		
Clozapine	For refractory dz	1% incidence of agranulocytosis mandates weekly CBC
Risperidone	First line	Minimal
Olanzapine	First line	Minimal

[a] Anticholinergic effects = dry mouth, blurry vision (miosis), urinary retention, constipation.
[b] Atypical agents have much lower incidence of movement disorders—see below.

PSYCHIATRY

TABLE 6-5 Antipsychotic-Associated Movement Disorders

DISORDER	TIME COURSE	CHARACTERISTICS
Acute dystonia	4 hr → 4 days	• Sustained muscle spasm anywhere in the body but often in neck (torticollis), jaw, or back (opisthotonos) • Tx = immediate IV diphenhydramine
Parkinsonism	4 days → 4 mo	• Cog-wheel rigidity, shuffling gait, resting tremor • Tx = benztropine (anticholinergic)
Tardive dyskinesia	4 mo → 4 yr	• Involuntary, irregular movements of the head, tongue, lips, limbs & trunk • Tx = immediately change medication or ↓ doses because effects are often permanent
Akathisia	Any time	• Subjective sense of discomfort → restlessness: pacing, sitting down & getting up • Tx = lower medication doses
Neuroleptic malignant syndrome	Any time	• Life-threatening muscle rigidity → fever, ↑ BP/HR, rhabdomyolysis appearing over 1–3 days • Can be easily misdiagnosed as ↑ psychotic Sx • Labs → ↑ WBC, ↑ creatine kinase, ↑ transaminases, ↑ plasma myoglobin, as well as myoglobinuria • Tx = supportive: immediately stop drug, give dantrolene (inhibits Ca release into cells), cool pt to prevent hyperpyrexia

     c. Compliance to drugs can be improved with **depot** form of haloperidol, which administers a month's supply of drug in 1 IM injection

  3. Psychotherapy can improve social functioning

     a. Behavioral Tx teaches social skills that allow pts to deal more comfortably with other people

     b. Family-oriented Tx teaches family members to act in more appropriate, positive fashion

D. Px

  1. Schizophrenia is a chronic, episodic dz, recovery from each relapse typically leaves pt below former baseline function

  2. Presence of negative Sx (e.g., flat affect) marks poor Px

  3. High-functioning prior to psychotic break marks better Px

IV. Anxiety Disorders

A. PANIC DISORDER

  1. Si/Sx = mimic MI: chest pain, palpitations, diaphoresis, nausea, marked anxiety, escalate for 10 min, remain for about 30 min (rarely longer than an hour)

  2. Occurs in younger pts (average age 25)—good way to distinguish from MI

  3. DDx = myocardial infarction, drug abuse (e.g., cocaine, amphetamines), phobias (see below)

  4. Dx is by exclusion of true medical condition & drug abuse

  5. Panic attacks are unexpected, so if pt consistently describes panic Sx in a specific setting, phobia is a more likely diagnosis

  6. Tx

     a. TCAs (clomipramine & imipramine) are best studied

     b. More recently SSRIs have been shown to have efficacy

c. Benzodiazepines work immediately, have ↑ risk of addiction

d. Therefore, start benzodiazepine for immediate effects, add a TCA or SSRI, taper off the benzodiazepine as the other drugs kick in

e. Cognitive/behavior TX & **respiratory training** (to help patients recognize & overcome desire to hyperventilate) are helpful

B. AGORAPHOBIA

1. Sx = fear of being in situations where it would be very difficult to get out of should a panic attack arise

2. Theorized that pts develop panic disorder because they've had enough unexpected attacks to know that it can come at any time—& wouldn't it be embarrassing if it happened while sitting in the mezzanine watching a sold-out performance of *Tosca*? (It would certainly be more interesting.)

3. Dx = clinical, look for evidence of social/occupational dysfunction

4. Tx (for phobias in general)

   a. β-blockers useful for prophylaxis in phobias related to performance

   b. **Exposure desensitization** = exposure to noxious stimulus in increments, while undergoing concurrent relaxation Tx

C. OBSESSIVE COMPULSIVE DISORDER (OCD)

1. **Obsessions ≡ recurrent thought; compulsions ≡ recurrent act**

2. Sx = obsessive thought causes anxiety & the compulsion is a way of temporarily relieving that anxiety (e.g., pt worries whether he/she locked the door & going back to see it's locked relieves the anxiety), but because relief is only temporary the pt performs compulsion repeatedly

3. Obsessions commonly involve **cleanliness/contamination** (washing hands), doubt, symmetry (elaborate rituals for entering doorways, arranging books, etc.) & sex

4. Dx = pt should be disturbed by their obsessions & **should recognize their absurdity** in contrast to obsessive compulsive personality disorder, where pt sees nothing wrong with compulsion

5. Tx = SSRIs (first line) or clomipramine, psychotherapy in which the pt is literally forced to overcome their behavior

D. POSTTRAUMATIC STRESS DISORDER (PTSD)

1. Dx requires a traumatic, violent incident that effectively scars the person involved; the experiences of Vietnam vets are emblematic of this disorder

2. Sx

   a. **Pt relives the initial incident via conscious thoughts or dreams**

   b. Due to resultant subjective & physiologic distress, the pt avoids any precipitating stimuli & **hence often avoids public places & activities**

   c. Pt may suffer restricted emotional involvement/responses & may experience a detachment from others

   d. **Depression is common, look for moodiness, diminished interest in activities & difficulties with sleeping & concentrating**

3. DDx = **acute stress disorder**

   a. Dx also requires a traumatic incident, but Sx are more immediate (within 4 wk of the event) & limited in time (<4 wk)

   b. The Sx are different; imagine being so traumatized that you are in a daze, where nothing seems real & you have trouble remembering what has happened (commonly seen in victims of sexual assault)

4. Tx

    a. Use of tricyclics (imipramine & amitriptyline) is well-supported by clinical trials, SSRIs have also been used

    b. **Beware of giving benzodiazepines due to a high association of substance abuse with PTSD!**

    c. Psychotherapy takes two approaches

        1) Exposure therapy, the idea being to confront one's demons by "reliving" the experience (either step-wise or abruptly)

        2) Relaxation techniques, think of the two modalities as attacking the source vs. controlling the symptoms

5. Px = variable, but the predictive factors are similar to schizophrenia: abrupt Sx & strong premorbid functioning lead to better outcomes

E. GENERALIZED ANXIETY DISORDER

1. Sx = worry for most days for at least 6 mo, irritability, inability to concentrate, insomnia, fatigue, restlessness (just think of a medical student or intern preparing for the USMLE!)

2. DDx = specific anxieties, including separation anxiety disorder, anorexia nervosa, hypochondriasis

3. **Dx requires evidence of social dysfunction** (e.g., poor school grades, job stagnation, or marital strains) to rule out "normal" anxiety

4. Tx = psychotherapy due to chronicity of the problem

    a. Cognitive-behavioral Tx = teaching pt to recognize his/her worrying & find ways to respond to it through behavior & thought patterns

    b. **Biofeedback** & **relaxation** techniques, in particular, can help the pt deal with physical manifestations of anxiety, e.g., heart rate

    c. Pharmacotherapy includes buspirone or β-blockers (works for peripheral Sx, e.g., tachycardia, but not worry itself)

V. Personality Disorders

A. GENERAL CHARACTERISTICS

1. Sx = pervasive pattern of maladaptive behavior causing functional impairment, consistent behavior can often be traced back to childhood

2. Typically present to psychiatrists because behavior is causing significant problems for others, e.g., colleagues at work, spouse at home, **or for the medical staff in the inpatient or clinic setting (typical USMLE question)**

3. **Pts usually see nothing wrong with their behavior (ego-syntonic)**, contrast with pts who recognize their hallucinations as abnormal (ego-dystonic)

4. Ego defenses

    a. Unconscious mental process that individuals resort to in order to quell inner conflicts & anxiety that are unacceptable to the ego

    b. Examples include "splitting" & "projection"

5. Tx = psychotherapy, medication used for peripheral Sx (e.g., anxiety)

B. CLUSTERS

1. **Cluster A** = paranoid, schizoid & schizotypal personalities, often thought of as **"weird" or "eccentric"**

2. **Cluster B** = borderline, antisocial, histrionic & narcissistic personalities, **"dramatic"** & **"aggressive"** personalities
3. **Cluster C** = avoidant, dependent & obsessive-compulsive personalities, **"shy"** & **"nervous"** personalities

C.

TABLE 6-6   Specific Personality Disorders

DISORDER	CHARACTERISTICS
Paranoid (Cluster A)	• Negatively misinterpret the actions, words, intentions of others • Often utilize **projection** as ego defense (attributing to other people impulses & thoughts that are unacceptable to their own selves) • **Do not hold fixed delusions** (delusional disorder), **nor do they experience hallucinations** (schizophrenia)
Schizoid (Cluster A)	• Socially withdrawn, introverted, with little external affect • Do not form close emotional ties with others (often feel no need) • Are, however, able to recognize reality
Schizotypal (Cluster A)	• **Believe in concepts not considered real by the rest of society (magic, clairvoyance)**, display the prototypical ego defense: **fantasy** • Not necessarily psychotic (can have brief psychotic episodes) • Like schizoids, they are often quite isolated socially • **Often related to schizophrenics (unlike other cluster A disorders)**
Antisocial (Cluster B)	• Violate the rights of others, break the law (e.g., theft, substance abuse) • Can also be quite seductive (particularly with the opposite sex) • **For Dx the pt must have exhibited the behavior by a certain age (15—think truancy) but must be a certain age (at least 18—adult)** • **A popular USLME topic; you may have to differentiate it from conduct disorder (bad behavior, but Dx of children/adolescents)**
Borderline (Cluster B)	• Volatile emotional lives, swing wildly between idealizing & devaluing other people: (**splitting** ego defense = people are very good or bad) • **Also commonly asked on USMLE**, typical scenario is a highly disruptive hospitalized pt; on interview, he (but usually she) says some nurses are incompetent & cruel but wildly praises others (including you) • Exhibit self-destructive behavior (scratching or cutting themselves) • Ability to **disassociate**: they simply "forget" negative affects/experiences by covering them with overly exuberant, seemingly positive behavior
Histrionic (Cluster B)	• Require the attention of everyone, use sexuality & physical appearance to get it, exaggerate their thoughts with dramatic but vague language • Utilize disassociation & **repression** (block feelings unconsciously)—don't confuse with **suppression** (feelings put aside consciously)
Narcissistic (Cluster B)	• Feel entitled—strikingly so—because they are the best & everyone else is inferior, handle criticism very poorly
Dependent (Cluster C)	• Can do little on their own, nor can they be alone
Avoidant (Cluster C)	• Feel inadequate & are extremely sensitive to negative comments • Reluctant to try new things (e.g., making friends) for fear of embarrassment
Obsessive-compulsive (Cluster C)	• Preoccupied with detail: rules, regulations, neatness • Isolation is a common ego-defense: putting up walls of self-restraint & detail-orientation that keep away any sign of emotional affect

PSYCHIATRY

D. **OTHER EGO DEFENSES**
  1. Acting out = transforming unacceptable feeling into actions, often loud ones (tantrums)
  2. Identification = patterning behavior after someone else's

3. Intellectualization = explaining away the unreasonable in the form of logic
4. Rationalization = making the unreasonable seem acceptable (e.g., upon being fired, you say you wanted to quit anyway)
5. Reaction formation = set aside unconscious feelings & express exact opposite feelings (show extra affection for someone you hate)
6. Regression = resorting to child-like behavior (often seen in the hospital)
7. Sublimation = taking instinctual drives (sex) & funneling that energy into a socially acceptable action (studying)

VI. Somatoform and Factitious Disorders

A. DEFINITIONS

1. Somatoform disorder = **lack of conscious manipulation of somatic Sx**
2. Factitious disorder = **consciously faking** or manipulating Sx for purpose of "assuming the sick role," **but not for material gain**
3. Malingering = consciously faking Sx **for purpose of material gain**

B. FACTITIOUS DISORDER

1. Pt may mimic any Sx, physical or psychological, to assume the sick role
2. **The patient is not trying to avoid work or win a compensation claim**
3. Munchausen syndrome = factitious disorder with predominantly physical (not psychologic) symptoms
4. Munchausen by proxy = pt claiming nonexistent symptoms in someone else under their care, e.g., parents bringing in their "sick" children
5. DDx = malingering
6. **HINT: the USLME will very likely present a scenario involving nurses or other health care workers as the pts (often involving an episode of apparent hypoglycemia), look for evidence of factitious disorder (e.g., low C-peptide levels suggesting insulin self-injection)**
7. Dx is by exclusion of real medical condition
8. Tx is nearly impossible; when confronted pts often become angry, deny everything, tell you how horrible you are & move on to someone else

C. SOMATOFORM DISORDERS

1. Somatization disorder
   a. Often female pts with problems starting before age 30, with history of frequent visits to the doctor for countless procedures & operations (often exploratory), & often history of abusive/failed relationships
   b. Sx = somatic complaints involving different systems, particularly gastrointestinal (nausea, diarrhea), neurologic (weakness) & sexual (irregular menses), with no adequate medical explanation on the basis of exam/lab findings
   c. Dx = rule out medical condition & material or psychologic gain
   d. Tx = **continuity of care**
      1) Schedule regular appointments so pt can express his or her Sx
      2) Perform physical exam but do not order laboratory tests
      3) As the therapeutic bond strengthens, strive to establish awareness in the pt that psychologic factors are involved & if successful in doing so, arrange a psychiatric consult—but if done too early or aggressively, pt may be reluctant or resentful
2. Conversion disorder

a. Sx are neurologic, not multisystem, & are not consciously faked
b. Sensory deficits often fail to correspond to any known pathway, e.g., a stocking-&-glove sensory deficit that begins precisely at the wrist, studies will reveal intact neurologic pathways, & pts rarely get hurt, e.g., patients who are "blind" will not be colliding into the wall
c. Dx requires identification of a stressor that precipitated the Sx as well as exclusion of any adequate medical explanation (**NOTE:** in some studies 50% of pts who received this Dx were eventually found to have nonpsychiatric causes of illness, e.g., brain tumors & multiple sclerosis. Bummer!)
d. Tx = supportive, Sx resolve within days (less than a month), **do not tell pt that they are imagining their Sx, but suggest that psychotherapy may help with their distress**
e. Px = the more abrupt the symptoms, the more easily identified the stressor & the higher the premorbid function, the better the outcome
3. Hypochondriasis
a. Sx = preoccupation with disease, pt does not complain of a large number of Sx but misinterprets them as evidence of something serious
b. Tx = regular visits to MD with every effort not to order lab tests or procedures, psychotherapy should be presented as a way of coping with stress, **again, do not tell patients that they are imagining their Sx**
4. Body dysmorphic disorder
a. Sx = concern with body, **pt usually picks 1 feature, often on the face, & imagines deficits that other people do not see;** if there are slight imperfections, the pt exaggerates them excessively
b. Look for a significant amount of emotional & functional impairment
c. Tx = SSRIs may be helpful in some cases, surgery is not recommended

VII. Child and Adolescent Psychiatry

A. AUTISM & ASPERGER'S SYNDROME

1. Autism is the prototypic **pervasive developmental disorder**, pervasive because the disorder encompasses so many areas of development: language, social interaction, emotional reactivity
2. The expression "living in his own world" captures this tragic disorder; the autistic child fails to develop normal interactions with others & seems to be responding to internal stimuli
3. Si/Sx
a. Becomes evident before 3 yr old, often much earlier
b. The baby does not seem to be concerned with the mother's presence or absence & makes no eye contact, as the baby becomes older, deficiencies in language (including repetitive phrases & made-up vocabulary) & abnormal behavior become more obvious
c. Look for the behavioral aspects; the child often has a strange, persistent fascination with specific, seemingly mundane objects (vacuum cleaners, sprinklers) & may show stereotyped, ritualistic movements (e.g., spinning around)
d. Autistic children have an inordinate need for constancy
4. Think of Asperger's syndrome as autism **without** the language impairment
5. **Contrary to older thought, poor parenting/bonding is not a cause of autism!— parents need reassurance about this**

PSYCHIATRY

B. DEPRESSION

1. Depression may present slightly differently depending on the age group
   a. Preschool children may be hyperactive & aggressive
   b. Adolescents show boredom, irritability, or openly antisocial behaviors
2. One should still look for the same symptoms as described for adult depression: depressed mood, anhedonia, neurovegetative changes, etc.
3. Tx
   a. Unlike adult depression, the use of antidepressants is much more controversial, with far less data supporting its effectiveness
   b. **Note:** children's mood disorders are especially sensitive to psychosocial stressors, so family therapy is a major consideration

C. SEPARATION ANXIETY

1. Look for a child that seems a bit too attached to his parents or any other figures in his life; the child is worried that something will happen to these beloved figures or that some terrible event will separate them
2. Si/Sx = sleep disturbances (nightmares, inability to fall asleep alone) & somatic Sx during times of separation (headaches, stomach upset at school)
3. Tx = desensitizing therapy (gradually increasing the hours spent away from Mom & Dad), in some cases imipramine is used

D. OPPOSITIONAL DEFIANT/CONDUCT DISORDER

1. Differentiate the 2 by words & action
2. Oppositional defiant disorder Si/Sx ("bark")
   a. Pts are argumentative, temperamental & defiant, more so with people they know well (they may seem harmless to you)
   b. Big surprise that they are often friendless & perform poorly in school
3. Conduct disorder Si/Sx ("bite")
   a. Pts bully others, start fights, may show physical cruelty to animals, violate/destroy other people's property (fire-setting), steal things & stay out past curfews or run away
   b. They do not feel guilty for any of this
   c. A glimpse into the child's family life often reveals pathology in the form of substance abuse or negligence
4. Oppositional defiant disorder may lead to conduct disorder, but the two are not synonymous
5. Tx = providing a setting with strict rules & expected consequences for violations of them

E. ATTENTION-DEFICIT HYPERACTIVITY DISORDER (ADHD)

1. Si/Sx can be divided into the components suggested by their name
   a. Attention-deficit Sx = inability to focus or carry out tasks completely & being easily distracted by random stimuli
   b. Hyperactivity Sx are more outwardly motor; the child is unable to sit still, talks excessively & can never "wait his turn" in group games
2. Dx requires that Sx have been present since before 7 yr old
3. Tx = methylphenidate, an amphetamine
   a. Parents & teachers notice improvement in the child's behavior
   b. Because of concerns about impeding the child's growth, drug holidays are often taken (e.g., no meds over weekends or vacations)

    c. Children with ADHD also do better with an extremely structured environment featuring consistent rules & punishments

    d. Px is variable, some children show remissions of their hyperactivity, but quite a few continue to show Sx through adolescence & adulthood; children with ADHD have a higher likelihood of developing conduct disorders or antisocial personalities

F. Tourette's Disorder

1. Tics are involuntary, stereotyped, repetitive movements or vocalizations
2. **Tourette's Dx requires both a motor tic & a vocal tic present for ≥1 yr**
3. **The vocal tics are often obscene or socially unacceptable (coprolalia)**, which is a cause of extreme embarrassment to the patient
4. Tx = haloperidol, effective, but not required in mild cases
5. Psychotherapy is unhelpful in treating the tics per se, but can be helpful in dealing with the emotional stress caused by the disorder

G. Anorexia & Bulimia Nervosa

1. Eating disorders are by no means limited to children—but because they often start in adolescence, they are worth mentioning here
2. In both disorders exists a profound disturbance in body image & its role in the person's sense of self-worth
3. Anorexia Si/Sx
    a. **By definition anorexic patients are below their expected body weight** because they do not eat enough, often creating elaborate rituals for disposing of food in meal settings, e.g., cutting meat into tiny pieces & rearranging them constantly on the plate
    b. **Amenorrhea occurs 2° to weight loss**
4. Bulimia Si/Sx
    a. More common than anorexia, **characterized by binge eating**: consuming huge amounts of food over a short period, with a perceived lack of control
    b. This may be accompanied by active purging (vomiting, laxative use)
    c. **Unlike anorexics, who by definition have decreased body weight, bulimics often have a normal appearance**
    d. **Abrasions over the knuckles** (from jamming the fingers into the mouth to induce vomiting) & **dental erosion** suggest the Dx
5. Tx
    a. Hospitalization may be required for anorexia to restore the pt's weight to a safe level, which the pt will often resist
    b. Because of vomiting, monitoring serum electrolytes is essential; the most worrisome consequence is cardiac dysfunction—as exemplified by singer Karen Carpenter, whose battle with anorexia led to her untimely death
    c. Psychotherapy is the mainstay of Tx for both diseases
6. Overall, anorexia nervosa has a relatively poor prognosis, with persistent preoccupations with food & weight; bulimics fare slightly better

VIII. Drugs of Abuse

A. Introduction

1. Always consider drug abuse when a pt's life seems to be going down the tubes, e.g., deteriorating family relations, work performance, financial stability

2. Generally (with many exceptions), withdrawal Sx are the opposite of intoxication, dysphoria is characteristic of all of them—**withdrawal is a sign of physiologic dependence**
3. Individual drugs

TABLE 6-7   Drug Intoxications and Withdrawal

DRUG	INTOXICATION SI/SX	WITHDRAWAL
Alcohol	Disinhibition, ↓ cognition Screen for alcoholism with CAGE • C–feeling the need to **cut** down • A–feeling **annoyed** when asked about drinking • G–feeling **guilty** for drinking • E–need a drink in the morning **(eye-opener)**	Tremor, seizures, delirium tremens (high mortality! → prevent with benzo's)
Cocaine/Amphetamine	Agitation, irritability, ↓ appetite, formication, ↑ or ↓ BP & HR, cardiac arrhythmia or infarction, stroke, seizure, nosebleeds	Hypersomnolence, dysphoria ↑ appetite
Heroin (opioids)	Intense, fleeting euphoria, drowsy, slurred speech, ↓ memory, pupillary constriction, ↓ respiration **The triad of ↓ consciousness, pinpoint pupils & respiratory depression should always lead to a suspicion of opioids**	Nausea/vomiting, pupillary dilation & insomnia
Benzodiazepine & barbiturates	Respiratory & cardiac depression	Agitation, anxiety, delirium
Phencyclidine (PCP)	Intense psychosis, violence, rhabdomyolysis, hyperthermia	
LSD	Sensation is enhanced, colors are richer, music more profound, tastes heightened	

IX. Miscellaneous Disorders

A. DISORDERS OF SEXUALITY & GENDER IDENTITY
1. Sexual identity is based on biology, e.g., men have testes
2. Gender identity is based on self-perception, e.g., biological male perceives himself as a male
3. **Children have a firm conception of their gender identity very early (before age 3)**
4. Sexual orientation is who the person is attracted to; **remember that homosexuality is not a psychiatric disorder** (it used to be, until taken off the DSM in the 1970s) & that treating crises of sexual orientation should focus on accepting one's orientation, not changing it to conform to social "norms"

B. DISASSOCIATIVE DISORDER (MULTIPLE PERSONALITY DISORDER)
1. This was a hot diagnosis in the late 1970s (replaced in 1980s by borderline personality) & a perennial favorite of the movies (think: *Three Faces of Eve, Sybil,* & more recently, *Primal Fear*). The older name says it all: a patient seemingly possesses different personalities that can each take control at a given time. A patient's history

may give some history of childhood trauma, e.g., abuse. Treatment focuses on gradual integration of these personalities.

2. The main differentials are **dissociative amnesia** & **dissociative fugue**. Amnesia is a syndrome of forgetting a great deal of personal information; fugue refers to the syndrome of sudden travel to another place, with inability to remember the past & confusion of present identity. *Neither case involves shifting between different identities.*

C. Adjustment Disorder

1. This refers to any behavioral or emotional Sx that occur in response to stressful life events in excess of what is normal

2. Obviously has a catch-all quality to it; **this will be a frequent answer option on the USMLE**

3. **Dx requires the Sx to come within 3 mo of the stressor** (so they do not have to be immediate) & **they must disappear within 6 mo of the disappearance of the stressor**

4. Bereavement may seem to be a type of adjustment disorder (the stressor being death), but they are separate diagnoses

5. Depending on the setting, adjustment disorder may appear as depression or anxiety—so how to tell the difference? It isn't easy, but remember: **axis I disorders such as major depression & generalized anxiety take precedence**

D. Impulsive-Control Disorders

1. Pt is unable to resist the drive to perform certain actions **harmful to themselves or others**

2. Note the emotional response: these individuals **feel anxiety before the action & gratification afterward**

3. *Intermittent explosive disorder*
   a. Discrete episodes of aggressive behavior far in excess of any possible stressor
   b. The key term is **episodic**; antisocial personalities also commit aggressive behaviors, but their aggression is present between outbursts of such behavior

4. *Kleptomania*: the impulse to steal
   a. The object of theft is not needed for any reason (monetary or otherwise)
   b. The kleptomaniac often feels guilty after stealing

5. *Pyromania*: purposeful fire-setting
   a. There is often a fascination with fire itself that distinguishes this from the antisocial personality/conduct disorders, where the fire-setting is purposeful, e.g., revenge, & not the failure to resist an impulse

6. *Trichotillomania*: hair-pulling, resulting in observable hair loss

TABLE 6-8

DSM-IV Classification	
AXIS I	Clinical disorders
AXIS II	Personality disorders/mental retardation
AXIS III	Medical conditions
AXIS IV	Social and environmental factors
AXIS V	Level of functioning

7. Neurology

Brad Spellberg

I. Infarct

A. Terminology

1. Stroke ≡ a sudden, nonconvulsive focal neurologic deficit
2. TIAs ≡ deficit lasting ≤24 hr (usually <1 hr) & resolve completely
3. Emboli sources = **carotid atheroma (most common)**, cardiac & fat emboli, marantic endocarditis (metastasizing cancer cells)
4. Lacunar infarct = small infarct in deep gray matter, strongly associated with hypertension & atherosclerosis
5. Watershed infarcts occur at border of areas supplied by different arteries (e.g., MCA-ACA), often following prolonged hypotension

B. Presentation (See Figures 7-1 and 7-2)

1.

Table 7-1   Presentation of Stroke

Sign/Symptom	Artery	Region (Lobe)
Amaurosis fugax (monocular blind)	Carotid (emboli)	Ophthalmic artery
Drop attack/Vertigo/CN palsy/coma	Vertebrobasilar (emboli)	Brain stem
Aphasia	Middle cerebral	Dominant frontal or temporal[a]
Sensory neglect & apraxia[b]	Middle cerebral	Nondominant frontal or temporal[a]
Hemiplegia	Middle or anterior cerebral	Contralateral parietal
Urinary incontinence & grasp reflex	Middle or anterior cerebral	Frontal
Homonymous hemianopia	Middle or posterior cerebral	Temporal or occipital

[a] Dominant = left in 99% of right-handers & >50% of left-handers.
[b] Apraxia = patient cannot follow command even if it is understood & the pt is physically capable of it.

2. Wernicke's aphasia (temporal lobe lesion) = receptive, pt speaks fluently but words do not make sense: **Wernicke's is wordy**
3. Broca's aphasia (frontal lobe lesion) = expressive, pt is unable to verbalize: **Broca's is broken**
4. Edema occurs 2–4 days postinfarct, watch for this clinically (e.g., ↓ consciousness, projectile vomiting, pupillary changes)
5. Decorticate (cortical lesion) posturing → flexion of arms
6. Decerebrate (midbrain or lower lesion) posturing → arm extension

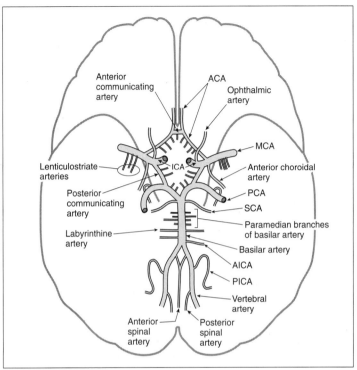

FIGURE 7-1   Circle of Willis. ACA = anterior cerebral artery; AICA = anterior inferior cerebellar artery; ICA = internal carotid artery; MCA = middle cerebral artery; PCA = posterior cerebral artery; PICA = posterior inferior cerebellar artery; SCA = superior cerebellar artery.
(Reproduced with permission from Pritchard TC and Alloway KD. Medical Neuroscience. Madison, Connecticut: Fence Creek Publishing, 1999: 78. © Fence Creek Publishing, LLC.)

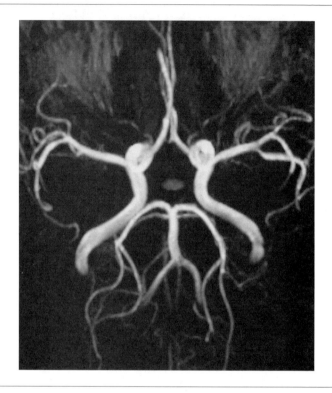

FIGURE 7-2   Magnetic resonance angiography (MRA). The arteries at the base of the brain, the circle of Willis, are very well shown by MRA without the use of any contrast agent.

C. DIFFERENTIAL DIAGNOSIS

1. Stroke, seizure, neoplasm, encephalitis, multiple sclerosis
2. Stroke causes = 35% local atheroembolic, 30% cardiac, 15% lacunar, 10% parenchymal hemorrhage, 10% subarachnoid hemorrhage, ≤1% other (e.g., vasculitis, temporal arteritis, etc.)
3. Dx = CT for acute, MRI for subacute infarct &/or hemorrhage (See Figure 7-3)
4. Rule out seizure → EEG, loss of bowel/bladder control & tongue injury
5. Lumbar puncture to rule out encephalitis & rule in intracranial bleed

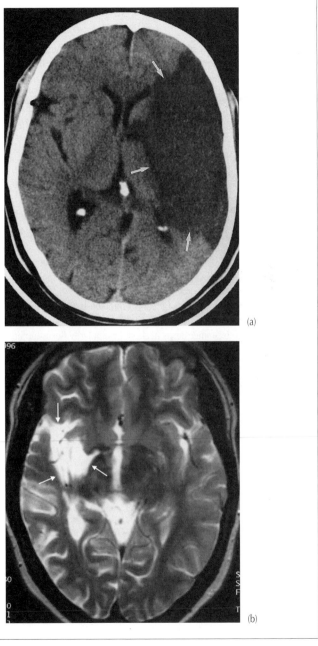

(a)

(b)

FIGURE 7-3 Cerebral infarction. (a) Unenhanced CT scan showing a low-density region of the left cerebral hemisphere conforming to the distribution of the middle cerebral artery (arrows). (b) MRI scan of another patient with a right middle cerebral artery territory infarct. The infarcted area (arrows) shows patchy high-signal intensity on this T2-weighted image. The arrows point to the anterior and posterior extent of the infarcted brain tissue.

D. TREATMENT

1. tPA within 3–6 hours of onset (preferably 1 hr) for occlusive dz only!
2. **Intracranial bleeding is an absolute contraindication to tPA use!**
3. Correct underlying disorder, e.g., hyperlipidemia, hypertension, diabetes, valve abnormality, coagulopathy, atrial fibrillation
4. For embolic strokes give aspirin/warfarin anticoagulation for prophylaxis
5. If carotid is 70% occluded & patient has Sx → endarterectomy

E. PROGNOSIS

1. 20–40% mortality at 30 days (20% atheroemboli, 40% bleed)
2. Less than 1/3 patients achieve full recovery of lifestyle
3. Atheroembolic strokes recur at 10%/yr

II. Infection & Inflammation

A. MENINGITIS

1. 50% due to *Streptococcus pneumonia*, 25% due to *Neisseria meningitidis, Hemophilus influenza* is rare now due to vaccination, *Listeria* seen in neonates, elderly and immunocompromised pts, and Group B *Strep* (*S. agalactiae*) and *E. coli* are the #1 and #2 causes of neonatal meningitis
2. Si = **meningismus** (pt cannot touch chin to chest), ⊕ **Kernig's sign** (pt is supine with hip and knees flexed at 90°, examiner cannot extend knee), ⊕ **Brudzinski's sign** (pt is supine, when examiner flexes neck, pt involuntarily flexes hip and knees)
3. CSF differential for meningitis

TABLE 7-2   CSF Findings in Meningitis

	CELLS	PROTEIN	GLUCOSE
Bacterial	↑ **neutrophils**	↑↑	↓↓ (≤2/3 serum)
Viral	↑ mononuclear	± ↑	**Nml**
Subacute	↑ mononuclear	↑	↓

4. Can be acute, subacute, chronic presentations
5. Acute
   a. Send CSF for Gram's stain, bacterial cultures, HSV PCR
   b. Treat all patients empirically by age until specific tests return

TABLE 7-3   Empiric Therapy for Meningitis by Age

AGE	REGIMEN	COMMON ETIOLOGIES
Neonates (≤1 mo)	**Ampicillin + cefotaxime**	*Streptococcus agalactiae, Listeria, Escherichia coli*
Children to teens	**Cefotaxime + vancomycin**[a]	*Streptococcus pneumonia, Neisseria meningitidis*
Adults	**Cefotaxime + vancomycin**[a]	*S. pneumonia* by far most common

• Add acyclovir to any pt with possible HSV.
[a] Due to increasing rate of β-lactam resistance *S. pneumonia*

   c. Of viral causes, only HSV (acyclovir) & HIV (AZT) can be treated—otherwise treatment is supportive

d.

TABLE 7-4 Bacterial Meningitis

ORGANISM	PATIENTS	CHARACTERISTICS	TREATMENT
Streptococcus pneumoniae	**#1 cause in adults**: old age, asplenia, poor health predispose	Can progress from otitis media, sinusitis, or bacteremia	Pen G (if susceptible) Second line = cefotaxime, third line = vancomycin
Neisseria meningitidis	≥1 yr old or in adults in epidemics in close populations (military barracks)	**Petechiae on trunk, legs, conjunctivae**—beware of Waterhouse-Friderichsen syndrome (adrenal infarct)	Pen G Rifampin or fluoroquinolone prophylaxis for close contacts
Hemophilus influenzae type B	Formerly #1 cause in children, until vaccine	Now rare, but can cause epiglottitis	Cefotaxime
Streptococcus agalactiae	**#1 cause in neonates**	Acquired at birth	Ampicillin
Escherichia coli	Common in neonates	Acquired at birth	Cefotaxime
Listeria monocytogenes	Elderly/neonates, AIDS, diabetes, steroids	Difficult CSF Gram's stain/ Cx, Dx → blood Cx	Ampicillin
Staphylococcus aureus	Trauma/Neurosurgery	Wound infxn from skin	Oxacillin/Vancomycin

6. Subacute/chronic meningitis
   a. Si/Sx = per acute but evolves over wk → mo, +/– fever
   b. DDx = fungal, mycobacterial, noninfectious, other rare dzs
   c. Send CSF for fungal Cx, cytology, India Ink, TB PCR
   d. Fungal meningitis
      1) DDx = *Cryptococcus, Coccidioides,* other more rare dz
      2) *Cryptococcus* **commonly seen in AIDS**
         a) **India Ink stain will show *Cryptococcus* in CSF**
         b) **Opening pressure is commonly elevated**
      3) *Coccidioides* **blastocysts seen on CSF cytology**
      4) Tx = IV amphotericin B (intrathecal may be necessary)
   e. TB meningitis
      1) Usually occurs in elderly by reactivation, grave Px
      2) Dx is made by TB PCR of the CSF
      3) Tx = **RIPE: R**ifampin + **I**NH + **P**yrazinamide + **E**thambutol
   f. Other causes = sarcoid, cancer, collagen-vascular dz, drug reactions

B. ENCEPHALITIS

1. Si/Sx = similar to meningitis, but focal findings are evident

TABLE 7-5   Encephalitis

ETIOLOGY	DISEASE	SI/SX	TX/PX
Toxoplasmosis	1) Transplacental congenital dz → hydrocephalus/ mental retardation	**Multiple ring enhancing lesions → focal neurologic deficits**	Bactrim
	2) Adults exposed via cat feces get dz if immunosuppressed—**Toxo is the #1 CNS lesion in AIDS**	Toxoplasmosis antibody test very sensitive	Prophylax if CD4 ≤200/μL
HSV	**#1 cause of viral encephalitis**	**Olfactory hallucinations, bloody CSF, personality changes** EEG/MRI → temporal lobe dz	Acyclovir
Syphilis	**Meningovascular disease** Parenchymal disease:	**Argyll-Robertson pupil**[a]	
	1) Tabes dorsalis = bilateral spinal cord demyelination	Pain, hypotonia, ↓ tone, ↓ DTRs ↓ proprioception, incontinence	IV penicillin
	2) Dementia paralytica = cortical atrophy, neuron loss, gliosis	Sx = psychosis, dementia, personality change	
PML[b]	Usually in AIDS, caused by JC virus	Diffuse neurologic dz	None, death inevitable

[a] Pupil accommodates but doesn't react to direct light.
[b] PML = progressive multifocal leukoencephalopathy.

C. ABSCESS

1. Si/Sx = headache, fever, ↑ ICP, focal neurologic findings
2. Risk factors = congenital R-L shunt (lung filtration bypassed), otitis, paranasal sinusitis, metastases, trauma & immunosuppression
3. Anaerobes & aerobes, gram-positive cocci & gram-negative rods can cause
4. Tx = antibiotics ⊕ **surgical drainage if >3 cm or if persists**
5. **Brain abscesses are invariably fatal if untreated**
6. Helminthic infections
   a. Cysticercosis (*Taenia solium*)
      1) Eggs transmitted by fecal-oral route
      2) **Encephalitis in Latin American immigrant is due to neurocysticercosis until proven otherwise**
      3) Tx = praziquantel ⊕ steroids (dead cyst → inflammation)
   b. Hydatid cysts (*Echinococcus*)
      1) Acquired by dog feces, can cause focal Sx & seizure
      2) If cysts rupture they can cause fatal anaphylaxis
      3) Tx = careful surgical excystation, mebendazole

III. Demyelinating Diseases

A. MULTIPLE SCLEROSIS (MS)

1. Unknown etiology, but ⊕ genetic & environmental predispositions, ↑ common in pts who lived first decade of life in northern latitudes

2. Si/Sx = relapsing asymmetric limb weakness, ↑ DTRs, nystagmus, tremor, scanning speech, paresthesias, optic neuritis, ⊕ Babinski sign

3. Dx = history, MRI, lumbar puncture

4. MRI → periventricular plaques, multiple focal demyelination scattered in brain & spinal cord (lesions disseminated in space & time)

5. Lumbar puncture → ↑ CSF immunoglobulins manifested as multiple oligoclonal bands on electrophoresis

6. Tx = interferon-β, may induce prolonged remissions in some pts

7. Px
   a. Variable types of disease, long remissions sometimes seen
   b. But can progressively decline → death in only a few years

B. GUILLAIN-BARRÉ SYNDROME

1. Acute autoimmune demyelinating dz involving peripheral nerves

2. Si/Sx = muscle weakness & paralysis ascending up from lower limbs, ↓ reflexes, can cause bilateral facial nerve palsy

3. Most often preceded by gastroenteritis (classically *Campylobacter jejuni*), *Mycoplasma* or viral infection, immunization, or allergic reactions

4. Dx = Hx of antecedent stimuli (see above), CSF → albumin-cytologic dissociation (CSF protein ↑↑↑ without ↑ in cells seen)

5. Tx = plasmapheresis, IVIG, intubation for respiratory failure

6. Px is excellent for 80–90% of patients, will spontaneously regress

7. Respiratory failure & death can occur in remainder

C. CENTRAL PONTINE MYELINOLYSIS

1. Diamond-shaped region of demyelination in basis pontis

2. Due to rapid correction of hyponatremia & in liver dz

3. No Tx once condition has begun

4. Coma or death is a common outcome

IV. Metabolic & Nutritional Disorders

A. CARBON MONOXIDE POISONING

1. Seen in pts enclosed in burned areas, or during the start of a cold winter (people are using their new gas heaters) → bilateral pallidal necrosis

2. Si/Sx = headache, nausea, vomiting, delirium, cherry-red color of lips

3. Dx = elevated carboxyhemoglobin levels

4. Tx = hyperbaric oxygen (first line) or 100% O_2

B. THIAMINE DEFICIENCY

1. Usually 2° to alcoholism

2. Beriberi peripheral neuropathy due to Wallerian degeneration

3. Wernicke's encephalopathy: Wernicke's triad = confusion (confabulation), ophthalmoplegia, ataxia

4. Wernicke's is related to lesions of mamillary bodies

5. Tx: give thiamine prior to glucose (e.g., thiamine should be run in IV fluid without glucose) or will exacerbate mamillary body damage

C. B_{12} DEFICIENCY

1. Subacute degeneration of posterior columns & lateral corticospinal tract

2. Si/Sx = weakness & ↓ vibration sense (both worse in legs), paresthesias, hyper-

reflexia, ataxia, personality change, dementia—note, **neurological deficits can occur even if no hematologic abnormalities are present!**

3. Tx = B_{12} replacement (can use high-dose oral in lieu of injection)

D. WILSON'S DISEASE (HEPATOLENTICULAR DEGENERATION)
 1. Defect in copper metabolism → lesions in basal ganglia
 2. Si/Sx = extrapyramidal tremors & rigidity, psychosis, & manic-depression
 3. **Pathognomonic → Kayser-Fleischer ring around the cornea**
 4. Dx = ↓ serum ceruloplasmin
 5. Tx = penicillamine or liver transplant if drug fails

E. HEPATIC ENCEPHALOPATHY
 1. Seen in cirrhosis, may be due to brain toxicity 2° to excess ammonia & other toxins not degraded by malfunctioning liver
 2. Sx = hyperreflexia, **asterixis** (flapping of extended wrists), dementia, seizures, obtundation/coma
 3. Tx = lactulose, neomycin & protein restriction to ↓ ammonia-related toxins

F. TAY-SACHS DISEASE
 1. Hexosaminidase A defect → ↑ ganglioside GM2
 2. Si/Sx = **cherry-red spot on macula**, retardation, paralysis, blind
 3. Dx by biopsy of rectum, or enzymatic assay, no Tx

V. Seizures (Sz)

A. TERMINOLOGY
 1. Complex sz → loss of consciousness (LOC), simple sz does not
 2. Generalized sz = entire brain involved, partial sz = focal area
 3. Tonic sz → prolonged contraction, clonic sz → twitches
 4. Absence = complex generalized sz → brief LOC
 5. Grand mal = complex generalized tonic-clonic sz

B. PRESENTATION
 1. Hx of prior head trauma, stroke, or other CNS disease ↑ risk for sz
 2. Si/Sx = loss of bowel/bladder control, tongue maceration, postictal confusion/lethargy, focal findings indicate epileptogenic foci
 3. If pt has Hx of seizures, always check blood level of medication

C. TREATMENT
 1. Tx seizures if they recur or if pt has known epileptic focus

TABLE 7-6   Seizure Therapy

PARTIAL	GRAND MAL	ABSENCE	MYOCLONIC
Phenytoin*	Valproate*	Ethosuximide*	Valproate*
Carbamazepine*	Carbamazepine	Valproate	Clonazepam
Valproate	Phenytoin	Clonazepam	

*First-line choice.

2. Tx underlying cause: electrolyte, infxn, toxic ingestion, trauma, azotemia, stroke/bleed, delirium tremens, hypoglycemia, hypoxia
3. **Phenytoin causes gingival hyperplasia, hirsutism**
4. Carbamazepine causes leukopenia/aplastic anemia, hepatotoxic
5. Valproate causes neutropenia, thrombocytopenia, hepatotoxic
6. Stop Tx if no seizures for 2 yr & normal EEG

D. Status Epilepticus
1. Continuous seizing lasting >5 min
2. Tx with benzodiazepines for immediate control, followed by phenytoin loading & phenobarbitol for refractory cases
3. This is a medical emergency!

VI. Degenerative Diseases

A. Dementia vs. Delirium Differential

Table 7-7   Dementia versus Delirium

	Dementia	Delirium
Definition	Both cause global decline in cognition, memory, personality, motor, or sensory functions	
Course	Constant, progressive	Sudden onset, waxing/waning daily
Reversible?	Usually not	Almost always
Circadian?	Constant, no daily pattern	Usually worse at night (sun-downing)
Consciousness	Normal	Altered (obtunded)
Hallucination	Usually not	Often, classically visual
Tremor	Often not	Often present (i.e., asterixis)
Causes	Alzheimer's, multi-infarct, Pick's dz, alcohol, brain infxn/tumors, malnutrition (thiamine/B_{12} deficiency)	Systemic infection/neoplasm, drugs (**particularly narcotics & benzodiazepines**), stroke, heart dz, alcoholism, uremia, electrolyte imbalance, hyper/hypoglycemia
Treatment	Supportive—see below for specifics depending on the disease	Treat underlying cause, **control Sx with haloperidol instead of sedatives**—due to agitation pts are often given benzodiazepines or sedatives, but these drugs often exacerbate the delirium as they disorient the pt even more

B. Alzheimer's Disease (Senile Dementia of Alzheimer Type)
1. Most common cause of dementia—affects 5% of people over 70
2. Si/Sx = dementia, anxiety, hallucination/delusion, tremor
3. Occurs in Down's syndrome pts at younger ages (age 30–40)
4. Dx = clinical, with definitive diagnosis only possible at autopsy
5. Tx = anticholinesterase inhibitor can slow dementia, antidepressants & antipsychotics can be used for psychosis
6. Px = inevitable decline in function usually over about 10 yr

C. Multi-Infarct Dementia
1. Si/Sx = acute, step-wise ↓ in neurologic function, multiple focal deficits on exam, hypertension, old infarcts by CT or MRI

    2. Dx = clinical, radiographic

    3. Tx = prevent future infarcts by ↓ cardiovascular risks

D. PICK'S DISEASE

    1. Clinically resembles Alzheimer's, more in women, younger age onset (50s)

    2. Predominates in frontal (more personality changes seen) & temporal lobes

    3. Dx = MRI → symmetrical frontal or temporal atrophy, confirm by autopsy

    4. Tx/Px = as per Alzheimer's

E. PARKINSON'S DISEASE

    1. Parkinson's disease = idiopathic Parkinsonism, mid- to late-age onset

    2. Parkinsonism

        a. **Syndrome of tremor, cog-wheel rigidity, bradykinesia, classic shuffling gait, mask-like facies**, ± dementia due to loss of dopaminergic neurons in substantia nigra

        b. DDx = Parkinson's disease, severe depression (bradykinesia & flat affect), intoxication (e.g., manganese, synthetic heroin), phenothiazine side effects, rare neurodegenerative diseases

    3. Dx = clinical, rule out other causes

    4. Tx

        a. Sinemet (levodopa = carbidopa) best for bradykinesia

        b. Anticholinergics (benztropine/trihexyphenidyl) for tremor

        c. Amantadine → ↑ dopamine release, effective for mild dz

        d. Surgical pallidotomy for refractory cases

    5. Px = typically progresses over years despite treatment

F. HUNTINGTON'S CHOREA

    1. Si/Sx = progressive choreiform movements of all limbs, ataxic gait, grimacing → dementia, usually in 30s–50s (can be earlier or later)

    2. Autosomal CAG triplet repeat expansion in HD gene → atrophy of striatum (especially caudate nucleus), with neuronal loss & gliosis

    3. Dx = MRI → atrophy of caudate, ⊕ family history

    4. Tx/Px = supportive, death inevitable

G. AMYOTROPHIC LATERAL SCLEROSIS (LOU GEHRIG'S DISEASE, MOTOR NEURON DISEASE)

    1. Si/Sx = **upper & lower motor neuron dz** → muscle weakness with fasciculations (anterior motor neurons) progressing to denervation atrophy, hyperreflexia, spasticity, difficulty speaking/swallowing

    2. Dx = clinical Hx & physical findings

    3. Tx/Px = supportive, death inevitable, usually from respiratory failure

8. Dermatology

Carlos Ayala

I. Terminology

1. Macule = flat discoloration, <1 cm in diameter
2. Papule = elevated skin lesion, <1 cm in diameter
3. Plaque = elevated skin lesion, >1 cm in diameter
4. Vesicle = small fluid-containing lesion <0.5 cm in diameter
5. Wheal = like a vesicle but occurs transiently as in urticaria (hives)
6. Bulla = large fluid-containing lesion, >0.5 cm in diameter
7. Lichenification = accentuated skin markings in thick epidermis due to scratching
8. Keloid = an irregular raised lesion resulting from scar tissue hypertrophy
9. Petechiae = flat, pinhead, nonblanching, red-purple lesion caused by hemorrhage into the skin: seen in any cause of thrombocytopenia
10. Purpura = larger than petechiae
11. Cyst = closed epithelium-lined cavity or sac containing liquid or semi-solid material
12. Hyperkeratosis = ↑ thickness of stratum corneum (seen in chronic dermatitis)
13. Parakeratosis = hyperkeratosis with retention of nuclei in stratum corneum & thinning of stratum granulosum (usually seen in psoriasis)
14. Steroids

TABLE 8-1 Use of Topical Steroids

POTENCY	DRUG	USE FOR DISEASE ON . . .
Low	1% hydrocortisone	Face, genitals, skin folds (prevent atrophy/striae), also use in children for dz on body
Moderate	0.1% triamcinolone	Body/extremities, or ↑ dz on face, genitals, skin folds
High	Fluocinonide (Lidex)	Thick skin (palms/soles), or ↑ body dz, **do not use on face**
Very High	Diflorasone	Thick skin, or if very severe on body

Carrier substance: lotion = low potency; cream = mid potency; ointment = high potency.

DERMATOLOGY

II. Infections

A. ACNE
1. Inflammation of pilosebaceous unit caused by secondary *Propionibacterium acnes* infection of blocked pore
2. Si/Sx = open comedones (blackheads) & closed comedones (whiteheads) on face, neck, chest, back, & buttocks, can become inflamed & pustular (See Color Plate 4)
3. Tx = topical antibiotics, Retin-A, benzoyl peroxide, systemic antibiotics, if acne is scarring consider Accutane

B. IMPETIGO
1. Superficial skin infection of epidermis

243

2. Si/Sx = honey-crusted lesions or vesicles occurring most often in children around the nose & mouth, can be bullous or nonbullous (See Color Plate 5)
3. Common organisms include *Staphylococcus aureus* & *S. pyogenes*
4. Tx = Keflex or oxacillin for 7–10 days

C. FOLLICULITIS
1. Si/Sx = erythematous pustules commonly noted around beard area
2. *S. aureus* most common, *Pseudomonas aeruginosa* causes "hot tub" folliculitis (organism lives in warm water), also fungi & viruses
3. Tx = local wound care, Keflex only if severe

D. SUBCUTANEOUS INFECTIONS
1. Cellulitis
   a. Si/Sx = spreading subcutaneous infxn with classic signs of inflammation: *rubor* (red), *calor* (hot), *dolor* (pain) & *tumor* (swelling)
   b. *Staphylococcus* & *Streptococcus* most common etiologies
   c. Tx = oxacillin or Keflex
2. Abscess
   a. Local collection of pus, often with fever, ↑ white count
   b. Tx = incision & drainage (I&D), can add Keflex
3. Furuncle (boil) & carbuncle
   a. Furuncle = pus collection in 1 hair follicle, often caused by *S. aureus*
   b. Carbuncle = pus collection involving many hair follicles
   c. Tx = I&D, add Keflex or oxacillin if severe
4. Paronychia
   a. Infxn of skin surrounding nail margin that can extend into surrounding skin & into tendons within hand
   b. Commonly caused by *S. aureus*, also *Candida*
   c. Tx = warm compress, I&D if area is purulent, add Keflex if severe
5. Necrotizing fasciitis
   a. Infxn along fascial planes with severe pain, fever, ↑ white count, local inflammation may be deceptively absent but pt will appear very ill
   b. Caused by *S. pyogenes* (group A Strep) or *Clostridium perfringens*
   c. Tx = **immediate, extensive surgical débridement, add penicillin & clindamycin to help prevent further spread**
   d. Px = ↑↑↑ mortality unless débridement is rapid & extensive

E. SCARLET FEVER
1. *S. pyogenes* (group A *Strep* = GAS) is the cause
2. Si/Sx
   a. **"Sunburn with goose bumps"** rash, finely punctate, erythematous but blanches with pressure, initially on trunk, generalizes within hours
   b. Sandpaper rough skin, **strawberry tongue**, beefy-red pharynx, circumoral pallor
   c. **Pastia's lines = rash, most intense in creases of axillae & groin**
   d. Eventual desquamation of hands & feet as rash resolves
   e. Systemic Sx include fever, chills, delirium, sore throat, cervical adenopathy, all of which appear at same time as rash
3. Complications include rheumatic fever & glomerulonephritis
4. Tx = penicillin

F. Hidradenitis Suppurativa

1. Si/Sx = plugged apocrine glands presenting as inflamed masses in groin/axilla, become secondarily infected
2. Tx = surgical débridement & antibiotics

G. Rose Spots

1. **Rose spots** = small pink papules in groups of 1–2 dozen on trunk, found in 30% of pts with typhoid fever (*Salmonella typhi*)
2. Typhoid fever Si/Sx
   a. High fever, myalgias, abdominal tenderness, splenomegaly
   b. **Classic pulse-fever dissociation** = high fever with relative bradycardia (also seen in brucellosis)
3. **Tx for chronic aSx typhoid fever (carrier state like "Typhoid Mary") is cholecystectomy because *S. typhi* resides in the gallbladder**

H. Erythrasma

1. Si/Sx = irregular erythematous rash found along major skin folds (axilla, groin, fingers, toes & breasts) (See Color Plates 6 and 7)
2. Commonly seen in adult diabetics, caused by *Corynebacterium* spp.
3. Dx = Wood's lamp of skin → **coral-red fluorescence, KOH prep negative**
4. Tx = erythromycin

III. Common Disorders

A. Psoriasis

1. Si/Sx = pink plaques with silvery-white scaling **occurring on extensor surfaces such as elbows & knees** (see Color Plate 8) (also scalp, lumbosacral, glans penis, intergluteal cleft), & **fingernail pitting**, can be associated with arthritis (see Color Plates 9 and 10)
2. Classic finding = **Auspitz sign** → removal of overlying scale causes pinpoint bleeding due to thin epidermis above dermal papillae
3. Classic finding = **Koebner's phenomenon** → psoriatic lesions appear at sites of cutaneous physical trauma (skin scratching, rubbing, or wound)
4. Dx = clinical, biopsy is gold standard
5. Tx = topical steroids (first line), PUVA (second line) = **P**soralens + **UVA** light, methotrexate & cyclosporin (third line)

B. Eczema (Eczematous Dermatitis)

1. Family of superficial, intensely pruritic, erythematous skin lesions
2. Atopic dermatitis
   a. Si/Sx = an "itch that rashes," rash 2° to scratching chronic pruritus, commonly found on the face in infancy, later in childhood can present on the flexor surfaces such as antecubital & popliteal fossa
   b. Atopy = inherited predisposition to asthma, allergies & dermatitis
   c. Dx is clinical
   d. Tx = avoid irritants or triggers, keep skin moist with lotions, use steroids & antihistamines for Sx relief of itching & inflammation
3. Contact dermatitis
   a. Si/Sx = linear pruritic rash at site of contact

b. Caused by delayed type hypersensitivity reaction after exposure to poison ivy, poison oak, nickel, or chemicals

c. Dx is clinical, history of exposure crucial

d. Tx = as per atopic dermatitis

4. Seborrheic dermatitis

a. Si/Sx = erythema, scaling, white flaking (dandruff) in areas of sebaceous glands (face, scalp, groin, axilla & external ear)

b. Called "cradle cap" in infants

c. Dx = clinical & KOH prep to rule out fungal infection

d. Tx = selenium shampoo on face & trunk, steroids for severe dz

C. URTICARIA (HIVES)

1. Common disorder caused by mast cell degranulation & histamine release

2. Si/Sx = transient papular wheals, intensely pruritic, surrounded by erythema, **dermographism** (write word on the skin & it remains imprinted as erythematous wheals) (See Color Plate 11)

3. Most lesions are IgE-mediated (type I hypersensitivity) but exercise, certain chemicals in sensitive pts & inhibitors of prostaglandin synthesis (e.g., aspirin) can also cause IgE-independent reactions

4. Dx = skin testing or aspirin or exercise challenge

5. Tx = avoidance of triggers, antihistamines, steroids, epinephrine

6. Can cause respiratory emergency requiring intubation

D. HYPOPIGMENTATION

1. Vitiligo

a. **Loss of melanocytes** in discrete areas of skin, appearing as sharply demarcated depigmented patches (See Color Plate 12)

b. Occurs in all races but most apparent in darkly pigmented pts

c. Chronic condition that may be autoimmune in nature

d. Associated with thyroid dz in 30% of pts, especially women

e. Tx = mini-grafting or total depigmentation

f. Px = some patients remit over long term, others never do

2. Albinism

a. **Melanocytes are present** but fail to produce pigment due to tyrosinase deficiency

b. Si/Sx = white skin & eyelashes, nystagmus, iris translucency, ↓ visual acuity, decreased retinal pigment & strabismus

c. Tx = avoid sun exposure, sunscreens

d. Px = the oculocutaneous form predisposes to skin cancer

3. Pityriasis alba

a. Nonpathological areas of hypopigmentation on face or upper extremities

b. Can be 2° to prior infection or inflammation, often regress over time

c. Differentiated from tinea versicolor by KOH prep

E. HYPERPIGMENTATION

1. Freckle (ephelis) is caused by normal melanocyte number but ↑ melanin within basal keratinocytes, darkens with sun exposure

2. Lentigo is pigmented macules caused by melanocyte hyperplasia that, unlike freckles, do not darken with sun exposure

3. Nevocellular nevus
   a. Common mole, benign tumor derived from melanocytes
   b. Variations of nevi
      1) Blue nevus = black-blue nodule present at birth, often mistaken for melanoma
      2) Spitz nevus = red-pink nodule, often seen in children, confused with hemangioma or melanoma
      3) Dysplastic nevus = atypical, irregularly pigmented lesion with ↑ risk of transformation into malignant melanoma
      4) Dysplastic nevus syndrome is autosomal dominant inherited dz
   c. Dx = biopsy, Tx = full excision
4. Melasma (chloasma)
   a. A mask-like hyperpigmentation on face seen in pregnancy
   b. Sunlight accentuates pigmentation, which typically fades postpartum
   c. Tx = minimize facial exposure to sun, or hydroquinone cream (works for any hyperpigmentation)
5. Hemangioma
   a. Group of "birthmarks," capillary hemangiomas present at birth
   b. Port-wine stains (purple-red on face or neck)
      1) Can be associated with Sturge-Weber syndrome (See Phakomatoses below, Section V)
      2) Must screen for glaucoma & CNS dz (CT scan)
      3) Tx = laser therapy, will not regress spontaneously
   c. Strawberry hemangiomas (bright raised red lesions) are benign, most disappear on their own
   d. Cherry hemangiomas (benign small red papule) Tx with laser therapy
6. Xanthoma
   a. Yellowish papules, often accumulations of foamy histiocytes
   b. Can be idiopathic or associated with familial hyperlipidemia
   c. If seen on eyelids they are called "xanthelasma"
   d. Tx = ↓ hyperlipidemia, surgically excise papules as needed
7. Pityriasis rosea
   a. Erythematous maculopapular rash with scale apparent in center
   b. Often preceded by a "herald patch" on trunk
   c. **Can appear on back in a Christmas tree distribution**
   d. Tx = sunlight, otherwise spontaneously remits in 6–12 wk
8. Erythema nodosum
   a. Inflammation of subcutaneous fat (panniculitis) & adjacent vessels
   b. Characteristic lesions are **tender red nodules occurring on the lower legs** & sometimes forearms
   c. Usually resolves in 6–8 wk, Tx directed at underlying cause
   d. Common causes
      1) Infections = *Mycoplasma*, *Chlamydia*, *Coccidioides immitis*, *Mycobacterium leprae* & others
      2) Drugs = sulfonamides & contraceptive pills
      3) Inflammatory Bowel Disease, sarcoidosis, rheumatic fever

        4) Pregnancy
9. Dermatomyositis
    a. An autoimmune disorder sometimes seen with polymyositis·
    b. Presents with **heliotropic (reddish-purple) patches on eyelids** & erythematous scaly rash on hands
    c. Tx = high-dose steroids
10. Seborrheic keratosis
    a. Black or brown benign plaques, appear to be stuck onto skin surface
    b. Commonly seen in elderly & runs in families
    c. Can be mistaken for melanoma
    d. Tx = liquid nitrogen freezing, usually too many to treat
11. Acanthosis nigricans
    a. Black velvety plaques on flexor surfaces & intertriginous areas
    b. Seen in obesity & endocrine disorders (e.g., diabetes)
    c. Can mark underlying malignancy (e.g., GI/GU, lymphoma)
12. Bronze diabetes = 1° hemochromatosis
    a. Familial defect causing intestinal hyperabsorption of iron
    b. **Classic triad: ↑ skin pigmentation, cirrhosis, diabetes mellitus**
    c. Other Sx = cardiomyopathy, pituitary failure & arthropathies
    d. **Clinical pearl: hemochromatosis is the likely Dx in any patient with osteoarthritis involving the MCP joints**
    e. Dx = transferrin saturation (iron/TIBC) ≥ 50%
    f. Tx = phlebotomy, which improves survival if started early

F. VERRUCAE (WARTS)
1. Verruca vulgaris = hand wart
2. Verruca plana (flat wart) smaller than vulgaris, seen on hands & face
3. Human papilloma virus (HPV) types 1–4 cause skin & plantar warts
4. HPV 6 & 11 cause anorectal & genital warts (condyloma acuminatum)
5. HPV 16, 18, 31, 33, 35 cause cervical cancer
6. Condylomata lata are flat warts caused by *Treponema pallidum* (syphilis)

IV. Cancer

TABLE 8-2   Skin Cancer

DISEASE	SI/SX	TX	PX
Basal cell carcinoma	Most common skin cancer, classic "**rodent ulcer**" seen on face, with **pearly translucent borders & fine telangiectasias**, not usually found on lips (See Color Plate 13)	Excision	Excellent— almost never metastasize
Squamous cell carcinoma	Common in elderly, appears as erythematous nodules on sun-exposed areas that eventually ulcerate & crust, **frequently preceded by actinic keratosis = rough epidermal lesions on sun-exposed areas such as lower lip, ears & nose** (See Color Plate 14)	Excision, radiation	Metastasize more than basal cell but not as much as melanoma

TABLE 8-2   *Continued*

DISEASE	SI/SX	TX	PX
Malignant melanoma	Seen in lightly pigmented individuals with ↑ sun exposure—diagnose with **ABCDEs** (See Color Plate 15) **A**symmetry = malignant, benign = symmetrical **B**order = irregular, benign = smooth **C**olor = multicolored, benign = 1 color **D**iameter >6 mm, benign = <6 mm **E**levation = raised above skin, benign = flat **E**nlargement = growing, benign = not growing	Excision, chemo if mets likely	High rate of metastasis → **#1 skin cancer killer, risk of mets ↑ with depth of invasion on biopsy**
Kaposi's sarcoma	Connective tissue cancer caused by human herpes virus 8, appears as red/purple plaques or nodules on skin & mucosa, frequently affects lungs & GI viscera, almost exclusively seen in AIDS patients (See Color Plate 16)	HIV drugs, chemo	Benign unless damages internal organs
Cutaneous T-cell lymphoma	**"Mycosis fungoides," presents with erythroderma (total body erythematous & pruritic rash), rash can precede malignancy by years,** leukemic phase of disease called "Sézary syndrome"	PUVA, topical chemo, radiation	7–10 yr life expectancy without Tx

V. Neurocutaneous Syndromes (Phakomatoses)

1. Tx is supportive depending upon individual signs & symptoms
2.

TABLE 8-3   Neurocutaneous Syndromes (Phakomatoses)

DISEASE*	CHARACTERISTICS
Tuberous sclerosis	Ash leaf patches (hypopigmented macules), Shagreen spots (leathery cutaneous thickening), adenoma sebaceum of the face, **seizures, mental retardation**
Neurofibromatosis (NF)	Si/Sx = **café-au-lait spots** (see Color Plate 1), neurofibromas, meningiomas, acoustic neuromas, kyphoscoliosis—NF 2 causes bilateral acoustic neuromas
Sturge-Weber syndrome	Si/Sx = **port-wine hemangioma of face** in CN V distribution, mental retardation, seizures
von Hippel-Lindau syndrome	Si/Sx = multiple hemangiomas in various organs, ↑ frequency of renal cell CA & polycythemia (↑ erythropoietin secretion)

*All are autosomal dominant except Sturge-Weber, which has no genetic pattern.

VI. Blistering Disorders

A. PEMPHIGUS VULGARIS (PG)

1. PG is a rare autoimmune disorder, **affecting 20–40-yr-olds**
2. Si/Sx = **flaccid epidermal bullae** that easily slough off leaving large denuded areas of skin (Nikolsky's sign), ↑ risk of 2° infxn

DERMATOLOGY

3. DDx = bullous pemphigoid
4. Dx = skin biopsy → **immunofluorescence surrounding epidermal cells** showing "tombstone" fluorescent pattern
5. Tx = high-dose oral steroids, antibiotics for infection
6. Px = **often fatal if not treated**

B. BULLOUS PEMPHIGOID (BP)
1. Common autoimmune disease affecting **mostly the elderly**
2. Resembles PG but much less severe clinically
3. Si/Sx = **hard, tense bullae** that do not rupture easily & usually heal without scarring if uninfected (See Color Plate 17)
4. Dx = skin biopsy → immunofluorescence as a **linear band along the basement membrane, with ↑ eosinophils** in dermis
5. Tx = oral steroids
6. Px = much better than PG

C. ERYTHEMA MULTIFORME
1. A hypersensitivity reaction to drugs, infections, or systemic disorders such as malignancy or collagen vascular disease
2. Si/Sx = **diffuse, erythematous target-like lesions** in many shapes (hence name "multiforme"), often accompanying a herpes eruption
3. **Stevens-Johnson syndrome = a severe febrile form (sometimes fatal) → hemorrhagic crusting also affects lips & oral mucosa**
4. Dx = clinical, hx of herpes infection or drug exposure
5. Tx = stop offending drug, prevent eruption of herpes with acyclovir

D. PORPHYRIA CUTANEA TARDA
1. Autosomal dominant defect in heme synthesis (50% ↓ in uroporphyrinogen decarboxylase activity in RBC & liver)
2. Si/Sx = blisters on sun-exposed areas of face & hands (see Color Plate 18), ↑ hair on temples & cheeks, **no abdominal pain** (differentiates from other porphyrias)
3. Dx = Wood's lamp of urine → **urine fluoresces with distinctive orange-pink color due to ↑ levels of uroporphyrins**
4. Tx = sunscreen, phlebotomy, chloroquine, no alcohol
5. Px = remitting/relapsing, exacerbations due to viral hepatitis, hepatoma, alcohol abuse, estrogen, sunlight

VII. Vector Borne Diseases

A. BACILLARY ANGIOMATOSIS (PELIOSIS HEPATIS)
1. Si/Sx = weight loss, abdominal pain, **rash = red or purple vascular lesions**, from papule to hemangioma-sized, located anywhere on skin & disseminated to any organ
2. DDx = Kaposi's sarcoma, cherry hemangioma
3. **Almost always seen in HIV ⊕ patients or homeless population**
4. Caused by *Bartonella* spp., leading to dysregulated angiogenesis
5. **Cat-scratch disease caused by *B. henselae* transmitted by kitten scratches, trench fever caused by *B. quintana* spread by lice**
6. Dx = histopathology with silver stain, visualization of organisms in lesion, blood culture & PCR can also be done
7. Tx = erythromycin

8. Px = excellent with Tx, some pts require lifelong suppressive Tx

B. LYME DISEASE
1. Si/Sx = fever, chills, headaches, lethargy, photophobia, meningitis, myocarditis, arthralgia & myalgias
2. **Classic rash = erythema chronicum migrans → erythematous annular plaques with a red migrating border & central clearing & induration**
3. Dx = PCR for *Borrelia burgdorferi* DNA, or skin biopsy of migrating edge looking for causative spirochete
4. Tx = spray skin & clothes with DEET or permethrin, wear long pants in woods to prevent tick bite (*Ixodes dammini* & *Ixodes pacificus*)
5. Once infected → high-dose penicillin or ceftriaxone for 2–4 wk

C. ROCKY MOUNTAIN SPOTTED FEVER
1. Si/Sx = acute onset fever, headache, myalgias, classic rash
2. **Rash = erythematous maculopapular, starting on wrists & ankles then moving toward palms, soles & trunk**
3. Rash may lead to cutaneous necrosis due to DIC-induced occlusion of small cutaneous vessels with thrombi
4. Dx = by Hx (exposure to outdoors or tick bite, *Dermacentor* spp.), serologies for *Rickettsia rickettsii*, skin biopsy
5. Doxycycline or chloramphenicol

VIII. Parasitic Infections

A. SCABIES
1. SiSx = erythematous, **markedly pruritic papules & burrows located intertriginous areas** (e.g., finger & toe webs, groin), lesions contagious (See Color Plate 19)
2. Dx = microscopic identification of *Sarcoptes scabiei* mite in skin scrapings (See Figure 8-1)
3. Tx = pt & all close contacts apply Permethrin 5% cream to entire body for 8–10 hr then repeat in 1 wk, wash all bedding in hot water the same day
4. Lindane cream is less effective, associated with adverse effects in kids
5. Symptomatic relief of hypersensitivity reaction to dead mites may be treated with antihistamines & topical steroids

B. PEDICULOSIS CAPITIS (HEAD LOUSE)
1. Si/Sx = can be asymptomatic, or pruritus & erythema of scalp may be noted, common in school-aged children
2. Dx = microscope exam of hair shaft, nits may fluoresce with Wood's lamp
3. Permethrin shampoo or gel to scalp, may need to repeat

C. PEDICULOSIS PUBIS ("CRABS")
1. Si/Sx = very **pruritic papules in pubic area**, axilla, periumbilically in males, along eyelashes, eyebrows & buttocks
2. Dx = microscopic identification of lice, rule out other STDs
3. Tx = apply Permethrin 5% shampoo for 10 min then repeat in 1 wk

D. CUTANEOUS LARVA MIGRANS (CREEPING ERUPTION)
1. Si/Sx = erythematous, pruritic, **serpiginous thread-like lesion** marking burrow of migrating nematode larvae, often on back, hands, feet, buttocks
2. Organism = hookworms: *Ancylostoma, Necator* & *Strongyloides*

3. Dx = Hx of unprotected skin lying in moist soil or sand, Bx of lesion
4. Tx = ivermectin orally or thiabendazole topically

IX. Fungal Cutaneous Disorders

TABLE 8-4   Fungal Cutaneous Disorders

DISEASE	SI/SX	DX	TX
Tinea	• Erythematous, pruritic, scaly, well-demarcated plaques (See Color Plate 20) • Black dots may be seen on scalp of patients with tinea capitis	Clinical or KOH prep	Topical antifungal (oral needed for tinea capitis)
Onycho-mycosis	• Fingernails or toenails appear thickened, yellow, degenerating	Clinical or KOH prep	PO itraconazole or fluconazole
Tinea versicolor	• Caused by *Pityrosporum ovale* • Multiple sharply marginated hypopigmented macules on face & trunk noticed in summer because macules will not tan (See Color Plate 21)	KOH prep → yeast & hyphae with classic **spaghetti & meatball appearance**	Selenium sulfide shampoo daily on affected areas for 7 days
Candida	• Erythematous scaling plaques, often in intertriginous areas (groin, breast, buttocks, web of hands) (See Color Plate 22) • Oral thrush → cottage-cheese-like white plaques on mucosal surface • Can extend to esophagus & cause dysphagia & odynophagia	KOH prep → budding yeast & pseudohyphae	Topical Nystatin or oral fluconazole

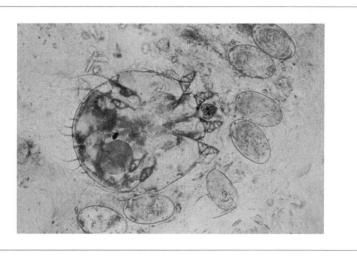

FIGURE 8-1   *Sarcoptes scabiei,* the scabies mite. Female with eggs.

9. Ophthalmology

Carlos Ayala

I. Eyes

A. CLASSIC SYNDROMES OR SYMPTOMS
1. Amblyopia
   a. Decreased vision secondary to failure of development of the pathway between the retina & visual cortex before age 7
   b. Usually affects one eye, can be secondary to cataract, severe refractive error, or strabismus
   c. Si/Sx = esotropia (inwardly rotated "crossed eyes") or exotropia (outwardly rotated "walled eyes"), diplopia & refractive error not correctable with lenses
   d. Tx = early correction of cause of visual acuity disturbance
2. Bitemporal hemianopsia (See Figure 9-1)
   a. Unable to see in bilateral temporal fields
   b. Usually caused by a pituitary tumor
3. Internuclear ophthalmoplegia
   a. **Classically found in multiple sclerosis**
   b. Lesion of median longitudinal fasciculus (MLF)
   c. Si/Sx = inability to adduct the ipsilateral eye past midline on lateral gaze (inability to perform conjugate gaze)
   d. Caused by lack of communication between contralateral CN VI nucleus & the ipsilateral CN III nucleus
4. Parinaud's syndrome
   a. Midbrain tectum lesion → bilateral paralysis of upward gaze
   b. Commonly associated with pineal tumor
5. Marcus-Gunn pupil
   a. Due to afferent defect of CN II, pupil will not react to direct light but will react consensually when light is directed at the normal contralateral eye
   b. **Characterized by ⊕ swinging flashlight test**
      1) Swing penlight quickly back & forth between eyes
      2) Denervated pupil will not constrict to direct stimulation & **instead will actually appear to dilate when light is shone in it** because it is dilating back to baseline when consensual light is removed from other eye
6. Argyll-Robertson pupil
   a. **Pathognomonic for 3° syphilis (neurosyphilis)**
   b. Pupils constrict with accommodation but do not constrict to direct light stimulation (pupils accommodate but do not react)
7. Lens dislocation
   a. Occurs in homocystinuria, Marfan's & Alport's syndromes
   b. Lens **dislocates superiorly in Marfan's (mnemonic:** Marfan's patients are tall, their lenses dislocate upward), inferiorly in homocystinuria & variably in Alport's syndrome

253

8. Kayser-Fleischer ring
   a. **Pathognomonic for Wilson's disease**
   b. Finding is a ring of golden pigment around the iris
9. Pterygium
   a. Fleshy growth from conjunctiva onto nasal side of cornea
   b. Associated with exposure to wind, sand, sun & dust
   c. Tx = cosmetic removal unless impairing vision
10. Pinguecula (See Color Plates 23 and 24)
    a. Benign yellowish nodules on either side of the cornea
    b. Commonly seen in patients > 35
    c. Rarely grows & requires no treatment
11. Subconjunctival hemorrhage
    a. Spontaneous onset of a painless, bright red patch on sclera
    b. Benign, self-limited condition usually seen after overexertion
12. Retrobulbar neuritis
    a. Caused by inflammation of the optic nerve, usually unilateral
    b. **Seen in multiple sclerosis, often is the initial sign**
    c. Si/Sx = rapid loss of vision & pain upon moving eye, spontaneously remitting within 2–8 wk, each relapse damages the nerve more, until eventually blindness results
    d. Funduscopic exam is nonrevealing
    e. Tx = corticosteroids
13. Optic neuritis
    a. Inflammation of optic nerve within the eye
    b. Causes include viral infection, multiple sclerosis, vasculitis, methanol, meningitis, syphilis, tumor metastases
    c. Si/Sx = variable vision loss & ↓ pupillary light reflex
    d. **Funduscopic exam reveals disk hyperemia**
    e. If pt is > 60 yr, biopsy temporal artery to rule out temporal arteritis
    f. Tx = corticosteroids

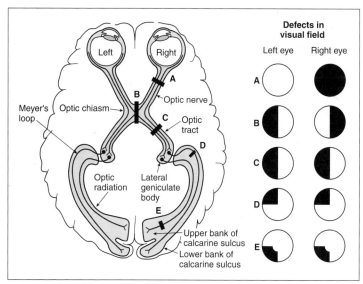

FIGURE 9-1 Visual field deficits. Lesions in the visual system are correlated with specific visual field deficits. (A) Blindness in the right eye. (B) Bitemporal heteronymous hemianopsia. (C) Left homonymous hemianopsia. (D) Superior quadrantic anopia. (E) Inferior quadrantic anopsia with macular sparing. (Reproduced with permission from Pritchard TC and Alloway KD. Medical Neuroscience. Madison, Connecticut: Fence Creek Publishing, 1999:307. © Fence Creek Publishing, LLC.)

B. PALPEBRAL INFLAMMATION

TABLE 9-1   Palpebral Inflammation (See Figures 9-2 and 9-3)

DISEASE	SI/SX	TX
Chalazion	• Inflammation of internal meibomian sebaceous gland • Presents with swelling on conjunctival surface of eyelid	None, self-limiting
Hordeolum (Stye)	• Infection of external sebaceous glands of Zeiss or Mol • Presents with tender red swelling at lid margin	Hot compress, can add antibiotics
Blepharitis	• Inflammation of eyelids & eyelashes due to infection (*S. aureus*) or secondary to seborrhea • Presents with red, swollen eyelid margins, with dry flakes noted on lashes • **Without Tx can extend along eyelid (cellulitis)**	Wash lid margins daily with baby shampoo, control scalp seborrhea with shampoo
Orbital cellulitis	• Can occur if blepharitis is left untreated (See Figure 9-3) • Also seen as complication of paranasal sinus infection • **Can spread to cavernous sinus leading to deadly thrombosis & meningitis**	Treat emergently with IV nafcillin or cephalosporin

OPHTHAL-MOLOGY

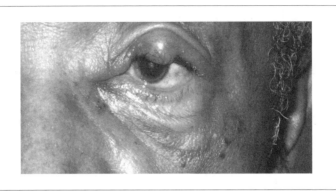

FIGURE 9-2   Stye (hordeolum).

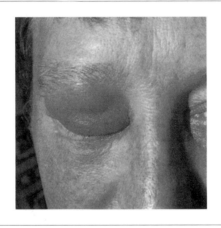

FIGURE 9-3   The appearance of a patient with preseptal cellulitis.

C. RED EYE

1. **Assess pain, visual acuity, type of eye discharge, pupillary abnormalities in all patients**
2. DDx

TABLE 9-2   Red Eye

DISEASE	SI/SX	CAUSE	TX
Bacterial conjunctivitis	• Minimal pain, no vision changes • **Purulent** discharge • No pupillary changes • **Rarely** preauricular adenopathy (only *N. gonorrhoeae*)	*S. pneumoniae, Staph.* spp., *N. gonorrhoeae, Chlamydia trachomatis* (in neonates, sexually active adults)	Topical sulfacetamide or erythromycin
Viral conjunctivitis	• Minimal pain, no vision changes • **Watery** discharge • No pupillary changes • **Often preauricular adenopathy** • **Often pharyngitis** (adenovirus)	Adenovirus most common, others = HSV, varicella, EBV, influenza, echovirus, coxsackie virus	No treatment required, self-limiting dz
Allergic conjunctivitis	• No pain, vision, or pupil changes • **Marked pruritus** • **Bilateral** watery eyes	Allergy/Hay fever	Antihistamine or steroid drops
Hyphema	• Pain, no vision changes • No discharge, no pupil changes • **Blood in anterior chamber of eye, fluid level noted** (See Figure 9-4)	Blunt ocular trauma	Eye patch to ↓ movement
Xerophthalmia	• Minimal pain, vision blurry, no pupillary changes, no discharge • **Bitot's spots** visible on exam (desquamated, keratinized conjunctival cells) • **Keratoconjunctivitis sicca** (Sjögren's disease) **Dx by Schirmer test** (place filter paper over eyelid, if not wet in 15 min → Dx)	Sjögren's disease or vitamin A deficiency	Artificial tears, vitamin A
Corneal abrasion	• **Painful, with photophobia** • No pupil changes • Watery discharge • Dx by fluorescein stain to detect areas of corneal defect	Direct trauma to eye (finger, stick, etc.)	Antibiotics, eye patch, examine daily
Keratitis	• **Pain**, photophobia, tearing • **Decreased vision** • **Herpes shows classic dendritic branching on fluorescein stain** (See Color Plates 25 and 26) • **Pus in anterior chamber (hypopyon) is a grave sign**	Adenovirus, HSV, *Pseudomonas, S. pneumoniae, Staph., Moraxella* (often in contact lens wearers)	**Emergency, immediate Ophtho consult** Tx = topical vidarabine for herpes
Uveitis	• Inflammation of the iris, ciliary body, &/or choroid • **Pain, miosis**, photophobia • **Flare & cells** seen in aqueous humor **on slit lamp examination** (See Figure 9-5)	Seen in seronegative spondyloarthropathy, inflammatory bowel disease, sarcoidosis, or infxn (CMV, syphilis)	Tx underlying dz
Angle closure glaucoma	• **Severe pain** • ↓ **vision**, halos around lights • **Fixed mid-dilated pupil** • **Eyeball firm to pressure** (See Figure 9-6)	↓ aqueous humor outflow via canal of Schlemm—mydriatics can also cause	**Emergency,** IV mannitol & acetazolamide, laser iridotomy for cure

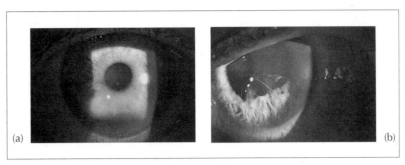

FIGURE 9-4   (a) A hyphema; (b) penetrating eye injury (notice the eyelashes in the anterior chamber and the distorted iris).

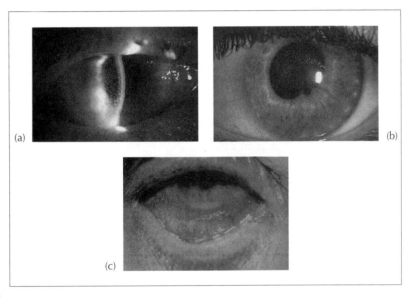

FIGURE 9-5   Signs of anterior uveitis; (a) keratic precipitates on the corneal endothelium; (b) posterior synechiae (adhesions between the lens and iris) give the pupil an irregular appearance; (c) a hypopyon, white cells have collected as a mass in the inferior anterior chamber.

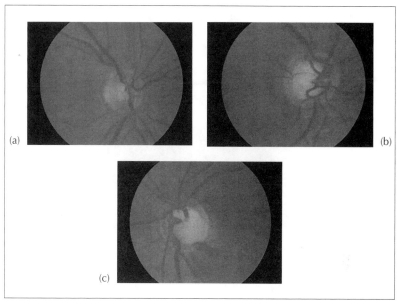

(a)   (b)

(c)

FIGURE 9-6   Comparison of (a) a normal optic disk; (b) glaucomatous optic disc; (c) a disc hemorrhage is a feature of patients with low-tension glaucoma.

D. DACRYOCYSTITIS (TEAR DUCT INFLAMMATION)

1. Infection of lacrimal sac, usually caused by *Staphylococcus aureus, Streptococcus pneumoniae, Hemophilus influenzae,* or *S. pyogenes*
2. Si/Sx = inflammation & tenderness of nasal aspect of lower lid, purulent discharge may be noted or expressed (See Figure 9-7)
3. Tx = Keflex

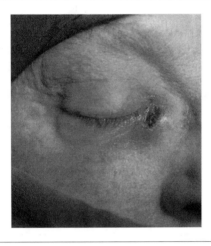

FIGURE 9-7   Dacrocystitis, unusually, in this case, pointing through the skin.

E. EYE COLORS
1. **Yellow eye** (icterus) from bilirubin staining of sclera (jaundice)
2. **Yellow vision** seen in digoxin toxicity
3. **Blue sclera** classically found in osteogenesis imperfecta & Marfan's disease [see Musculoskeletal, Sections II.D & IV.G]
4. **Opaque eye** due to cataract
    a. Opacity of lens severe enough to interfere with vision
    b. Causes = congenital, diabetes (sorbitol precipitation in lens), galactosemia (galactitol precipitation in lens), Hurler's disease [see Appendix A]

F. RETINA (See Color Plate 27)
1. Diabetic retinopathy
    a. Occurs after about 10 yr of diabetes
        1) Background type
            a) Flame hemorrhages, microaneurysms & soft exudates (cotton-wool spots) on retina (See Color Plates 28 and 29)
            b) Tx is strict glucose & hypertension control
        2) Proliferative type
            a) More advanced dz, with neovascularization easily visible around fundus (hyperemia) & hard exudates (See Color Plate 30)
            b) Tx is photocoagulation (laser ablation of blood vessels in the retina) that slows disease progression but is not curative
2. Age-related macular degeneration (AMD)
    a. AMD causes painless loss of visual acuity
    b. Dx by altered pigmentation in macula
    c. Pts often retain adequate peripheral vision
    d. Tx = antioxidants and laser therapy

3. Retinal detachment
    a. Presents with painless, dark vitreous floaters, flashes of light (photopsias), blurry vision, eventually progressing to a curtain of blindness in vision as detachment worsens
    b. Tx = urgent surgical reattachment
4. Retinitis pigmentosa (See Figure 9-8)
    a. Slowly progressive defect in night vision (often starts in young children) with ring-shaped scotoma (blind-spot) that gradually increases in size to obscure more vision
    b. Disease is hereditary with unclear transmission mode
    c. May be part of the Laurence-Moon-Biedl syndrome
    d. There is no treatment
5. Classic physical findings of retina
    a. **Leukocoria** = absent red reflex, actually appears white, seen in retinoblastoma (See Figure 9-9)
    b. **Roth spots** = small hemorrhagic spots with central clearing in retina associated with endocarditis
    c. **Copper wiring, flame hemorrhages, A-V nicking** seen in subacute hypertension &/or atherosclerosis
    d. **Cotton-wool spots** (soft exudates) seen in chronic HTN
    e. Papilledema appears as disk hyperemia, blurring, & elevation, associated with ↑ intracranial pressure
    f. "Sea fan" neovascularization in sickle cell anemia
    g. Wrinkles on retina seen in retinal detachment
    h. **Cherry-red spot on macula** seen in Tay-Sachs, Niemann-Pick disease, central retinal artery occlusion
    i. Hollenhorst plaque = yellow cholesterol emboli in retinal artery
    j. Brown macule on retina = malignant melanoma (most common intraocular tumor in adults) (See Figure 9-10)

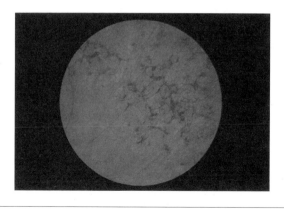

FIGURE 9-8   The clinical appearance of peripheral retina in retinitis pigmentosa.

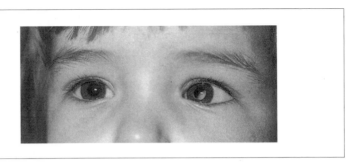

FIGURE 9-9 Left leukocoria.

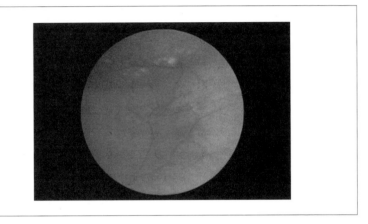

FIGURE 9-10 The clinical appearance of a choroidal melanoma.

10. Radiology

Michael Gentry

I. Introduction

1. This section will cover common causes for radiologic findings presented in the clinical vignettes on the USMLE as well as on rounds. Where useful, the causes will be divided into categories using the mnemonic **VINDICATE**

   V = Vascular
   I = Inflammatory/Infectious
   N = Neoplastic
   D = Degenerative
   I = Idiopathic/Intoxication
   C = Congenital
   A = Autoimmune
   T = Trauma
   E = Endocrine

II. Helpful Terms and Concepts

A. LUCENT VS. SCLEROTIC LESIONS
On plain film, a lucency is a focal area of bone or tissue that has a decreased density, usually resulting from a pathological process. A lucent bone lesion may appear like a dark, punched-out hole in the surrounding, normal bone. In contrast, sclerotic bone lesions appear denser than the surrounding bone. Thus, a sclerotic mass presents as whiter and more intense than its surroundings.

B. HYPODENSE VS. HYPERDENSE
Similar to that on plain films, tissue density on CT can be characterized by how light or dark it appears relative to surrounding, normal parenchyma. Hypodense lesions appear darker than normal tissue and hyperdense lesions are brighter. Air- or fluid-filled lesions such as cysts and abscesses are common hypodense lesions.

C. RING-ENHANCEMENT
This refers to a bright intensity that can be observed surrounding many lesions on both CT and MRI. This usually indicates local edema around a mass lesion and in the brain it can indicate breakdown of the blood-brain barrier.

D. RADIOPAQUE
The more radiopaque an object is, the brighter it appears on plain film. Dental fillings, bullets, and metal prostheses are very radiopaque so they appear white on plain film.

E. RADIOLUCENT
The more radiolucent an object is, the darker it appears on plain film.

III. Common Radiologic Studies

RADIOLOGY

263

TABLE 10-1   Common Radiologic Studies

STUDY	INDICATIONS
CT vs. MRI	• CT → faster, less expensive, greater sensitivity for acute head trauma, better for detection of spinal cord compression • MRI → better visualization of soft tissue, allows multiplanar imaging (axial, coronal, sagittal & obliques), no ionizing radiation
Endoscopic retrograde cholangio-pancreatography (ERCP)	Pancreatitis 2° to choledocholithiasis, cholestatic jaundice
Ultrasound (Utz)*	Abdominal aortic aneurysm, gallbladder disease, renal & adrenal masses, ectopic pregnancy, kidney stones
Carotid doppler Utz	Carotid artery stenosis, assessing flow dynamics
Intravenous pyelogram (IVP)	GU obstruction
Kidney, ureter, bladder (KUB) x-ray*	Kidney stones, solid abdominal masses, abdominal free air
Lateral decubitus chest plain film	To determine whether a suspected pleural effusion will layer

*Note 80/20 rule: gallstones diagnosed 80% of the time & kidney stones 20% of the time by Utz. Kidney stones diagnosed 80% of the time & gallstones only 20% of the time by x-ray.

IV. An Approach to a Chest X-Ray (See Figure 10-1)

A = **A**irway—is trachea midline? & **A**lignment—symmetry of clavicles

B = **B**ones—look for fractures, lytic lesions, or defects

C = **C**ardiac silhouette—normally occupies < $\frac{1}{2}$ chest width

D = **D**iaphragms—flattened (e.g., COPD)?, blunted angles (effusion)?, elevated (airspace consolidation)?

E = **E**xternal soft tissues—lymph nodes (especially axilla), subQ emphysema, other lesions

F = **F**ields of the lung—opacities, nodules, vascularity, bronchial cuffing, etc.

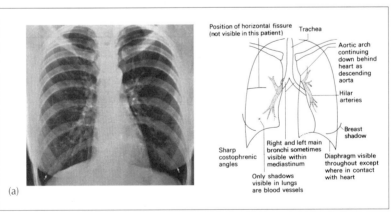

(a)

FIGURE 10-1   Normal chest. (a) PA view. The arrows point to the breast shadows of this female patient. (b) Lateral view. Note that the upper retrosternal area is of the same density as the retro-cardiac areas, and the same as over the upper thoracic vertebrae. The vertebrae are more transradiant (i.e., blacker) as the eye travels down the spine, until the diaphragm is reached. Ao = aorta; T = Trachea.

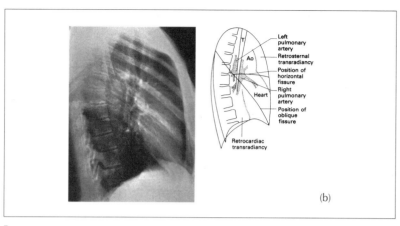

(b)

FIGURE 10-1   *Continued*

V. Common Radiologic Findings

TABLE 10-2   Common Radiologic Findings

FINDING/DESCRIPTION	DIFFERENTIAL DIAGNOSIS	
Hair-on-end skull sign on plain film Caused by new bone formation that occurs perpendicular to the skull table, resulting in a thin, spiked appearance, as if bony hairs growing out of skull (See Figure 10-2)	• Congenital • Sickle cell anemia • Osteosarcoma	
Hypodense cerebral masses on CT (See Figure 10-3)	**Neoplastic:** • Glioma • Prolactinoma • Craniopharyngiomas	**Infectious:** • Pyogenic abscess • Tuberculoma • Hydatid cyst
Multiple contrast-enhancing lesions on CT or MRI	**Neoplastic:** • Metastases (See Figure 10-4) ◊ Breast CA & bronchogenic lung CA most common ◊ Also malignant melanoma, prostate, lymphoma	**Infectious:** • Bacterial abscess • Toxoplasmosis • Cysticercosis **Vascular:** • Infarct **Degenerative:** • Demyelinating disease
Nonsclerotic skull lucency	**Infectious:** • TB • Syphilis • Osteomyelitis **Neoplastic:** • Multiple myeloma	• Metastases **Trauma:** • Burr hole **Endocrine:** • Hyperparathyroidism

RADIOLOGY

TABLE 10-2 *Continued*

FINDING/DESCRIPTION	DIFFERENTIAL DIAGNOSIS	
Sclerotic bone lesions (See Figures 1-16 and 10-5)	**Infectious:** • Osteomyelitis (presents with periosteal reaction) • Syphilis **Congenital:** • Fibrous dysplasia • Tuberous sclerosis **Vascular:** • Healing fracture callus	**Neoplastic:** • Metastases—primarily prostate & breast • Lymphoma • Multiple myeloma—usually presents with multiple lesions (See Figure 1-17) • Osteosarcoma
"Bone within bone" sign	**Endocrine:** • Growth arrest & recovery • Paget's disease • Osteopetrosis	**Intoxication:** Heavy metal poisoning
Inferior surface rib notching	**Vascular:** • Coarctation of the aorta—**classic finding** • Superior vena cava obstruction	**Congenital:** • Chest wall A-V malformation
Ivory vertebral body Sclerotic change in a single vertebra	**Neoplastic:** • Sclerotic metastases • Lymphoma	**Endocrine:** • Paget's disease
Honeycomb lung Fibrotic replacement of lung parenchyma with thick-walled cysts	**Idiopathic:** • Idiopathic interstitial fibrosis • Histiocytosis X • Sarcoidosis **Congenital:** • Cystic fibrosis • Tuberous sclerosis • Neurofibromatosis	**Autoimmune:** • Scleroderma • Rheumatoid arthritis **Intoxication:** • Allergic alveolitis • Asbestosis • Bleomycin • Nitrofurantoin • Cyclophosphamide
Ground glass opacities on lung CT Hazy, granular increase in density of lung parenchyma that usually implies an acute inflammatory process	**Inflammation:** • Interstitial pneumonia • Hypersensitivity pneumonitis • *Pneumocystic carinii* pneumonia (See Figure 1-9) • Alveolar proteinosis	
Water-bottle-shaped heart on PA plain film	Pericardial effusions with more than 250 mL of fluid	
Pulmonary edema Classically, severe pulmonary edema appears as **a bat's-wing shadow**	**Vascular:** • Congestive heart failure **Inflammatory:** • Adult respiratory distress syndrome (See Figure 1-5) • Mendelson's syndrome	**Intoxication:** Smoke inhalation **Trauma:** Near drowning
Blunting of costophrenic angles 300–500 mL of fluid is needed before blunting of the lateral costophrenic angles becomes apparent (See Figures 10-6 and 10-7)	Pleural effusion	

TABLE 10-2 *Continued*

FINDING/DESCRIPTION	DIFFERENTIAL DIAGNOSIS	
Kerley B lines (See Figure 10-8) Interlobar septa on the peripheral aspects of the lungs that become thickened by disease or fluid accumulation	**Vascular:** • Left ventricular failure • Lymphatic obstruction	**Inflammatory:** • Sarcoidosis Lymphangitis carcinomatosa
Multiple lung small soft tissue Densities <2 mm	**Inflammatory:** • Sarcoidosis • Miliary TB • Fungal infection • Parasites • Extrinsic allergic alveolitis	**Neoplastic:** Metastases **Endocrine:** Hemosiderosis
Lung nodules >2 cm Ghon complex—calcified granuloma classic for TB, found at lung base along hilum (See Figures 10-9 and 1-6)	**Neoplastic:** • Metastases • Primary lung CA • Benign hamartoma **Intoxication:** • Silicosis **Idiopathic:** • Histiocytosis X	**Inflammatory:** • Sarcoidosis • TB • Wegener's • Fungal infections • Abscess
Hilar adenopathy (See Figure 1-24)	**Inflammatory:** • Sarcoidosis (bilateral, eggshell calcification) • Amyloidosis **Intoxication:** • Silicosis	**Neoplastic:** • Bronchogenic CA (unilateral) • Lymphoma
Ring shadow Annular opacity with central lucency (See Figure 10-10)	**Infectious:** • TB (apex) • Lung abscess • Fungal • Amebiasis	**Neoplastic:** • Bronchogenic carcinoma • Metastases • Lymphoma **Autoimmune:** • Rheumatoid lung dz
Unilaterally elevated diaphragm (See Figure 10-11)	**Trauma:** • Phrenic nerve palsy **Congenital:** • Pulmonary hypoplasia scoliosis	**Vascular:** • Pulmonary embolism
Bilaterally elevated diaphragm	• Obesity • Pregnancy • Fibrotic lung dz	
Steeple sign Narrowed area of subglottic trachea	Parainfluenza virus (croup)	
Thumb sign	Epiglottitis classically caused by *Haemophilus influenzae*	
Pneumoperitoneum Free air under the diaphragm on an upright chest film or upright abdomen **Double wall sign on abdominal plain film** The appearance of the outer & inner walls of bowel is almost pathognomonic for pneumoperitoneum	**Inflammatory:** • Perforation ◊ Ulcer ◊ Diverticulitis ◊ Appendicitis ◊ Toxic megacolon ◊ Infarcted bowel	Also can be: • Peritoneal dialysis • Pneumomediastinum that has tracked inferiorly • Diaphragmatic rupture

RADIOLOGY

TABLE 10-2 *Continued*

FINDING/DESCRIPTION	DIFFERENTIAL DIAGNOSIS	
Gasless abdomen on abdominal plain film (See Figure 10-12)	• Obstruction • Severe ascites • Pancreatitis	
Filling defects in stomach on upper GI series	• Gastric ulcer • Gastric cancer	

Dilated small bowel (See Figures 10-12 and 10-13)	• Mechanical obstruction
	  ◊ Postsurgical
	  ◊ Incarcerated hernia
	  ◊ Intussusception
		• Paralytic ileus
		Inflammatory:
		• Celiac sprue
		• Scleroderma

Coffee bean sigmoid volvulus (See Figure 10-14)	• Large bowel obstruction • Paralytic ileus	
String sign on barium swallow Narrowing of the terminal ileum caused by thickening of the bowel wall	• Crohn's disease	
Lead pipe sign on barium enema Smooth, narrowed colon without haustra	• Inflammatory bowel dz (See Figure 10-15)	
Apple core lesion Circumferential growth in the bowel lumen	• Colon cancer	
Liver calcifications	**Inflammatory:** • Granuloma • Hydatid cyst	**Neoplastic:** • Hepatoma
Gas in portal vein Linear lucencies that reach within 2 cm of liver capsule	**Vascular (seen in adults):** • Mesenteric infarct • Air embolism	**Inflammatory (children):** • Necrotizing enterocolitis
Unilateral cystic renal mass Hypodensities with thin walls	**Inflammatory:** • Renal abscess • Hemodialysis-induced cyst • Hydatid cyst	**Congenital:** • Bilateral renal cysts • Polycystic kidney dz **Neoplastic:** • Renal cell carcinoma
String of beads on renal arteriogram Multiple dilatations alternating with strictures of both renal arteries	• Fibromuscular dysplasia	

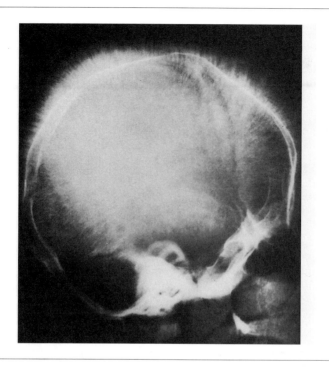

FIGURE 10-2   "Hair-on-end" appearance.

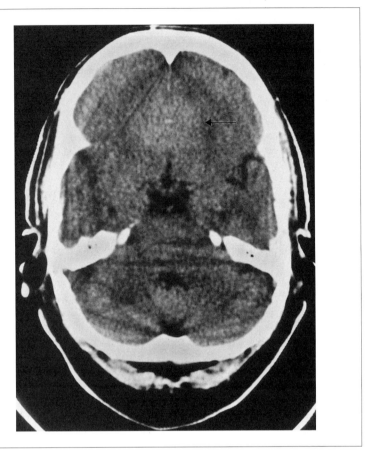

FIGURE 10-3   Hypodense mass on CT.

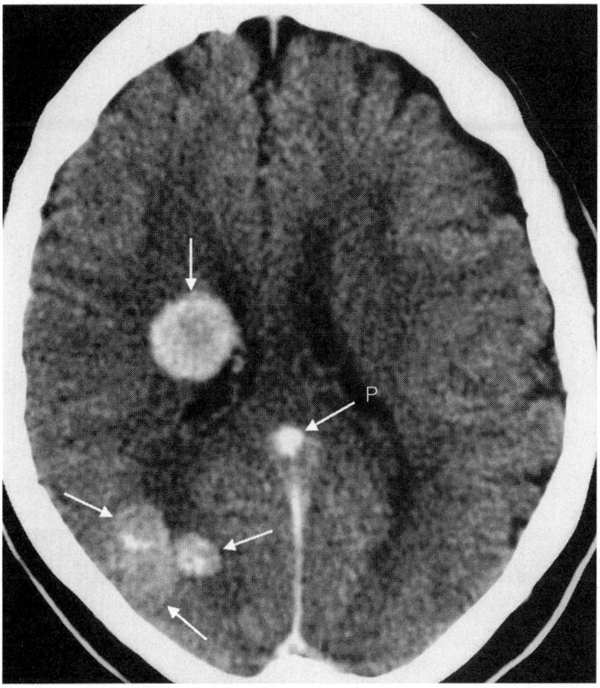

FIGURE 10-4   Metastases (arrows). (P = pineal.)

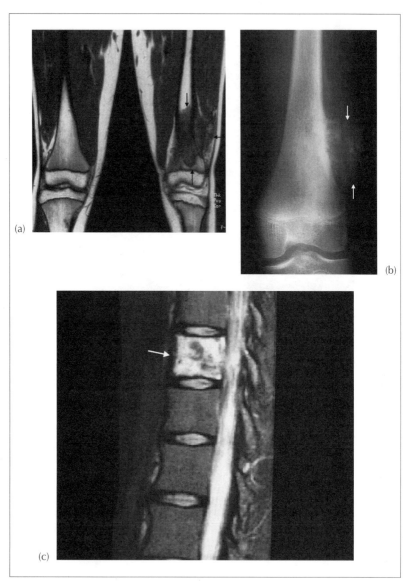

FIGURE 10-5 MRI imaging of bone tumors. (a) T1-weighted scan of osteosarcoma in the lower shaft and metaphysis of the left femur. The extent of tumor (arrows) within the bone and the soft-tissue extension are both very well shown. This information is not available from the plain film (b), although the plain film provides a more specific diagnosis, because the bone formation within the soft-tissue extension (arrows) is obvious. (c) T2-weighted scan of lymphoma in the T10 vertebral body (arrow). The very high signal of the neoplastic tissue is very evident even though there is no deformity of shape of the vertebral body.

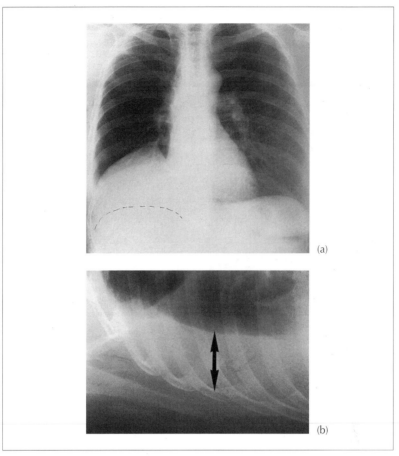

(a)

(b)

FIGURE 10-6   Large right subpulmonary effusion (the patient has had right mastectomy). Almost all the fluid is between the lung and the diaphragm. The right hemidiaphragm cannot be seen. (a) Its estimated position has been penciled in. (b) In the lateral decubitus view, the fluid moves to lie between the lateral chest wall and the lung edge (arrows).

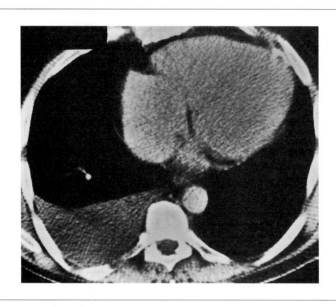

FIGURE 10-7   CT of pleural fluid. The right pleural effusion is of homogeneous density, with a CT number between zero and soft tissue. Its well-defined, meniscus-shaped border with the lung is typical.

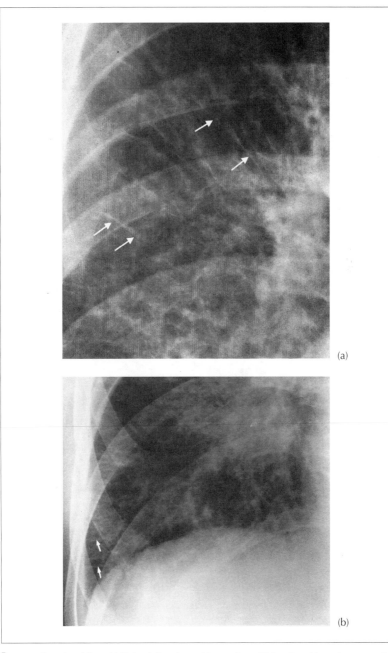

(a)

(b)

FIGURE 10-8   Septal lines. (a) Kerley A lines (arrows) in a patient with lymphangitis carcinomatosa. (b) Kerley B lines in a patient with pulmonary edema. The septal lines (arrows) are thinner than the adjacent blood vessels. The B lines are seen in the outer centimeter of lung where blood vessels are invisible or very difficult to identify.

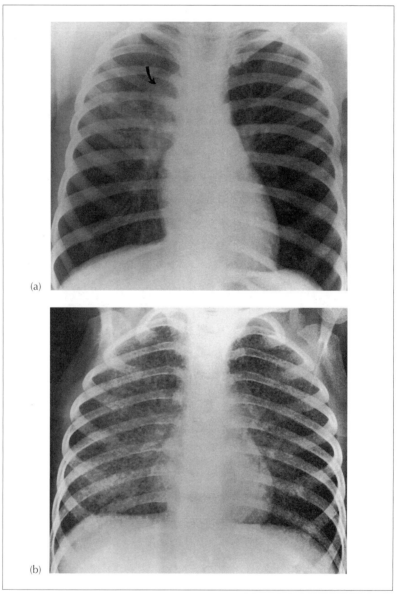

(a)

(b)

FIGURE 10-9   Tuberculosis. (a) The primary complex. This 7-year-old child shows ill-defined consolidation in the right lung together with enlargement of the draining lymph nodes (arrow). (b) Miliary tuberculosis. The innumerable small nodular shadows uniformly distributed throughout the lungs in this young child are typical of miliary tuberculosis. In this instance, no primary focus of infection is visible.

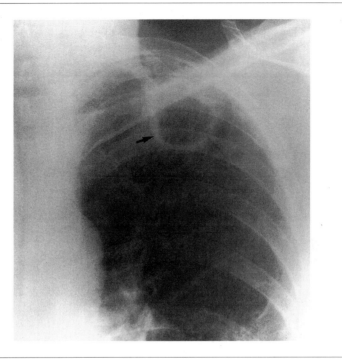

FIGURE 10-10   Fungus infection. The cavity (arrow) in this patient from the southeastern US was due to North American blastomycosis. Note the similarity to tuberculosis. Other fungi, e.g., histoplasmosis, can give an identical appearance.

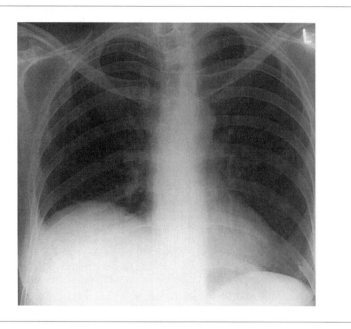

FIGURE 10-11   Elevated right diaphragm.

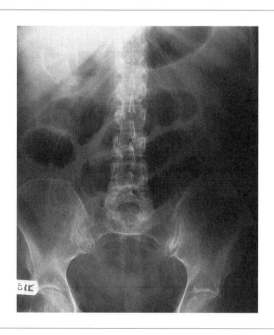

FIGURE 10-12   Small bowel obstruction: distended small bowel and absence of gas shadows in the colon.

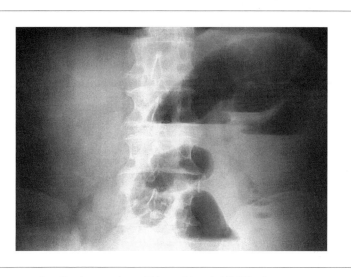

FIGURE 10-13   Erect film demonstrating multiple small bowel air/fluid levels.

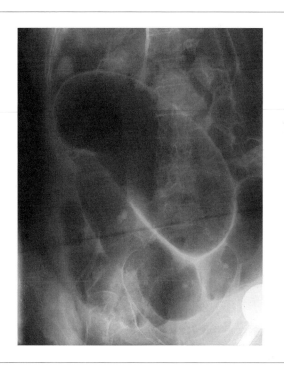

FIGURE 10-14   Sigmoid volvulus with a grossly distended sigmoid.

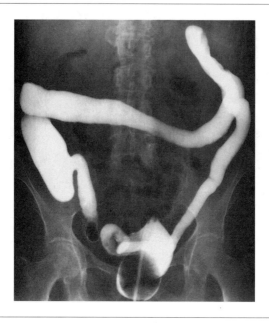

FIGURE 10-15   Ulcerative colitis. With long-standing disease the haustra are lost and the colon becomes narrowed and shortened, coming to resemble a rigid tube. Reflux into the ileum through an incompetent ileocecal valve has occurred.

Appendix A. Zebras and Syndromes

DISEASE	DESCRIPTION/SX
Achondroplasia	Autosomal dominant dwarfism due to early epiphyseal closure → shortening & thickening of bones. Si/Sx = leg bowing, hearing loss, sciatica, infantile hydrocephalus. Patients can live normal lifespans.
Adrenoleuko-dystrophy	X-linked recessive defect in long-chain fatty acid metabolism due to a peroxisomal enzyme deficiency. Causes rapidly progressing central demyelination, adrenal insufficiency, hyperpigmentation of skin, spasticity, seizures & death by age 12.
Albers-Schönberg disease (osteopetrosis)	↑↑ skeletal density due to osteoclastic failure → multiple fractures due to ↓ perfusion of thick bone, also causes anemia due to ↓ marrow space & blindness, deafness & cranial nerve dysfunction due to narrowing & impingement of neural foramina.
Alkaptonuria	Defect of phenylalanine metabolism causing accumulation of homogentisic acid. Presents with black urine, ochronosis (blue-black pigmentation of ear, nose, cheeks) & arthropathy due to cartilage binding homogentisic acid.
Alport's syndrome	X-linked hereditary collagen defect causing sensorineural hearing loss, lens dislocation, hematuria (glomerulonephritis).
Ataxia-Telangiectasia	DNA repair defect affects B & T lymphocytes. Autosomal recessive disease usually appears by age 2. Physical signs include ataxia of gait, telangiectasias of skin & conjunctiva, & recurrent sinus infections.
Banti's syndrome	"Idiopathic portal HTN." Splenomegaly & portal HTN following subclinical portal vein occlusion. Insidious onset, occurring years after initial occlusive event.
Bartter's syndrome	Kidney disease that causes Na, K & Cl wasting. Despite increased levels of renin, the blood pressure remains low.
Beckwith-Wiedemann syndrome	Autosomal dominant fetal overgrowth syndrome of macrosomia, microcephaly, macroglossia, organomegaly, omphalocele, distinctive lateral earlobe fissures, hypoglycemia associated with hyperinsulinemia, ↑ incidence of Wilms' tumor.
Bernard-Soulier syndrome	Autosomal recessive defect of platelet GpIb receptor (binds to vWF), presents with chronic, severe mucosal bleeds & giant platelets on blood smear.
Binswanger's disease	Subacute subcortical dementia caused by small artery infarcts in periventricular white matter. Usually seen in long-standing hypertension, but is rare.
Bruton's agamma-globulinemia	X-linked block of B-cell maturation, causing ↓ B cell levels & immunoglobulin levels. Presents with recurrent bacterial infections in infants >6 mo of age.
Caisson's disease	Decompression sickness ("the bends") caused by rapid ascent from deep-sea diving. Sx occur from 30 min to 1 hr = joint pain, cough, skin burning/mottling.
Caroli's disease	Segmental cystic dilation of intrahepatic bile ducts complicated by stones & cholangitis, can be cancer precursor.
Charcot-Marie-Tooth disease	Autosomal dominant peroneal muscular atrophy causing foot drop & stocking-glove decrease in vibration/pain/temperature sense & DTRs in lower extremities. Histologically → repeated demyelination & remyelination of segmental areas of the nerve. Patients may present as children (type 1) or adults (type 2).
Chediak-Higashi syndrome	Autosomal recessive defect of microtubule function of neutrophils, leads to decreased lysosomal fusion to phagosomes. Presents with recurrent *Staphylococcus* & *Streptococcus* infections, albinism, peripheral & cranial neuropathies.
Cheyne-Stokes respirations	A central apnea seen in CHF, ↑ ICP, or cerebral infection/inflammation/trauma: cycles of central apnea followed by regular crescendo-decrescendo breathing (amplitude first waxes & then wanes back to apnea): Biot's is an uncommon variant seen in meningitis in which the cycles consist of central apnea followed by steady amplitude breathing that then shuts back off to apnea.

DISEASE	DESCRIPTION/SX
Chronic granulomatous disease	Phagocytes lack respiratory burst or NADPH oxidase, so can engulf bacteria but are unable to kill them. Presents with recurrent infections with *Aspergillus* & *S. aureus* infections. Tx = recombinant interferon-γ.
Cystinuria	Autosomal recessive failure of tubular resorption of cystine & dibasic amino acids (lysine, ornithine, arginine), clinically see cystine stones. Tx = hydration to ↑ urine volume, alkalinization of urine with bicarbonate & acetazolamide.
de Quervain's tenosynovitis	Tenosynovitis causing pain on flexion of thumb (motion of abductor pollicis longus).
Diamond-Blackfan syndrome	"Pure red cell aplasia," a congenital or acquired deficiency in the RBC stem cell. Congenital disorder is sometimes associated with abnormal facies, cardiac & renal abnormalities. Tx = steroids.
DiGeorge's syndrome	Embryologic defect in development of pharyngeal pouches 3 & 4 → thymic aplasia that causes T-cell deficiency, & parathyroid aplasia. Most commonly presents with tetany due to hypocalcemia secondary to hypoparathyroidism, & recurrent severe viral, fungal, or protozoal infections.
Dressler's syndrome	Acute pericarditis, develops within 2–4 wk after acute MI or heart surgery, may be due to autoimmune reaction to myocardial antigens.
Ehlers-Danlos syndrome	Autosomal dominant defect in collagen synthesis, variable expressivity. Si/Sx = loose joints, pathognomonic ↓ skin elasticity, mitral regurgitation, genu recurvatum of knee (fixed in hyperextension), aortic dilation.
Ehrlichiosis	Rickettsial family member, *Ehrlichiosis canis*, causes acute febrile illness, malaise, myalgia, severe headache but with no rash. The protracted illness presents with leukopenia, thrombocytopenia & renal failure. It is contracted by tick bites.
Ellis-van Creveld	Syndrome of polydactyly + single atrium.
Erb's paralysis	Waiter's tip—upper-brachial plexopathy (C5,6).
Evan's syndrome	IgG autoantibody-mediated hemolytic anemia & thrombocytopenia, associated with collagen-vascular dz, TTP, hepatic cirrhosis, leukemia, sarcoidosis, Hashimoto's thyroiditis. Tx = prednisone & intravenous immunoglobulin.
Fabry's disease	X-linked defect in galactosidase, Sx = deficient trunk skin lesions, corneal opacity, renal/cardiac/cerebral disease that are invariably lethal in infancy or childhood.
Fanconi's anemia	Autosomal recessive disorder of DNA repair. Presents with pancytopenia, ↑ risk of malignancy, short stature, bird-like facies, café-au-lait spots, congenital urogenital defects, retardation, absent thumb.
Fanconi syndrome	Dysfunction of proximal renal tubules, congenital or acquired (drugs, multiple myeloma, toxic metals), presenting with ↓ reabsorption of glucose, amino acids, phosphate, & bicarbonate. Associated with RTA type II, clinically see glycosuria, hyperphosphaturia, hypophosphatemia (vitamin D–resistant rickets), aminoaciduria (generalized, not cystine specific), systemic acidosis, polyuria, polydipsia.
Farber's disease	Auto recessive defect in ceramidase, causing ceramide accumulation in nerves, onset within months of birth, death occurs by age 2.
Felty's syndrome	Rheumatoid arthritis plus splenomegaly & neutropenia, often with thrombocytopenia.
Fibrolamellar carcinoma	Variant of hepatocellular carcinoma. Occurs in young people (20–40 yr), is not associated with viral hepatitis or cirrhosis. Has a good Px. Histologically shows nests & cords of malignant hepatocytes separated by dense collagen bundles.
Fitz-Hugh-Curtis syndrome	Chlamydia or gonorrhea perihepatitis as a complication of pelvic inflammatory disease. Presents with right upper quadrant pain & sepsis.
Galactosemia	Deficient galactose-1-phosphate uridyl transferase blocks galactose conversion to glucose for further metabolism, leading to accumulation of galactose in many tissues. Sx = failure to thrive, infantile cataracts, mental retardation, cirrhosis. Rarely due to galactokinase deficiency, blocking the same path at a different step.
Gardner's syndrome	Familial polyposis syndrome with classic triad of desmoid tumors, osteomas of mandible or skull & sebaceous cysts.

DISEASE	DESCRIPTION/SX
Gaucher's disease	The most frequent cause of lysosomal enzyme deficiency in Ashkenazi Jews. Autosomal recessive deficiency in β-glucocerebrosidase. Accumulation of sphingolipids in liver, spleen & bone marrow. Can be fatal if very expensive enzyme substitute (alglucerase) not administered.
Glanzmann's thrombasthenia	Autosomal recessive defect in GpIIbIIIa platelet receptor that binds fibrinogen, inhibiting platelet aggregation, presents with chronic, severe mucosal bleeds.
Glycogenoses	Genetic defects in metabolic enzymes causing glycogen accumulation. Si/Sx = hepatosplenomegaly, general organomegaly, exertional fatigue, hypoglycemia. Type I = von Gierke's disease, type II = Pompe's disease, type III = Cori's disease, type V = McCardle's disease.
Hartnup's disease	Autosomal recessive defect in tryptophan absorption at renal tubule. Sx mimic pellagra = the 3 D's: Dermatitis, Dementia, Diarrhea (tryptophan is niacin precursor). Rash is on sun-exposed areas, can see cerebellar ataxia, mental retardation & psychosis. Tx = niacin supplements.
Hepatorenal syndrome	Renal failure without intrinsic renal dz, occurring during fulminant hepatitis or cirrhosis, presents with acute oliguria & azotemia, typically progressive & fatal.
Holt-Oram syndrome	Autosomal dominant atrial septal defect in association with finger-like thumb or absent thumb, & cardiac conduction abnormalities & other skeletal defects.
Homocystinuria	Deficiency in cystine metabolism. Sx mimic Marfan's = lens dislocation (downward in homocystinuria as opposed to upward in Marfan's), thin bones, mental retardation, hypercoagulability & premature atherosclerosis → strokes & MIs.
Hunter's disease	X-linked lysosomal iduronidase deficiency, less severe than Hurler's syndrome. Sx = mild mental retardation, cardiac problems, micrognathia, etc.
Hurler's disease	Defect in iduronidase, causing multiorgan mucopolysaccharide accumulation, dwarfism, hepatosplenomegaly, corneal clouding, progressive mental retardation & death by age 10.
Isovalinic acidemia	"Sweaty-foot odor" disease. Caused by a defect in leucine metabolism, leads to buildup of isovaline in the bloodstream, producing characteristic odor.
Job's syndrome	B-cell defect causing hyper-IgE levels but defects in other immunoglobulin & immune functions. Presents with recurrent pulmonary infections, dermatitis, excess teeth (pts unable to shed their baby teeth), frequent bone fractures, classic "gargoyle facies," IgE levels 10- to 100-fold higher than normal.
Kasabach-Merritt	An expanding hemangioma trapping platelets, leading to systemic thrombocytopenia.
Keshan's disease	Childhood cardiomyopathy 2° to selenium deficiency, very common in China.
Klippel-Trénaunay-Weber syndrome	Autosomal dominant chromosomal translocation → prematurity, hydrops fetalis, hypertrophic hemangioma of leg & Kasabach-Merritt thrombocytopenia.
Klumpke's paralysis	Clawed hand—lower brachial-plexopathy (C8, T1) affecting ulnar nerve distributions, often presents with Horner's syndrome as well.
Leigh's disease	Mitochondrially inherited dz → absent or ↓↓ thiamine pyrophosphate. Infants or children present with seizures, ataxia, optic atrophy, ophthalmoplegia, tremor.
Lesch-Nyhan syndrome	Congenital defect in HPRT → gout, urate nephrolithiasis, retardation, choreiform spasticity & self-mutilation (patients bite off their own fingers & lips). Mild deficiency → Kelley-Seegmiller syndrome = gout without nervous system Si/Sx.
Leukocyte adhesion deficiency	Type I due to lack of β$_2$-integrins (LFA-1), type II due to lack of fucosylated glycoproteins (selectin receptors). Both have plenty of neutrophils in blood but can't enter tissues due to problems with adhesion & transmigration. Both present with recurrent bacterial infections, gingivitis, poor wound healing & delayed umbilical cord separation.
Lhermitte sign	Tingling down the back during neck flexion, occurs in any craniocervical disorder.
Liddle's disease	Disease mimics hyperaldosteronism. Defect is in the renal epithelial transporters. Si/Sx = HTN, hypokalemic metabolic alkalosis.

DISEASE	DESCRIPTION/SX
Li-Fraumeni's syndrome	Autosomal dominant inherited defect of p53 leading to primary cancers of a variety of organ systems presenting at an early age.
Maple syrup urine disease	Disorder of branched chain amino acid metabolism (valine, leucine, isoleucine). Sx include vomiting, acidosis & pathognomonic maple-like odor of urine.
Marchiafava-Bignami syndrome	Overconsumption of red wine → demyelination of corpus callosum, anterior commissure & middle cerebellar peduncles. Possibly anoxic/ischemic phenomenon.
Marfan's disease	Genetic collagen defect → tall, thin body habitus, long & slender digits, pectus excavatum, scoliosis, aortic valve dilation → regurgitation, aortic dissection, mitral valve prolapse, joint laxity, optic lens dislocations & blue sclera. Think about Abe Lincoln when considering this disease, tall & thin.
Melanosis coli	Overzealous use of laxatives causing darkening of colon, but no significant dz.
Mendelson's syndrome	Chemical pneumonitis following aspiration of acidic gastric juice, patient presents with acute dyspnea, tachypnea & tachycardia, with pink & frothy sputum.
Meralgia paresthetica	A condition common to truckers, hikers & overweight individuals who wear heavy backpacks or very tight-fitting belts compressing inguinal area. This causes patients to have a diffuse unilateral pain & paresthesias along anterior portion of upper thigh, corresponding to lateral femoral cutaneous nerve. Typically self-limiting, but can treat with steroids for refractory disease.

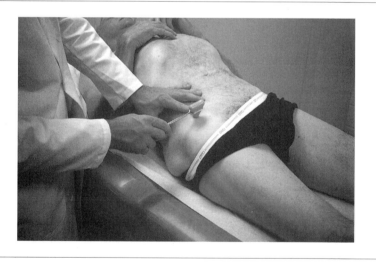

FIGURE A-1   Meralgia paresthetica.

DISEASE	DESCRIPTION/SX
Minamata disease	Toxic encephalopathy from mercury poisoning, classically described from fish eaten near Japanese mercury dumping site.
Molluscum contagiosum	Poxvirus skin infection causing umbilicated papules, transmitted by direct contact, often venereal. The central umbilication is filled with semi-solid white material that contains inclusion bodies & is highly characteristic for the disease.
Monckeberg's arteriosclerosis	Calcific sclerosis of the media of medium-sized arteries, usually radial & ulnar. Occurs in people over 50, but it does NOT obstruct arterial flow since intima is not involved. It is unrelated to other atherosclerosis & does not cause dz.
Munchausen's syndrome	A factitious disorder in which the pt derives gratification from feigning a serious or dramatic illness. Munchausen's by proxy is when the pt derives gratification from making someone else ill (often a mother injures her child for attention).
Niemann-Pick's disease	Autosomal recessive defect in sphingomyelinase with variable age onset (↑ severe dz in younger pt) → demyelination/neurologic Sx, hepatosplenomegaly, xanthoma, pancytopenia.
Noonan's syndrome	Autosomal dominant with Sx similar to Turner's syndrome → hyperelastic skin, neck webbing, ptosis, low-set ears, short stature, pulmonary stenosis, AS defect, coarctation of aorta, small testes. Presents in males, X & Y are both present.
Ortner's syndrome	Impingement of recurrent laryngeal nerve by the enlarging atrium in mitral regurgitation, leading to hoarseness.
Osteogenesis imperfecta	Genetic disorder of diffuse bone weakness due to mutations resulting in defective collagen synthesis. Multiple fractures 2° to minimal trauma = brittle bone disease. Classic sign = blue sclera, due to translucent connective tissue over choroid.
Peliosis hepatis	Rare primary dilation of hepatic sinusoids. Associated with exposure to anabolic steroids, oral contraceptives & danazol. Irregular cystic spaces filled with blood develop in the liver. Cessation of drug intake causes reversal of the lesions.
Plummer-Vinson syndrome	Iron deficiency syndrome with classic triad of esophageal web, spoon nail & iron deficiency anemia. Webs produce dysphagia, will regress with iron replacement.
Polycystic kidney disease	Autosomal dominant bilateral dz, Si/Sx = onset in early or middle adult life with hematuria, nephrolithiasis, uremia, 33% of cases have cysts in liver, 10–20% of cases have intracranial aneurysms, hypertension is present in 50% of pts at Dx. Juvenile version is autosomal recessive, much rarer than adult type; almost all cases have cysts in liver & portal bile duct proliferation = "congenital hepatic fibrosis."
Poncet's disease	Polyarthritis that occurs DURING active TB infection but no organisms can be isolated from the affected joints, is thought to be autoimmune-mediated disease.
Pott's disease	Tubercular infection of vertebrae (vertebral osteomyelitis) leading to kyphoscoliosis secondary to pathologic fractures.
Potter's syndrome	Bilateral renal agenesis; incompatible with fetal life, mother has oligohydramnios because fetus normally swallows large quantities of amniotic fluid & then urinates it out, but fetus cannot excrete swallowed fluid because it has no kidneys.
Prinzmetal's angina	Variant angina occurring at rest due to vasospasm, EKG → ST elevation instead of depression. Tx = calcium channel blockers.
Refsum's disease	Autosomal recessive defect in phytanic acid metabolism → peripheral neuropathy, cerebellar ataxia, retinitis pigmentosa, bone disease & ichthyosis (scaly skin).
Rett's syndrome	Congenital retardation secondary to ↑ serum ammonia levels, more common in females. Sx = autism, dementia, ataxia, tremors.
Schafer's disease	Defect in hexosaminidase B, in contrast to the A component of the enzyme that is defective in Tay-Sachs. Px is better for Schafer's.
Schindler's disease	Defect in N-acetylgalactosaminidase.
Schmidt's syndrome	Hashimoto's thyroiditis with diabetes &/or Addison's disease (autoimmune syndrome).

DISEASE	DESCRIPTION/Sx
Sweet's syndrome (See Color Plate 31)	Recurrent painful reddish-purple plaques & papules associated with fever, arthralgia & neutrophilia. Occurs more commonly in women, possibly due to hypersensitivity reaction associated with *Yersinia* infection. Can also be seen in following URI or along with leukemia. Tx = prednisone, antibiotics if associated with *Yersinia* infection.
Syndrome X	Angina relieved by rest (typical) with a normal angiogram. Caused by vasospasm of small arterioles, unlike Prinzmetal's angina, which is vasospasm of large arteries.
Tay-Sachs disease	Autosomal recessive defect in hexosaminidase A, causing very early onset, progressive retardation, paralysis, dementia, blindness, cherry-red spot on macula & death by 3–4 yr. Common in Ashkenazi Jews.
Tropical spastic paraparesis	Insidious lower extremity paresis caused by HTLV, which is endemic to Japan & the Caribbean, transmitted like HIV, via placenta, body fluids & sex. Presents with mild sensory deficits, marked lower extremity hyperreflexia, paralysis, urinary incontinence.
Turcot's syndrome	Familial adenomatous polyposis with CNS medulloblastoma or glioma.
Usher syndrome	Most common condition involving both hearing & vision impairment. Autosomal recessive dz → deafness & retinitis pigmentosa (a form of night blindness).
Verner-Morrison syndrome	VIPoma = vasoactive intestinal polypeptide overproduction. Leads to pancreatic cholera, increased watery diarrhea, dehydration, hypokalemia, hypo/ achlorhydria.
Von Recklinghausen's disease	Diffuse osteolytic lesions caused by hyperparathyroidism causing characteristic "brown tumor" of bone due to hemorrhage. Can mimic osteoporosis on x-rays.
Wiskott-Aldrich syndrome	X-linked recessive defect in IgM response to capsular polysaccharides like those of *S. pneumoniae*, but pts have ↑ IgA levels. Classic triad = recurrent pyogenic bacteria infections, eczema, thrombocytopenia. Bloody diarrhea is often first Sx, then URIs; leukemia & lymphoma are common in children who survive to age 10.
Xeroderma pigmentosa	Defect in repair of DNA damage caused by UV light (pyrimidine dimers). Patients highly likely to develop skin cancers. Only Tx is avoidance of sunlight.

Appendix B. Toxicology

TOXIN	SI/SX	DX	ANTIDOTE
Acetaminophen	Nausea/vomiting within 2 hr, ↑ liver enzymes, ↑ prothrombin time at 24–48 hr	Blood level	N-acetylcysteine within 8–10 hr
Alkali agents	Derived from batteries, dishwasher detergent, drain cleaners, ingestion causes mucosal burns → dysphagia & drooling	Clinical	Milk or water, then NPO
Anticholinergic	**Dry as a bone, mad as a hatter, blind as a bat, hot as a hare** (delirium, miosis, fever)	Clinical	Physostigmine
Arsenic	Mees lines (white horizontal stripes on fingernails), capillary leak, seizures	Blood level	Gastric lavage & dimercaprol
Aspirin	Tinnitus, respiratory alkalosis, **anion gap metabolic acidosis with normal S_{OSM}**[a]	Blood level	Bicarbonate, dialysis
Benzodiazepine	Rapid onset of weakness, ataxia, drowsiness	Blood level	Flumazenil
β-Blockers	Bradycardia, heart block, obtundation, **hyperkalemia, hypoglycemia**	Clinical	Glucagon, IV calcium
Carbon monoxide	Dyspnea, confusion, coma, **cherry-red color of skin**, mucosal cyanosis	Carboxy-Hgb[b]	100% O_2 or hyperbaric O_2
Cyanide	In seconds to minutes → trismus, **almond-scented breath**, coma	Blood level	Amyl nitrite ⊕ Na thiosulfate
Digoxin	**Change in color vision, supraventricular tacyhcardia with heart block**, vomiting	Blood level[c]	Anti-digoxin Fab-antibodies
Ethylene glycol	**Calcium oxalate crystals in urine, anion gap metabolic acidosis with high S_{OSM}**[a]	Blood level	Ethanol drip, fomepizole[d]
Heparin	Bleeding, thrombocytopenia	Clinical	Protamine
Iron	Vomiting, bloody diarrhea, acidosis, CXR → radiopaque tablets	Blood level	Deferoxamine
Isoniazid	Confusion, peripheral neuropathy	Blood level	Pyridoxine
Lead	**Microcytic anemia with basophilic stippling**, ataxia, retardation, peripheral neuropathy, **purple lines on gums**	Blood level	EDTA, penicillamine
Mercury	**"Erethism" = ↓ memory, insomnia, timidity, delirium (mad as a hatter)**	Blood level	Ipecac, dimercaprol
Methanol	**Anion gap metabolic acidosis with high S_{OSM}**,[a] **blindness, optic disk hyperemia**	Blood level	Ethanol drip, bicarbonate
Opioids	CNS/respiratory depression, miosis	Blood level	Narcan
Organophosphate	Incontinence, cough, wheezing, dyspnea, miosis, bradycardia, heart block, tremor	Blood level	Atropine, pralidoxime
Phenobarbital	CNS depression, hypothermia, miosis, hypotensions	Blood level	Charcoal, bicarbonate
Quinidine	Torsades des pointes (ventricular tachycardia)	Blood level	IV magnesium
Theophylline	First Sx = hematemesis, then CNS → seizures or coma, cardiac → arrhythmias, hypotension	Blood level[c]	Ipecac, charcoal, cardiac monitor
Tricyclics	Anticholinergic Sx, QRS >100 ms, torsades des pointes	Blood level	Bicarbonate drip
Warfarin	Bleeding	↑ PT	Vitamin K

[a] S_{OSM} = serum osmolality; [b] carboxyhemoglobin; [c] correlates in acute but not chronic toxicity; [d] see N Engl J Med 1999, 340:832–838.

Appendix C. Vitamins and Nutrition

Nutrient	Deficiency	Excess
B₁ (thiamine)	Dry beriberi → neuropathy Wet beriberi → high-output cardiac failure Either → Wernicke-Korsakoff's syndrome	
B₂ (riboflavin)	Cheilosis (mouth fissures)	
B₃ (niacin)	Pellagra → dementia, diarrhea, dermatitis Also seen in Hartnup's disease (dz of tryptophan metabolism)	
B₅ (pantothenate)	Enteritis, dermatitis	
B₆ (pyridoxine)	Neuropathy (frequently caused by isoniazid therapy for TB)	
B₁₂ (cyanocobalamin)	Pernicious anemia (lack of intrinsic factor) → neuropathy, megaloblastic anemia, glossitis	
Biotin	Dermatitis, enteritis (caused by ↑ consumption of raw eggs, due to the avidin in the raw eggs blocking biotin absorption)	
Chromium	Glucose intolerance (cofactor for insulin)	
Copper	Leukopenia, bone demineralization	
Folic acid	Neural tube defects, megaloblastic anemia	
Iodine	Hypothyroidism, cretinism, goiter	
Iron	Plummer-Vinson syndrome = esophageal webs, spoon nails	Hemochromatosis → multiorgan failure (bronze diabetes)
Selenium	Myopathy (Keshan's disease, see Appendix A)	
Vitamin A	Metaplasia of respiratory epithelia (seen in cystic fibrosis due to failure of fat-soluble vitamin absorption), xerophthalmia, night blindness (lack of retinal in rod cells), acne, Bitot's spots, frequent respiratory infections (respiratory epithelial defects)	Pseudotumor cerebri (can be caused by consuming polar bear livers), headache, nausea, vomiting, skin peeling
Vitamin C	Scurvy: poor healing, hypertrophic bleeding gums, easy bruising, deficient osteoid mimicking rickets	
Vitamin D	Rickets in kids, osteomalacia in adults	Kidney stones, dementia, constipation, abdominal pain, depression
Vitamin E	Fragile RBCs, sensory & motor peripheral neuropathy	
Vitamin K	Clotting deficiency	
Zinc	Poor wound healing, decreased taste & smell, alopecia, diarrhea, dermatitis, depression (similar to pellagra)	
Calories	**Marasmus** = total calorie malnutrition → pts look deceptively well, but immunosuppressed, poor wound healing, impaired growth	
Protein	**Kwashiorkor** = protein malnutrition → edema/ascites, immunosuppression, poor wound healing, impaired growth & development	

Questions

1. A 60-year-old man dressed in combat fatigues is arrested by the police in a public square after screaming that he was "going to act like Rambo and kill all you VC commies!" The initial police investigation reveals that he had served one tour of duty in Vietnam with the Marines and was honorably discharged. A police psychiatrist is called in to interview the man. During the interview, the man sits proud and arrogantly looks down upon all his interrogators, accusing them of being "in cahoots with the Reds" and that "nothing you do to me today will make me talk" as he had been one of the handful of Americans to escape the infamous POW prison known as the "Hanoi Hilton." The man further boasts that he was a member of the Marine's elite Force Recon and had been a sniper credited with the most confirmed kills during his tour of duty. He further adds that if they do not release him soon, "Rambo is going to come looking for me."

    Meanwhile, police detectives learn that the man had adjusted well to civilian life after Vietnam. He was married, had many friends, had no criminal record, and was working as an accountant. However, a review of his military record reveals that while he had indeed served a tour in Vietnam as a Marine, he had been an embassy guard and had never come under direct fire, his tour concluding well before the Tet offensive; neither had he ever been a prisoner of war. He had never undergone sniper training, and had never been asked to join the elite Force Recon.

    When the man's wife is contacted by police, she is both very distressed and relieved because her husband had gone on a week-long business conference out of town and forgotten to take his lithium with him. He had not been in touch with her for several days, and his coworkers on this trip had told her that he had disappeared after acting a little bit out of his normal self. She is relieved that someone has found him.

    Which of the following is the most probable diagnosis for this colorful gentleman?

    A. Posttraumatic stress disorder

    B. Manic episode

    C. Generalized anxiety disorder

    D. Panic disorder

    E. Antisocial personality disorder

2. A 35-year-old man with no significant past medical history presents to your clinic complaining of "ugly toe nails." On exam, it as apparent that he has onychomycosis involving the nails of both feet.

    Which of the following would be the most efficacious treatment to prescribe, considering the elimination of the infection at the lowest toxicity level?

    A. Topical terbinafine

    B. Topical tolnaftate

    C. Topical econazole

D. Oral itraconazole

E. Oral griseofulvin

3. Parents of Eastern European background call their family physician because their 8-month-old son's coordination seems to be off. The parents bring their boy in to the physician's office and, on examination, the physician finds some muscular flaccidity, motor incoordination, and decreased mental and visual acuity. The parents become particularly concerned because both have cousins in Europe who had children with some sort of disorder that resulted in the children's paralysis and vegetative state by age 2, and death before age of 5.

This child is afebrile, and no nuchal rigidity is noted. Exam of the abdomen is negative for hepatosplenomegaly. However, funduscopic exam is positive for a particular finding.

Which of the following classical findings did the clinician observe on the retina?

A. Grayish-white ovoid lesions with irregular, wool-like margins of varying sizes, some just slightly smaller than the size of the disc

B. Small hemorrhagic spots each with a central white area

C. A normal-appearing disc with gray-folded elevations of the retina; over the elevations, the blood vessels appear tortuous whereas elsewhere they appear normal

D. Elevated, edematous discs with blurred margins and tortuous engorged veins

E. A cherry-red spot on the macula

4. An 82-year-old woman with a past medical history of hypertension, presents with weight loss, headache, and generalized weakness. Head CT is obtained and reveals multiple enhancing masses. Of the following, which is the most likely diagnosis (see Figure 10-4)?

A. Glioblastoma multiforme

B. Primary CNS lymphoma

C. Cerebrovascular accident

D. Cerebral metastases

E. Meningioma

5. An 18-year-old man presents with left wrist pain after falling on his hand during a basketball game. Physical examination reveals tenderness of the anatomic "snuff box" and pain response to both passive and active wrist motion. Plain radiograph of the wrist is shown below.

Based on the clinical and radiographic information, which of the following is the correct diagnosis and treatment for this condition (see figure below)?

A. Wrist sprain, ibuprofen for pain control

B. Wrist sprain, oxycodone for pain control

C. Scaphoid fracture, orthopedic consultation and thumb splint for 10 weeks

D. Scaphoid fracture, oxycodone for pain control

E. Triquetrum fracture, orthopedic consultation and thumb splint for 10 weeks

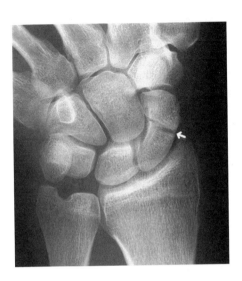

6. A 32-year-old G2P2 woman presents to the clinic and reports she has not menstruated for 3 months. She is a slender, athletically built, successful businesswoman.
   Which of the following is the most likely cause?

   A. Turner's syndrome

   B. Asherman's syndrome

   C. Tumor

   D. Anxiety

   E. Pregnancy

   F. Anorexia

7. A 70-year-old man who recently immigrated to the United States from a developing country presents with complaints of "electrical" radiating leg pain. He also reports sharp abdominal pains with nausea and vomiting, paroxysms of cough, and bladder and rectal spasms. On physical exam, a wide-based gait is observed. Laboratory results include a positive VDRL. Pupillary exam would reveal which of the following?

   A. Bilaterally nonreactive pupils

   B. A left pupil that is larger than the right and reacts minimally to bright light but responds more to accommodation; administration of methacholine drops to both eyes results in a prompt constriction of the left pupil with no response in the right

C. A left pupil that is smaller than the right accompanied by left upper-lid droop; administration of 4% cocaine in both eyes dilates the right pupil but not the left

D. Small pupils that are unreactive to a bright light but do accommodate to light

E. Bilateral pinpoint pupils

8. A 27-year-old woman presents to your office for a routine physical examination. She states that she is generally healthy and does not take any medications. She has no specific health concerns or new symptoms. Her heart rate is 70 beats per minute. Her weight of 60 kg is unchanged from the previous year. However, her blood pressure is found to be 160/95 mm Hg in each arm. One year ago, her blood pressure was recorded as 120/75 mm Hg. Physical examination reveals a high-pitched epigastric bruit. A pregnancy test is negative.

Serum electrolytes are as follows.

Na:	144.0 meq/L
K:	2.8 meq/L
HCO$_3$:	34.0 meq/L
BUN:	15.0 mg/dL
Creat:	1.0 mg/dL

Which of the following is the most likely diagnosis?

A. Primary (essential) hypertension

B. Aortic coarctation

C. Renal artery stenosis

D. Pheochromocytoma

E. Hyperthyroidism

9. A 20-year-old male college student is brought to the ED by his housemates when they found him this morning very lethargic. They deny they had been drinking or using drugs as this was the last day before their final exam period. The patient is lethargic but still able to answer questions. He states that he has been getting very little sleep this week because he has been cramming for exams. He denies taking any medications or herbal supplements to stay awake but admits drinking a lot of coffee (6 cups a day) this week. He also denies using any illicit drugs, which is confirmed by his housemates.

On exam, he has a fever of 101°, BP 125/65, HR 90. He reacts with pain during the exam as his head and neck are examined. Nuchal rigidity is quite prominent. While lying the patient flat, lifting the leg elicits neck pain. A panel of blood tests, including CBC and CHEM7, are drawn.

Which of the following is the next diagnostic step?

A. Go directly to a lumbar puncture

B. Perform a funduscopic exam

C. PPD for possible *Mycobacterium* meningitis

D. Order viral cultures and wait for positive results before initiating antiviral therapy

E. Order a head MRI

10. A 68-year-old man presents to the emergency room with nausea, vomiting, and abdominal pain and distension. He has not passed gas or had a bowel movement for more than 24 hours. He denies previous surgeries of any kind or serious medical illnesses. An abdominal plain film shows multiple, dilated loops of small bowel. A nasogastric tube is placed and IV fluids are administered.

Which of the following is the most likely cause of small bowel obstruction in this patient?

A. Peritoneal adhesions

B. Hernia

C. Neoplasm

D. Crohn's disease

E. Gallstone ileus

11. A 16-year-old presents with the complaint of being "really itchy down there" and "smelling funky." She denies any discharge ("I don't LOOK down there!") or dysuria. She denies sexual activity.

On physical examination, you note no erythema. You do, however, note some green discharge on the vaginal walls. You should treat with

A. fluconazole for the patient.

B. fluconazole for the patient and her partner.

C. metronidazole for the patient.

D. metronidazole for the patient and her partner.

E. yogurt douche for the patient.

12. You have been asked to evaluate a patient for possible alcohol abuse and dependence. You utilize the CAGE questionnaire to do a quick assessment. A more rigorous assessment is indicated when the patient answers "yes" when asked if he or she has ever

A. Consumed more than 8 drinks at one sitting.

B. felt Angered for no apparent reason.

C. felt Guilty about drinking.

D. felt more Energized after a drink.

E. felt more Eloquent after drinking.

13. A 67-year-old woman out shopping with her daughter complains of sudden-onset headache, lightheadedness, and right-sided weakness. Her daughter finds that her mother cannot move her right side.

You are on duty in the ED when the patient is brought in. A fingerstick glucose reads 125. The patient has no known seizure history and no known head trauma.

Which assay should be ordered next?

A. PET scan

B. EEG

C. Head x-ray

D. Carotid dopplers

E. Noncontrast head CT

14. An overweight 48-year-old patient, who has had multiple incidences of vaginitis, presents with a global darkening of her skin color. The patient was previously on the Atkins diet but denies any abnormal eating habits now.
You recommend

A. insulin.

B. steroids.

C. hydroquinone cream.

D. increased exposure to sunlight.

E. phlebotomy.

F. full disclosure of diet.

15. An 88-year-old woman with a history of osteoporosis and dementia is admitted for treatment of a community-acquired pneumonia. During the course of the evening the patient becomes confused, frightened, begins to address people that are not present, and attempts to climb out of bed.
Administration of which of the following would *increase* this patient's fall risk?

A. Haloperidol

B. Fluphenazine

C. Thiothixene

D. Clozapine

E. Chlorpromazine

16. A 17-year-old male presents to your office after being injured during a football game. He describes being blocked on the lateral aspect of the knee while his foot was planted in the ground. He heard a pop and felt significant pain that required him to limp off the field and stop playing. Plain radiographs were negative for fracture. On physical examination, the knee is swollen and the lower leg is easily pulled forward from the upper leg when the patient is supine. The patient is scheduled for an MRI of the knee.
Based on the history and physical examination, which three structures are likely to have been damaged during this injury?

A. Anterior cruciate ligament (ACL), medial collateral ligament (MCL), and medial meniscus

B. ACL, posterior cruciate ligament (PCL), and medial meniscus

C. ACL, lateral collateral ligament (LCL), and lateral meniscus

D. MCL, LCL, and medial meniscus

E. MCL, LCL, and lateral meniscus

17. A 65-year-old man presents to the emergency room with nausea, vomiting, and a distended abdomen. He states that he has been unable to eat very much for several weeks and has not been passing gas. Abdominal plain film shows dilated loops of small bowel. A nasogastric tube is placed and IV fluids are administered. Over the next several days, the patient's symptoms improve. The nasogastric tube is removed and he is nearly ready for discharge. However, the patient is found to be persistently hypokalemic (K = 2.7 meq/L) despite attempts at PO and IV potassium replacement for several days. He does not take any medications.
    Which of the following is the proper course of action?

    A. Place a central line in order to replace potassium at a rate of 40 meq/hr for 12 hours.

    B. Place two peripheral IV catheters in order to replace potassium at a rate of 40 meq/hr for 12 hours.

    C. Begin treatment with a potassium-sparing diuretic such as spironolactone.

    D. Measure serum magnesium levels and replace magnesium if deficient.

    E. Administer calcium gluconate and obtain serial EKGs because the risk for cardiac arrhythmia is very high.

18. A male patient appears in your clinic inquiring whether or not he should receive a pneumonia vaccine.
    Which of the following profiles would indicate use of the vaccine?

    A. An otherwise healthy 35-year-old patient with no spleen

    B. A 50-year-old patient who works in a day care center

    C. A 21-year-old medical student with no medical problems

    D. A 60-year-old with well-controlled hypertension

    E. A 22-year-old with no medical conditions who plans to go to Afghanistan on a photo assignment

19. A 9-month-old previously happy baby is brought in by his maternal grandmother, in whose house he lives with his 15-year-old mother and 13-year-old maternal aunt. Grandmother is concerned because the child has started to cry when his paternal grandfather comes to visit.
    You suspect

    A. inadequate exposure to men.

    B. neglect.

    C. abuse.

    D. colic.

    E. normal development.

20. There are currently many different classes of antidepressants available. If a patient is newly diagnosed with a major depressive episode, and this patient has ongoing suicidal thoughts as well as a history of intentional drug overdose, which of the following antidepressants should absolutely be *avoided* as a first-line medication?

A. Fluoxetine

B. Sertraline

C. Buproprion

D. Imipramine

E. Paroxetine

21. A 78-year-old woman presents to the clinic with increasing shortness of breath on exertion. She has also fainted on two occasions and is often lightheaded after standing up rapidly. Physical examination reveals a midsystolic crescendo-decrescendo murmur at the right sternal border that radiates to the carotids. Peripheral pulses are weak and late when compared to heart sounds.

Which of the following is the proper course of action in this patient?

A. IV penicillin for treatment of presumed endocarditis with echocardiography to confirm the diagnosis

B. Atenolol 25 mg p.o. q.d. to relieve symptoms of congestive heart failure and echocardiography to confirm the diagnosis in the near future

C. Lisinopril 10 mg p.o. q.d. to relieve symptoms of congestive heart failure and echocardiography to confirm the diagnosis in the near future

D. Digitalis 1 mg p.o. × 1.0 and 0.1 mg p.o. q.d. to relieve symptoms of aortic stenosis with echocardiography in the near future

E. Echocardiography to confirm aortic stenosis and referral to a cardiac surgeon

22. A 4-year-old with Down's syndrome is brought by his parents to his primary care doctor because he has refused to walk.

On physical exam, the patient is afebrile. There is no calor, rubor, or tumor on the legs. There is full range of motion passively, bilaterally, although the patient is irritable with the exam. There is no change evidenced on x-ray. White count is elevated to 50,000.

This is most likely

A. septic arthritis.

B. toxic synovitis.

C. leukemia.

D. pauciarticular juvenile rheumatoid arthritis.

E. a fussy child.

23. A 78-year-old male has a past medical history significant only for gastro-esophageal reflux disease (GERD). He presents to clinic complaining of mild abdominal pain, chronic fatigue, and increasing dyspnea on exertion. He denies hematemesis or black or bloody stools. Physical examination reveals generalized and conjunctival pallor. Stool is guaiac negative.

Laboratory results are as follows.

Hemoglobin:	8.4 g/dL
MCV:	77.8 μm³
Ferritin:	5.2 μg/L

Upper endoscopy reveals mild gastritis but is otherwise unremarkable. Which of the following is the most appropriate next course of action?

A. Ferrous sulfate 325 mg p.o. q.d. and reassurance

B. Ferrous sulfate 2 g IV × 1 and reassurance

C. Bone marrow biopsy

D. Abdominal CT

E. Colonoscopy

24. A G3P0 at 12 weeks gestation presents to the clinic for her second prenatal visit. You had ordered labs on her first visit and, upon their review, you learn that the patient is rubella nonimmune.

You recommend

A. voluntary interruption of the pregnancy.

B. immediate vaccination.

C. the vaccine be withheld until after first trimester.

D. the vaccine be withheld until after second trimester.

E. the vaccine be withheld until after third trimester.

F. the vaccine be withheld until after delivery.

G. the vaccine be withheld until the patient leaves the hospital.

H. the vaccine be withheld until first postnatal visit.

25. A 40-year-old hospital worker reports to the hospital's outpatient clinic to request a prescription for sleeping pills. During the interview and history taking, it soon becomes evident that this woman has had insomnia for the past 4 weeks after the death of her mother. This loss occurred just a week after her brother was nearly killed in a motor vehicle collision. In addition, the patient reports that she has been under much financial pressure, working two jobs in order to help support her other brother and his family. This other brother was totally disabled and is unable to work due to injuries he sustained while riding a motorcycle. The patient reports that over the past 4 weeks she has been constantly tearful and crying and feeling depressed, has lost at least 10 pounds, has withdrawn from initiating all social contact with her friends though appreciates the support they have given her, has had trouble concentrating at work, has been unable to both fall asleep and stay asleep, and has strong feelings of guilt for not being present with her mother during her final moments of life. The patient denies any visual or auditory hallucinations as well as any suicidal or homicidal ideation.

According to the DSM-IV criteria, this patient would most appropriately be diagnosed as experiencing

A. a major depressive episode.

B. normal grief/bereavement.

C. an acute adjustment disorder.

D. a brief psychotic disorder.

E. posttraumatic stress disorder.

26. A 26-year-old medical student has been told he needs a repeat purified protein derivative (PPD) before he can be allowed to begin his third year of school. The student was born abroad where BCG vaccine was routinely administered and received at least two doses as a young child.

If this man's PPD comes back with a positive induration of 15 mm (*Candida* and mumps controls both positive), how would you interpret this data?

A. His BCG is providing ongoing immunity to tuberculosis.

B. He needs a chest X-ray to rule out active TB.

C. The result is ambiguous because PPDs are always positive in individuals who received BCG.

D. His BCG is providing weakening immunity with time as you would expect an induration >20 mm in an individual who received two doses of BCG.

E. He needs an HIV test because individuals who received BCG should never have a positive PPD.

27. A 52-year-old woman with a long history of active rheumatoid arthritis undergoes emergency appendectomy while visiting relatives. She does not remember the names of her current medications. Following the surgery, she becomes persistently hypotensive and tachycardic, with a blood pressure of 80/55 mm Hg and heart rate of 120 beats per minute. Her hypotension does not respond to multiple fluid boluses of lactated Ringer's solution. She is also severely fatigued and hyper-kalemic (K = 5.3 meq/L).

Which of the following is the proper course of action in this patient?

A. Continue giving normal saline rapidly; obtain urgent nephrology consultation

B. Blood cultures, broad-spectrum antibiotics, and activated protein C to treat sepsis

C. Emergency echocardiogram to evaluate for congestive heart failure

D. Immediate abdominal CT to evaluate for abscess

E. Serum cortisol level and immediate administration of hydrocortisone 300 mg IV and normal saline

28. JR, an 8-year-old prepubescent boy, presents with a recent pruritic, erythematous rash on his face. He denies any history of insect bites or any systemic symptoms. The boy's mother admits to washing his clothes with a new generic detergent.

The preferred treatment is

A. hydrocortisone 1.0%.

B. hydrocortisone 2.5%.

C. triamcinolone 0.025%.

D. triamcinolone 0.1%.

E. betamethasone 0.1%.

29. A 75-year-old man with a history of hypertension and glaucoma presents to the clinic for a routine exam. During the history taking, the clinic physician finds that the patient's wife of 50 years passed away a year ago. Since that time, he has had poor appetite, poor sleep, loss of weight, feelings of despair and hopelessness, and become socially withdrawn. In addition, the patient has lost his meticulousness with his medications, including his eye drops.

Gross challenge of the patient's visual field would likely reveal which of the following?

A. Loss of the periphery of both eye's visual fields

B. Loss of the central portion of the visual fields

C. Monocular blindness

D. Bitemporal hemianopsia

E. Loss of the right upper quadrant of both visual fields

30. A 4-year-old Moroccan boy waits in the ER waiting room. He sits quietly, leaning forward, and has audible inspiratory stridor. An x-ray shows the "thumbprint sign." When intubating this patient, you note a cherry-red epiglottis.

Administration of which of the following would mostly likely have *prevented* this boy's condition?

A. Hib vaccine

B. Flu vaccine

C. RSV vaccine

D. Pneumococcal vaccine

E. No vaccine—this condition is secondary to a foreign body aspiration

31. A 25-year-old pregnant woman undergoes routine prenatal screening ultrasound. During the test, the technician incidentally notes the presence of multiple, small gallstones. The patient has never had any pain or other symptoms related to gallstones but seeks a surgical opinion on whether or not she should have her gallbladder removed.

Which of the following would you advise?

A. Her lifetime risk of developing biliary colic is approximately 5%.

B. Her lifetime risk of biliary colic is approximately 20% and she should not undergo cholecystectomy unless symptoms develop.

C. Her risk of developing biliary colic within the next year is approximately 20%.

D. She should wait until after pregnancy before undergoing elective laparoscopic cholecystectomy.

E. She should undergo immediate laparoscopic cholecystectomy to prevent acute cholecystitis.

32. A 55-year-old man with hypercholesterolemia presents with an episode of right-sided hemiparesis. The patient is administered a continuous infusion of intravenous normal saline solution containing 5% dextrose. The symptoms resolve in 12 hours. Based on this description, the patient had, by definition, which of the following?

    A. Transient ischemic attack
    B. Stroke
    C. Simple partial seizure
    D. Hypoglycemia
    E. Migraine

33. A 68-year-old man reports mild, increasing fatigue over the past several months. Physical examination is notable for cervical and axillary lymphadenopathy and splenomegaly. A CBC is ordered and reveals a white blood cell count of 234,000/μL. Other cell lines are within normal range. A peripheral blood smear shows multiple small, mature leukocytes with "soccer ball" nuclei.

    Which of the following is *true* for the treatment of this patient?

    A. Early treatment with aggressive chemotherapy will likely be curative.
    B. Immediate bone marrow transplantation is indicated.
    C. The patient has a benign, infectious condition that will resolve spontaneously.
    D. Treatment should focus on reducing symptoms rather than on prolonging life.
    E. The patient will likely die within 3 months.

34. A 78-year-old man is brought to the emergency room after an hour of abdominal pain, light-headedness, nausea, and vomiting. He is unable to provide additional history due to waxing and waning consciousness. His blood pressure is 90/50 mm Hg with a heart rate of 130 beats per minute while supine. On physical examination, a large, pulsatile, mid-abdominal mass is detected.

    Which of the following is the correct immediate management of this patient?

    A. Assess for orthostatic blood pressure changes.
    B. Obtain STAT preliminary laboratory studies, including electrolytes, complete blood count, amylase, and lipase and admit for observation.
    C. Obtain a STAT plain radiograph of the abdomen to rule out a bowel perforation or obstruction.
    D. Obtain a STAT abdominal CT with contrast to evaluate for ruptured abdominal aortic aneurysm.
    E. Immediate notification of surgical service and transfer to the operating room for an emergency laparotomy.

35. A 22-year-old woman was arrested by police at a Broadway musical after suddenly screaming hysterically at the actors that there was a government plot to implant mind control devices into people's brains during the production and running onto the stage. The police investigation after the event revealed that the

woman's friends and coworkers had noticed slight behavioral changes a few weeks prior. The patient's family knew of no history of psychiatric disorders, and the patient was not on any psychiatric medications. A urine screen was negative for illicit drugs or alcohol. A preliminary medical exam was positive for the presence of resting and intention tremors, spasticity, and rigidity.

The etiology of this woman's symptoms was noted by which of the following physical findings of her eyes?

A. A ring of gold-brown pigment at the periphery of iris that is wider at the superior and inferior aspects than the medial and lateral aspects.

B. Redness of the conjunctiva of one eye; pressing the lower lid against the globe produces a bulge above the point of compression.

C. A raised, subconjunctival fatty structure growing in a horizontal band toward the pupil.

D. Dots visible in the cornea without signs of inflammation.

E. A gray band of opacity in the cornea 1.5 mm in width that is separated by a clear zone from the limbus.

36. A 28-year-old woman presents with soft, nonpainful, fleshy growths around her vulva and anus.

You should initiate treatment with

A. benzathine penicillin G.

B. a reminder to use condoms with every act of intercourse.

C. topical podophyllin or trichloracetic acid.

D. topical steroid.

E. surgery.

37. A 20-year-old man is giving his medical history to his new primary care physician. He is complaining of a week of fever, accompanied by cough, arthralgias, and mild, nonbloody diarrhea. He is not on any medication except for some acetaminophen for the fever. His review of systems is negative for hypertension, polyuria, polydipsia, fatigue, or weight changes. The patient does note, however, that when he was 8 years old, he had developed a 2-week-long period of fever.

During the physical, the patient's new primary care physician notes that the patient has a II/VI systolic ejection murmur heard best at the apex. The patient was not aware he had this condition. The physician also found that the patient has finger clubbing as well as swellings of the fingertips. These swellings are slightly tender to palpation.

A funduscopic exam would most likely reveal which of the following?

A. Elevated, edematous discs with blurred margins and tortuous engorged veins

B. Small hemorrhagic spots, each with a central white area

C. A normal-appearing disc with gray-folded elevations of the retina; over the elevations, the blood vessels appear tortuous whereas elsewhere they appear normal

D. The presence of extra, numerous, narrow, tortuous blood vessels superimposed over the normal vasculature

E. Grayish-white ovoid lesions with irregular, wool-like margins of varying sizes, some just slightly smaller than the size of the disc

38. An 18-year-old man presents to the emergency department with acute onset of testicular pain, nausea, and vomiting. He admits to multiple recent new sexual contacts. On examination, the testicle is extremely tender, swollen, and lying transversely in the scrotum. The cremasteric reflex is absent on the affected side. Doppler ultrasound to assess testicular blood flow is not immediately available. Which of the following is the proper course of action in this patient?

A. Discharge to home with a 7-day course of ciprofloxacin for epididymitis and ibuprofen for pain

B. Admit to the hospital with patient-controlled administration of IV narcotics and vigorous hydration

C. Immediate urological consultation for likely surgical decompression

D. Order CBC, electrolytes, and urinalysis prior to determining disposition of the patient

E. Order pelvic CT with contrast to evaluate for anatomic abnormalities of the kidneys or ureters

39. A 15-year-old girl comes to see you for a routine physical for school. At some point during the interview, she tells you that she is pregnant, has missed two periods, and tested positive on a home test kit. She asks that you not tell her parents. After the appointment, the girl's father, who is a long-time patient of yours, comes to your office to drive her home. He takes you aside and asks to speak to you in private. The father states that he is concerned that his daughter seems heavier than usual, has had some bouts of nausea with vomiting, and was wondering if she could be pregnant.
Which of the following would you do?

A. Because the patient is a minor, you are required to tell the father everything.

B. Because patient-doctor confidentiality can only be broken by order of a judge or in cases where someone's life is in immediate danger, you lie and tell him that his daughter could not possibly be pregnant.

C. Because not telling the father the truth would break the trust between physician and patient (here, the father), you tell the father that his daughter is pregnant but that he should not confront her with the knowledge.

D. You strike a balance between the need to maintain confidentiality with the daughter while upholding the trust between the father and yourself by stating that "even if she were, I couldn't tell you without her permission."

E. You tell the father that you want to call in a family counselor.

40. A 65-year-old nonsmoking man presents to the clinic complaining of itching and redness of his face and body. These symptoms worsen after taking a warm

shower. In addition, he has frequent headaches and occasional blurred vision. Physical examination reveals generalized plethora, engorged retinal veins, and splenomegaly. On peripheral blood smear, red cell morphology is normal, and many basophils are present. A CBC reveals the following.

hemoglobin:	22.2 g/dL
hematocrit:	64%
leukocytes:	12,000/µL
platelets:	221,000/µL

Of the following, which is the most likely diagnosis?

A. Chronic hepatic failure

B. Chronic renal failure

C. Idiopathic myelofibrosis

D. Essential thrombocythemia

E. Polycythemia vera

41. A 20-year-old man with no significant medical history presents to your office complaining of a headache. The headache is described as 9 out of 10 in intensity, occurs usually in the evening, lasts under 30 minutes, and seems to be localized around the patient's right eye. The patient also notes that some tearing and redness of the right eye occurs during these attacks. Drinking beforehand seems to worsen the symptoms. The patient denies any visual changes, history of allergic rhinitis, polyuria, polydipsia, weight change, or recent respiratory illness.

This patient most likely has which of the following?

A. Migraine

B. Cluster headache

C. Subarachnoid hemorrhage

D. Simple partial seizure

E. Hypoglycemic episode secondary to new onset diabetes

42. A 55-year-old man with a prior history of alcoholism presents to the emergency department complaining of new onset tremors. He claims that he has been alcohol abstinent for 10 years. A urine toxicology screen is negative for alcohol or illicit drugs. On physical exam, it is noted that the patient has tremors, difficulty with finger-to-nose tasks as well as fine motor functions, such as writing. In addition, the patient has spider angiomata and noted asterixis. A mental status exam is notable for a defect in short-term memory. The patient is afebrile, denies bowel or bladder incontinence, and his white blood cell count is normal.

Which of the following would be the next best test to order?

A. Serum ammonia level

B. Noncontrast head CT scan

C. EEG

D. Portable chest x-ray

E. EMG

43. A 75-year-old Caucasian woman presents to the emergency room after slipping on ice and falling onto her outstretched arms. She reports right wrist pain. Plain radiograph shows a distal radial (Colles') fracture (see figure 2-11). The patient weighs 105 pounds and is 5 feet tall. Her only medications are atenolol and hydrochlorothiazide for hypertension, which she has taken for many years. She is 25 years postmenopausal and has not taken hormone replacement therapy. She smoked 1 pack of cigarettes per day for 30 years but quit smoking 20 years ago.

    Which of the following patient attributes *decreases* her risk for osteoporosis?

    A. Caucasian race

    B. Postmenopausal status

    C. Thin build

    D. Hydrochlorothiazide use

    E. History of smoking

44. Your nurse fields a call from a parent of a 3-year-old patient, whose older sibling has been home from school with chicken pox. The parent wants to know if the younger child needs to stay home from day care.

    You ask the nurse to tell the parents

    A. there is no reason to keep the child out of day care.

    B. the patient may return to day care immediately but should be kept home while developing active lesions.

    C. the patient may return to day care after lesions start.

    D. the patient may return to day care after lesions crust over.

    E. the patient may return to day care after lesions clear.

45. A 64-year-old man presents with painless jaundice and recent depressed mood. Abdominal CT is shown below.

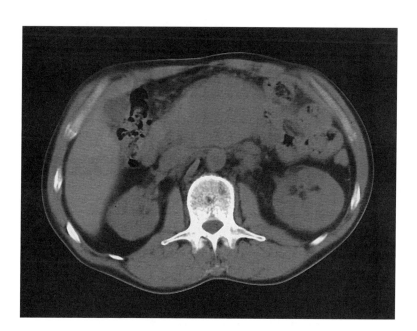

Which of the following is the most likely diagnosis?

A. Pancreatic adenocarcinoma

B. Pancreatic pseudocyst

C. Abdominal aortic aneurysm with compression of common bile duct

D. Splenic artery aneurysm with compression of common bile duct

E. Acute cholecystitis

46. An 11-year-old patient is in the clinic for a regular history and physical. He is concerned about how tall he will become and when puberty will start.
Which of the following will be the first indication of puberty?

A. Testicular enlargement

B. Pubic hair

C. Voice dropping

D. Growth spurt

E. Increased penile length

47. A new patient comes to your clinic for a routine cholesterol screening because his father had "some sort of heart disease." The patient notes that he has just had lunch 2 hours ago.
    Which of the initial screening tests listed below would you order?
    A. Total cholesterol and HDL
    B. LDL and triglycerides
    C. HDL and LDL
    D. Albumin and HDL
    E. VLDL and triglyceride

48. A 23-year-old male presents with a scaling rash on his elbows and knees. He also complains of dandruff that is not responsive to different treatment shampoos.
    Which of the following is(are) most likely involved as well?
    A. Palms and soles
    B. Fingernails
    C. Face
    D. Intertriginous areas
    E. Pulmonary (lungs)

49. A 75-year-old man with a 100-pack/year smoking history presents with 20 pound weight loss over the past 3 months, generalized weakness, and fatigue. He also reports occasional hemoptysis. A chest radiograph is obtained and shows hyperinflation consistent with emphysema but no focal abnormalities.
    In regards to further studies indicated for this patient, which of the following statements is correct?
    A. Absence of focal changes on chest radiograph essentially rules out the diagnosis of lung cancer.
    B. Routine screening of patients who smoke with chest radiography is effective in the early detection of lung cancer.
    C. High-resolution chest CT is indicated to further evaluate for malignancy.
    D. Head CT and full body CT are indicated to evaluate for malignancy.
    E. Screening for antibodies associated with paraneoplastic syndromes is indicated at this time.

50. A patient presents to your office one autumn afternoon inquiring if she should receive an influenza vaccine. Which of the following profiles would indicate giving the vaccine to your patient?
    A. She is 25 years old, with no medical problems who works in a publishing office.
    B. She is a 45-year-old federal judge with well-controlled hypertension.
    C. She is a 25-year-old medical student, with a documented allergy to chicken eggs.

D. She is a 66-year-old retired teacher who has emphysema.

E. She is 17 years old, with mild, intermittent asthma who is about to enter college.

51. A 4-year-old male, previously potty-trained, is just about ready to enter pre-K. He is now drinking a lot and has wet himself several times. When asked by his mom if everything is all right, he says he is being teased about having "bug eyes" by the other children at his new school.

Which of the following will most likely lead to the diagnosis of a histiocytosis X syndrome?

A. Splenomegaly

B. Hepatomegaly

C. Skull lesions

D. Hilar prominence

E. Sinus involvement

52. An 18-year-old woman is brought to the emergency room after ingesting a large number of unidentified pills. She complains of nausea, vomiting, and ringing in her ears. On physical examination, she is tachycardic, diaphoretic, and breathing rapidly and deeply. An arterial blood gas on room air reveals the following.

pH:	7.42
PO_2:	105 mm Hg
PCO_2:	24 mm Hg
HCO_3^-:	15 mg/dL

Serum electrolytes are as follows.

Na:	142 meq/L
K:	3.7 meq/L
Cl:	98 meq/L
HCO_3^-:	14 meq/L

Which of the following correctly interprets the clinical and laboratory data?

A. Metabolic alkalosis due to vomiting

B. Metabolic acidosis with respiratory compensation due to ingestion

C. Metabolic alkalosis with respiratory acidosis due to ingestion

D. Combined metabolic acidosis and respiratory alkalosis due to ingestion

E. Laboratory error because PO_2 cannot be greater than 100 mm Hg on room air

53. A 45-year-old woman with a history of Raynaud's syndrome and autoimmune thyroiditis presents to your clinic complaining of recent onset of itching and a slight

yellow tinge to her skin. She denies abdominal pain. Physical examination reveals slight jaundice but is otherwise unremarkable. Preliminary laboratory results are as follows.

AST (SGOT):	29 μ/L
ALT (SGPT):	25 μ/L
Alkaline phosphatase:	577 μ/L
Bilirubin (total):	2.2 mg/dL
Bilirubin (direct):	1.7 mg/dL
CBC:	normal

Which of the following tests should be ordered to evaluate this patient?

A. Infectious hepatitis serologies

B. Antimitochondrial antibodies and liver biopsy

C. Acetaminophen level

D. Direct Coombs' testing and serum haptoglobin

E. No further testing is indicated

54. A 65-year-old African American man has a history of benign prostatic hyperplasia and slow urinary stream. He develops increased frequency and dysuria. Urine microscopy shows 50–100 WBCs per high power field. Gram stain reveals gram negative rods. You administer a 3-day course of trimethoprim/sulfamethoxazole (Bactrim) to treat a urinary tract infection. However, 4 days later, the patient returns with fatigue. He notes a previous similar reaction to an antimalarial medication. Laboratory results are as follows.

Hemoglobin: 8.5 g/dL
Hematocrit: 25.5%
Haptoglobin (serum): 20 mg/dL (normal 50–220 mg/dL)

Which of the following diagnoses should be strongly considered?

A. Glucose-6-phosphate dehydrogenase deficiency

B. Sickle-cell anemia

C. Hereditary spherocytosis

D. Paroxysmal nocturnal hemoglobinuria

E. Folic acid deficiency

55. A 72-year-old man previously diagnosed as having emphysema and heart failure presents to the emergency room with increasing shortness of breath for the past 4 days. In addition, he notes increasing lower extremity swelling. On physical examination, the man is afebrile and his vital signs are within normal limits. Pulse oximetry reveals oxygen saturation of 86%. Lung examination is significant for accessory muscle use, prolonged expiratory phase, and scattered wheezes. In addition, he has jugular venous distension and 3+ pitting edema of the lower extremities. A

recent echocardiogram showed a left ventricular ejection fraction of 70%. His CXR shows hyperinflation without edema.

Which of the following treatments will offer the most immediate benefit for this patient?

A. Supplemental oxygen

B. Furosemide 40 mg IV × 1

C. Digoxin 1 mg p.o. × 1

D. Atenolol 25 mg p.o. × 1

E. Aspirin 325 mg p.o. × 1

56. A 28-year-old resident physician receives tuberculin skin testing as part of a routine health maintenance examination. He is generally healthy, HIV-negative, and has no known recent contacts with active tuberculosis. When read at 48 hours, the area of induration measures 6 mm. He has never received a BCG injection and prior tuberculin skin tests have not resulted in induration.

What is the diagnosis and course of action for this patient?

A. Negative tuberculin skin test; repeat in 1 to 2 years

B. Equivocal tuberculin skin test; obtain chest radiograph

C. Positive tuberculin skin test; obtain chest radiograph and treat with a 6-month course of isoniazid (INH)

D. Positive tuberculin skin test; treat for active tuberculosis with INH, ethambutol, pyrazinamide, and rifampin

E. Positive tuberculin skin test; treat only if symptoms develop

57. At a 20-week check of a 44-year-old G1P0, the patient reports that she is feeling basically fine but is still tired; she had expected that this feeling would have improved by the second trimester.

On physical examination, you note which one of the following, warranting a cardiology referral?

A. Diastolic murmur

B. S₃ gallop

C. Systolic ejection murmur

D. Increased S₂ split

E. Distended neck veins

58. A 25-year-old woman undergoes surgery to repair a torn anterior cruciate ligament. Her only medication is an oral contraceptive, which she continues to take during and after hospitalization. She has not been ambulatory since surgery. Her postoperative course is complicated by persistent fever of 38.1° to 39.2°C that began 4 days after surgery. In addition, she has reported two episodes of transient shortness of breath. She denies urinary symptoms. A chest radiograph and urinalysis are normal.

What is the appropriate next course of action?

A. Noncontrast chest CT to evaluate for atelectasis

B. Blood cultures to evaluate for bacteremia and initiation of broad-spectrum antibiotic therapy

C. Lower extremity ultrasound to evaluate for deep venous thrombosis ·

D. D-dimer level to evaluate for deep venous thrombosis

E. Repeat urinalysis to evaluate for urinary tract infection

59. A 42-year-old African American woman presents to the clinic with intermittent fever and cough. She does not smoke. Physical examination is unremarkable, with clear lungs to auscultation. The chest radiograph, shown below, reveals bilateral hilar adenopathy with eggshell calcification of lymph nodes. Levels of angiotensin converting enzyme (ACE) are elevated (see Figure 1-23).

Of the following, which is the most likely diagnosis?

A. Small cell lung cancer

B. Miliary tuberculosis

C. Left ventricular failure

D. Sarcoidosis

E. Extrinsic allergic alveolitis

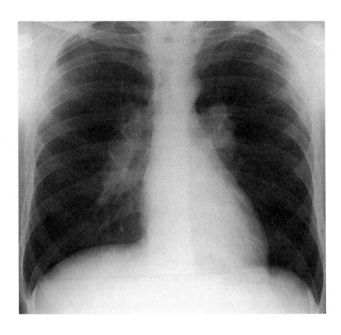

60. The mother of a 3-year-old patient calls because her child's temperature is 104°. He has no rash or other symptoms. The past medical history is significant only for recent adoption from Romania. The mother is concerned about preventing febrile seizures. Which of the following could you tell her?

   A. Give acetaminophen right away

   B. Give ibuprofen right away

   C. Give aspirin right away

   D. As long as the child is not drowsy after a seizure, he will be fine

   E. Febrile seizures occur as the temperature is rising, therefore, now that the temperature is already high, the child is not at as great a risk

61. An 85-year-old man with known coronary artery disease is admitted to the hospital because of hematemesis and hypotension. After fluid resuscitation with normal saline, upper endoscopy reveals an oozing gastric ulcer that is treated endoscopically. However, following endoscopy, the patient complains of left-sided chest pain, diaphoresis, and dyspnea. An EKG is obtained and is unchanged from admission, showing occasional premature ventricular complexes but no new ST-segment changes. The following additional laboratory values are obtained.

   Hemoglobin: 7.2 g/dL
   Hematocrit: 23.2%
   Cardiac troponin T: 0.65 µg/L (normal < 0.1 µg/L)

   Of the following interventions, which is indicated for this patient?

   A. Emergency administration of TPA (thrombolytic)

   B. Intravenous bolus of heparin followed by continuous heparin drip

   C. Emergency coronary artery bypass grafting

   D. Emergent transfusion of 4 units packed RBCs

   E. Lidocaine drip to prevent ventricular fibrillation

62. A 4-year-old female, new to your practice, comes for her first routine physical exam. You auscultate a continuous murmur. Further examination reveals the patient has a discrepancy on four extremity blood pressures, with lower levels in legs than arms. Before referring the patient to cardiology, you order a CXR and expect to find which of the following?

   A. Rib notching

   B. Egg-shaped heart

   C. Boot-shaped heart

   D. Hyperinflation

   E. Normal x-ray

63. A 42-year-old G5P5 presents at 36 weeks and complains of headache and leg swelling.

    On physical examination, you note a number of nonblanching patches on her legs and arms. You also note sock marks on her shins.

    Which of the following do you recommend?

    A. Referral to a shelter for abused women and their children

    B. Bed rest

    C. Avoidance of the sun

    D. Stricter discipline to ensure that the older children pick up their toys, so your patient won't fall so often

    E. Admission to the hospital for monitoring, labs, and likely delivery

64. The mother of a 6-week-old brings the baby in to your clinic for a chief complaint of constipation. The baby is formula-fed. The mother brings the baby in now because the child has seemed weak, less active, including feeding less actively, but has been drooling more. The patient has maintained normal urine output throughout.

    You advise this parent to

    A. learn about normal developmental stages.

    B. give the patient one-half a child-sized enema.

    C. return to the clinic if her baby worsens.

    D. send labs for urine organic acids

    E. take the patient to hospital to be admitted.

65. On a Friday before a long weekend, a G2P1 at 33 weeks returns early for a visit, complaining of sudden onset of shortness of breath, rapid heart rate, and chest pain. A normally calm woman, she is almost frenetic in your office. She also complains of leg swelling.

    On physical examination, you note the patient is anxious but has no active distress (NAD) with good skin color. Her lung fields are clear, without crackles or wheezes. Her abdomen is enlarged, consistent with her pregnancy. She has 2+ pitting edema in her legs, right > left.

    Which of the following applies in this situation?

    A. Recommend deep-breathing exercises

    B. Advise bed rest

    C. Tell the patient to increase her water consumption

    D. Offer reassurance

    E. Order a spiral CT

66. A 28-year-old female presents to your clinic. You note weight gain since her last visit. She brushes this off with a sheepish grin and apologizes for less exercise and poorer eating habits since starting a new job. She does complain of hirsutism and reports missing several periods. She had hoped this was because she was preg-

nant, but a urine β-hCG is negative. You run some labs and find she has increased testosterone and LH/FSH, and normal DHEA. You call her back to the office to explain that she needs

A. exercise and food-portion control.

B. hormonal contraceptives.

C. glucocorticoids.

D. mineralocorticoids.

E. exploratory surgery.

67. A 31-year-old patient comes in complaining of blistering on her skin. On physical exam, you realize that the pattern of distribution is consistent with areas of sun exposure. When you ask about sun exposure, the patient shows a picture of her at the beach with her family. You observe that all of the siblings are hirsute.
    Which of the following tests would most likely aid in the diagnosis?

A. Skin biopsy

B. Skin biopsy with immunofluorescence

C. Serum chromosomes

D. Wood's lamp of urine

E. Urine porphyrobilinogen

68. A 24-year-old female develops an acute bout of bloody diarrhea accompanied by a low-grade fever. She takes ciprofloxacin for several days and the diarrhea resolves. Within a few days after resolution, the patient begins to experience some weakness in her ankles, which makes it difficult to pick her feet up off the ground. Over the next several days the weakness spreads up her legs so that she cannot flex her hips. Two days later she develops the same weakness in her arms. She presents to the emergency room. The patient is profoundly weak in the lower extremities, and somewhat less weak in the upper extremities. She is areflexic in the lower extremities and hyporeflexic in the upper extremities. You perform a lumbar puncture and the CSF reveals: CSF WBC 2/μl, red cells 10/μl, protein 150 mg/dL, and glucose normal.
    Which of the following is the correct diagnosis?

A. Aseptic meningitis

B. Bacterial meningitis

C. Neurosyphilis

D. Guillain-Barré syndrome

E. Amyotrophic lateral sclerosis

69. A 34-year-old male with diffuse alveolar infiltrates on chest x-ray presents to the emergency room with severe hypoxia. Pulmonary function testing and arterial blood gas demonstrate the following: PCO_2 normal; large A-a difference; marked hypoxia, improving with oxygen administration; and decreased diffusion limited carbon monoxide (DLCO).

Which of the following is the cause of this patient's hypoxia?

A. Hypoventilation

B. Decreased FIO_2

C. Diffusion impairment

D. V/Q mismatch

E. Shunt

70. A 26-year-old medical student, born in Beverly Hills, California, attended private grade schools, a private high school, Harvard University as an undergraduate, and is now at an expensive, private medical school, receives a PPD test after a year of clinical clerkships. The patient currently lives in a penthouse apartment. He has no underlying illnesses and ran a triathlon last year.

How wide would the induration of his PPD response have to be at 48 hours for the test result to be considered positive?

A. 5 mm

B. 10 mm

C. 15 mm

D. 20 mm

E. It cannot be considered positive because the patient has no risks for TB

Answers

1. B

The key is the mention of the patient forgetting to take his lithium with him on this week-long conference. This fact, plus his haughtiness and grandiosity during the psychiatry interview, suggests mania as the cause.

A. A distractor, especially given the stereotype of all Vietnam veterans having posttraumatic stress disorder (PTSD). The reason this is not true in this patient is that he had never personally experienced or witnessed a traumatic event, such as coming under enemy fire or being held as a POW.

C. This is not correct because nothing suggests 6 months of excessive fatigue and worry prior to this event.

D. This is not correct; DSMIV criteria require at least four of each of the following: tachycardia/palpitations, sweating, trembling, shortness of breath, feeling of choking, chest pain, nausea, dizziness, derealization, fear of going crazy, fear of dying (definitely not true in this patient), paresthesia, and chills.

E. This might be suggested if the patient had disciplinary or legal infractions in the past; this patient had an honorable discharge and no criminal record.

2. D

Oral itraconazole and oral terbinafine given for several months are the most effective treatments for onychomycosis. Oral griseofulvin is less effective and is considered too toxic for routine use in this condition.

A. Topical terbinafine is effective for tinea pedis but, once infection is in the nail, topical agents show poor effectiveness.

B. Topical tolnaftate is also incorrect because topical agents are not effective for onychomycosis.

C. Topical econazole is incorrect for the same reasons given for answers A and B.

E. Oral griseofulvin, as mentioned in D, is too toxic for first-line use.

3. E

Tay-Sachs disease (GM2 gangliosidosis) is an autosomal recessive disorder due to the lack of the hexosaminidase alpha-subunit. This deficiency results in a lysosome storage defect in individuals who inherit two copies of the defective allele. Clinically, individuals who inherit two defective alleles are healthy at birth, but by age 6 months begin to show motor incoordination, muscular flaccidity, blindness, and dementia. All reach a vegetative state by age 3 and soon die. A characteristic cherry-red spot appears in the macula of afflicted children. In individuals of Ashkenazic descent, such as the parents of the above patient, the carrier rate is 1:30.

A. Cotton wool patches (soft exudates) are seen in hypertension, which is not present in this patient.

B. This describes the Roth spots of endocarditis.

C. The folded elevations of choice C describe a retinal detachment; the elevations being the detached portions of the retina.

D. This answer describes the effects of elevated intracranial pressure, which manifests in the fundus as papilledema

4. D

Cerebral metastases from unknown primaries are the most common cause of brain tumors in the elderly. In women, lung cancer and breast cancer are common causes of cerebral metastases.

A. Glioblastoma multiforme would not result in multiple discrete lesions.

B. Although primary CNS lymphoma may produce a similar appearance, with multiple enhancing lesions, it is far less common than metastatic disease.

C. Cerebrovascular accidents do not have this appearance of multiple discrete lesions.

E. Meningiomas may be multiple, discrete masses, but are located at the meninges rather than in the brain parenchyma.

5. C

The radiograph shows a scaphoid fracture, a potentially serious fracture because of the risk of avascular necrosis due to a single, distal blood supply. The correct treatment is thumb splint immobilization for 10 weeks. Orthopedic consultation is also indicated, since pin placement may reduce the risk of avascular necrosis.

A and B are incorrect because scaphoid fractures are often misdiagnosed as wrist sprains, but the radiograph clearly shows a scaphoid fracture.

D. Although pain control is necessary immobilization is important to promote adequate healing and prevent avascular necrosis.

E. The triquetrum is normal in this radiograph.

6. E

Pregnancy is actually the most likely cause of amenorrhea; it should always be the first consideration when a woman presents with a missing period.

This is a case of amenorrhea. The patient's amenorrhea should persist for 6 months since last menstruation to be classified as secondary amenorrhea. Primary amenorrhea is diagnosed when the patient has not menstruated by age 16 years.

A. Turner's syndrome would be a cause of primary amenorrhea.

B. Asherman's syndrome, wherein the uterine cavity gets scarred after a D&C, is the most common anatomical cause of secondary amenorrhea.

C. Tumors, anxiety, and anorexia are all additional causes of amenorrhea.

D. See C.

F. See C.

7. D

This patient has tertiary syphilis, a rarity in the United States today but still found in the developing world. Part of the spectrum of symptoms seen in advanced syphilis are the classic Argyll-Robertson pupils that do not react to light but do constrict when one asks the patient to track an object as it moves toward them. The pupils are usually, but not always, bilateral.

A. This may be caused by bilateral optic nerve lesions (or brain stem death, although obviously not applicable here).

B. This answer describes the Holmes-Adie pupil, which results from degeneration of ciliary ganglion cells (etiology unknown). Unlike the Argyll-Robertson pupil, this is usually unilateral.

C. This is a description of Horner's syndrome pupil, hinted at by the drooping eyelid. Whether the Horner's is due to a lesion above or below the superior cervical ganglion, the response to 4% cocaine is the same in that the affected pupil will not dilate. The use of an adrenaline eye drop solution can distinguish lesions above the ganglion (pupil will dilate in response to adrenaline) versus lesions below (no effect on the affected pupil).

E. This is typical for opiate overdose. Narcan will reverse the effect.

8. C

Renal artery stenosis should be strongly suspected when hypertension develops at an age younger than 30 or older than 50 years. A characteristic bruit or refractory hypertension makes the diagnosis more likely. In this patient, the most likely cause of renal artery stenosis is fibromuscular dysplasia. Atherosclerosis is the most common cause of renal artery stenosis in older patients. Hypokalemia due to hyperaldosteronism is often observed in renal artery stenosis.

A. Electrolyte abnormalities would not be expected in essential hypertension.

B. Aortic coarctation is an exceedingly rare cause of secondary hypertension in a person of this age.

D. Pheochromocytoma is a rare tumor that may cause secondary hypertension but is almost always accompanied by other symptoms (tachycardia, diaphoresis, anxiety, etc.)

E. Hyperthyroidism is usually accompanied by systemic symptoms such as weight loss, heat intolerance, and tachycardia.

9. B

A funduscopic exam to look for papilledema plus a head CT should be performed in cases of suspected meningitis *prior* to a lumbar puncture, to avoid the possible consequence of brain herniation if intracranial pressure is elevated. Antibiotics should be started as soon as possible.

A. This should not be done until ICP has been evaluated. Some texts state that LP may be done without a prior head CT if there are no neurological signs and funduscopic exam shows no papilledema but—at the very least—an ophthalmic exam must be done prior to a tap.

    C. This is an appropriate tertiary or quarternary test if one is considering *Mycobacterium* meningitis, but the test takes 48 hours to evaluate and is not appropriate in this setting.

    D. This answer is also inappropriate for the acute setting. Viral cultures can take weeks to months.

    E. An MRI is a slower exam than head CT and not considered a first-line scan before a CT.

10. B

In adult patients, the three most common causes of small bowel obstruction are, in order, peritoneal adhesions (due to past surgeries), incarcerated hernias, and neoplasm. In this patient without a history of abdominal surgery, incarcerated hernia becomes the most common cause. Physical examination should include a careful examination for hernias.

    A. This patient has no history of surgeries that would result in adhesions.

    C. Incarcerated hernias are more common than malignancies as a cause of small bowel obstruction.

    D. This patient would likely have a prior diagnosis of Crohn's disease, if present.

    E. Gallstone ileus is an extremely rare cause of small bowel obstruction.

11. D

The patient presents with trichomonal disease. One would expect to see the motile, flagellated organisms on a wet prep slide, with a vaginal pH > 6. The treatment of choice is metronidazole for the patient and her partner.

As much as we try to encourage a trusting and open relationship between teenaged patients and their physicians, a teenager should be offered treatment as though she were sexually active, even when she denies such activity.

    A. Fluconazole is the treatment of choice for Candida.

    B. It is not necessary to treat the partner of a patient with Candida.

    C. See D

    E. Some young women believe that douching will prevent STDs and yeast infections; this is not supported by the literature.

12. C

The CAGE questions are:

    1. Have you ever tried or felt the need to try to Cut down on your drinking?

    2. Have you been Annoyed by people asking you about your drinking?

    3. Have you ever felt Guilty about your drinking?

    4. Have you ever taken an Eye opener in the morning?

    Answering "yes" to at least one of the four suggests possible alcohol dependence and/or abuse and should lead to further inquiries. Answering yes to two questions gives an 80% sensitivity to the patient having an alcohol problem.

A, B, D, and E are not part of the CAGE questionnaire and are therefore incorrect.

13. E

A stroke must be ruled out. To evaluate for a potential intracranial bleed, a head CT, *without* contrast should be performed after a quick fingerstick to rule out hypoglycemia and a seizure history.

A. PET scans are used to evaluate brain activity centers and would not be appropriate in this emergent situation.

B. EEG would be used better for nonemergent evaluation of brain activity, especially in the case of seizures.

C. Head x-rays are no longer routinely performed because of the poor sensitivity and specificity of such a scan.

D. Carotid dopplers are best used for evaluating anterior blood flow going into the brain, not for intracranial flow itself.

14. A

This patient has bronze diabetes, or primary hemachromatosis, requiring early phlebotomy to improve patient survival. The classic triad indicating liver disease includes increased skin pigmentation, cirrhosis, and diabetes mellitus. Multiple bouts of vaginitis in a patient with acanthosis nigricans (skin darkening around the neck, flexor surfaces, and intertriginous areas) can be seen with diabetes.

B. Steroids are used for patients with dermatomyositis.

C. Hydroquinone cream can be used generically to lighten hyperpigmentation.

D. Sunlight can alleviate pityriasis rosea or psoriasis (for which one therapy is P-UVA).

E. Patients can get an orangey appearance with excessive consumption of beta-carotene-rich foods.

15. E

Chlorpromazine (brand name Thorazine) is considered a "low potency" neuroleptic (based on D_2 affinity) which, on the positive side, reduces the likelihood of Parkinsonian symptoms seen in the "high potentcy" neuroleptics but also increases the alpha-blocking effects, responsible for light-headedness and postural hypotension. Postural hypotension would *increase* the fall risk (and risk of hip fracture) in an elderly patient and should therefore be avoided in this patient population.

A. Haloperidol (Haldol) is considered to be a "high potency" neuroleptic and would be appropriate for sedating the above patient *without* increasing her risk of fall through postural hypotension.

B. Fluphenazine (Prolixin), is also considered to be a "high potency" neuroleptic and would be appropriate for sedating the above patient *without* increasing her risk of fall through postural hypotension.

C and D are not as good a choice as A or B because some orthostatic hypotension has been noted, but would still be better in the above patient than choice E.

16. A

These structures are known as the "unhappy triad" and are often injured during football games. High-impact force to the lateral knee stretches the structures that provide stability to the medial knee: the anterior cruciate ligament (ACL), medial collateral ligament (MCL), and medial meniscus. The anterior drawer sign indicates likely ACL injury and is present in this patient.

B. Posterior cruciate ligament is more often injured during bent-knee trauma such as motor vehicle accidents. The posterior drawer sign is present rather than the anterior drawer sign.

C. The lateral collateral ligament and lateral meniscus are unlikely to be damaged by trauma to the lateral knee. They are less often injured than the medial structures.

D and E are incorrect because damage to both collateral ligaments is rare during a single injury. The lateral collateral ligament is the least-injured knee ligament because it is under less tension than the medial collateral ligament.

17. D

Hypokalemia refractory to replacement is often due to hypomagnesemia, which promotes renal wasting of potassium. This is especially suspected in this patient with likely poor recent nutritional status due to small bowel obstruction. Replacement of magnesium is required in order for potassium replacement to be successful.

A. High levels of potassium through a central line can potentially lead to cardiac arrest.

B. This level of potassium replacement is excessive and would most likely damage the peripheral veins.

C. This is a reasonable long term therapy but would not be effective if magnesium is not replaced to normal levels.

E. This describes the correct management of hyperkalemia. Hypokalemia of this degree (K = 2.7 meq/L) does not put the patient at significant risk for arrhythmia, especially in the absence of digitalis therapy.

18. A

Asplenic patients are less effectively able to control infections from encapsulated organisms such as *Streptococcus pneumoniae*. The patient described would therefore be an appropriate recipient of the vaccine, even given his young age.

B. This patient is not at high-risk. The age cutoff is age 65+.

C. This is not a high-risk person, even though he works with patients.

D. Below the age cutoff, and the well-controlled hypertension is not a risk indication for the vaccine.

E. The colorful locale does not warrant administration of the vaccine.

19. E

The baby is showing stranger anxiety, which is a normal stage in development that starts between 6–12 months. This is the point when the child realizes who his or her primary caretakers are and shies away from others who are "new" (even relatively).

A. Has nothing to do with stranger anxiety.

B. In general, one would expect to see other manifestations of neglect, as well as less attachment to any figure or a general noncommittal response to any adult.

C. This behavior does not mean the child has been abused.

D. Colic, particularly in fussy babies, presents at about 3 weeks and lasts until about 3 months of age.

20. D

Imipramine is a TCA-class antidepressant. Agents in this class may cause fatal heart arrhythmias if taken in overdose.

A, B, and E are all SSRI, which are excellent first-line agents for depression.

C. Buproprion is a pure norepinephrine reuptake inhibitor. It may be used as a first-line agent except in patients with a seizure history.

21. E

This patient has symptoms and examination findings that are classic for aortic stenosis (AS). Digitalis may be effective for mild AS. Patients with severe AS require surgical valve replacement or, if unable to tolerate surgery, percutaneous balloon valvuloplasty. Echocardiography is useful to confirm the diagnosis of AS prior to referral to a cardiac surgeon.

A. This patient does not have evidence of endocarditis. In any case, blood cultures rather than echocardiography is the gold standard for the diagnosis of endocarditis.

B. Beta blockade is contraindicated in symptomatic aortic stenosis because it will likely increase symptoms by decreasing cardiac output.

C. Afterload reduction with an ACE-inhibitor will also exacerbate symptoms in aortic stenosis, as vasoconstriction is required to preserve adequate blood pressure.

D. This patient is too severely symptomatic for digitalis to result in any significant improvement.

22. C

Children with Down's syndrome are at an increased risk for leukemia.

A. One would expect a neutrophil predominance and elevated ESR with septic arthritis, as well as unilateral findings and a fever. The x-ray should show joint space widening.

B. Toxic synovitis would have a normal WBC and ESR.

D. Pauciarticular juvenile rheumatoid arthritis should not cause WBC elevation.

E. Fussiness would not elevate the WBCs.

23. E

Iron-deficiency anemia in adults must be assumed to result from occult gastrointestinal bleeding until proved otherwise. Colorectal cancer is an important cause of iron-deficiency anemia that should be ruled out in this patient by colonoscopy. Even if upper endoscopy reveals a possible source of bleeding, colonoscopy should also be performed to evaluate for iron-deficiency anemia. Since bleeding is likely to be intermittent, stool guaiac testing is insufficient to rule out colorectal cancer.

A and B are incorrect because iron replacement alone does not evaluate the cause of bleeding.

C. Bone marrow biopsy is unnecessary for the diagnosis of iron-deficiency anemia.

D. Abdominal CT is insensitive for the detection of colorectal cancer unless it has metastasized to the liver or outside the bowel lumen.

24. G

Rubella is one of the TORCH diseases. It is also a live vaccine, so it should not be given while the mother is pregnant or could be around other pregnant women. Thus, it is ideally given when the mother is leaving the hospital.

A. This is not an indication for a voluntary interruption of pregnancy.

25. B

This woman is experiencing normal grief because crying, weight changes, difficulty with concentration, insomnia, and social withdrawal are common to depression. These symptoms can also be associated with depression. This patient does not demonstrate any tendency toward suicide or homicidal ideation; neither does she admit visual nor auditory hallucinations. To distinguish between normal grief and depression, patients in depression tend to push away social contacts. Temporally, symptoms of grief are considered normal for up to 1 year.

A. Would be correct if this woman's symptoms continued well into the following year, especially if she had continuous suicidal thoughts or actively cut her social contacts.

C. DSM-IV requires that normal bereavement must first be excluded.

D. To be correct, there would have to be loss of reality testing, such as the presence of hallucinations or delusions, neither of which are present in this patient.

E. There would have to have been an actual experience of a traumatic event. This patient was not present at her mother's death.

26. B

BCG is not used in the United States. The only benefit of BCG is a reduction in the severity of tuberculosis in children who received it. BCG does not prevent TB.

A positive PPD, especially in someone who received it more than 5 years ago, should warrant a chest film to rule out active disease.

A. The benefits of BCG in ameliorating the symptoms of TB decline within 5 years.

C. The PPD will revert to negative after a few years.

D. The induration should not be that significant even in someone who received several doses.

E. BCG may produce an increase in induration if just a few years after administration.

27. E

Adrenal crisis is the most likely diagnosis in this patient with a history of rheumatoid arthritis likely treated with corticosteroids. Hypotension and mental status changes that do not respond to fluid challenge are the hallmark of this disease. Hyperkalemia may also be present. Immediate IV steroid administration is essential. Serum cortisol can confirm the diagnosis.

A. Fluids alone will not improve blood pressure in patients with adrenal insufficiency. These must be administered in conjunction with corticosteroids.

B. Whereas sepsis is a consideration, adrenal crisis is a more likely explanation for hypotension in this patient whose history probably included chronic corticosteroid use.

C. Signs and symptoms that indicate congestive heart failure are not present.

D. There is no reason to suspect abscess unless hypotension persists after adrenal insufficiency is treated.

28. A

This is likely a case of eczema or contact dermatitis. Either way, one does not want to write a prescription for a steroid cream stronger than hydrocortisone 1% for use on the face, due to the skin thinning tendencies (and resultant telangiectasias) of stronger steroids.

B. Hydrocortisone 2.5% is a Group VII steroid but obviously too strong.

C. Triamcinolone 0.025% is a Group VI steroid.

D. Triamcinolone 0.1% is a Group VI steroid but obviously too strong.

E. Betamethasone 0.1% is a Group V steroid.

29. A

Visual field loss in glaucoma is insidious because the patients often do not notice the loss of the peripheral visual field until late in the course of the disease.

B. This describes a central scotoma. This may occur if there is an occipital lesion corresponding to the central portion of the visual field, or if there is compression of the nerve bundles to both eyes, as the nerves corresponding to central vision are most vulnerable to extrinsic compression. Optic neuritis will also classically cause a central scotoma.

C. This explains a lesion of one optic nerve.

D. This is the classical presentation of a lesion of the optic chiasma, such as from a pituitary tumor.

E. This is due to a lesion of the left temporal lobe, where the optic radiations corresponding to the right upper quadrant visual field travel.

30. A

Epiglottis, caused by *Hemophilus influenzae* type b, has been far less common since the introduction of the Hib vaccine. Not all immigrant children, especially prior to entry into the school system, have had this vaccine. The "thumbprint sign" of the thickened epiglottis is diagnostic. The physicians may need to intubate, but if so, it should be done in the emergency room or operating room, so this patient does not need emergency breathing options.

B. Flu vaccine would be beneficial but not required; this is not linked to throat findings.

C. One can see the "steeple sign" on CXRs of patients with RSV.

D. Pneumococcus does not usually have this picture.

E. Children with foreign body aspiration have hyperinflated lungs on chest x-ray.

31. B

Asymptomatic gallstones are common and the vast majority of patients with them will not develop pain or other symptoms. However, there is a 2% to 3% yearly risk and 20% lifetime risk of developing biliary colic. There is no reason for surgical intervention unless symptoms arise.

A and C are incorrect because the *lifetime* risk of biliary colic is approximately 20%.

D and E are incorrect because surgical intervention is not indicated unless symptoms arise.

32. A

A transient ischemic attack (TIA) is a neurological deficit due to a cerebral circulation defect. Unlike a stroke, however, in a TIA the symptoms resolve in 24 hours.

B. The time duration was only 12 hours.

C. A simple partial seizure is certainly on the differential of strokelike symptoms; the postictal state following a seizure may sometimes result in Todd's paralysis.

D. Hypoglycemia can produce strokelike symptoms. However, if hypoglycemia had produced these symptoms, the administration of a dextrose solution would have reversed the symptoms in less than the 12 hours described.

E. Migraines can result in visual disturbances and dysarthria, but complete hemiparesis is uncommon.

33. D

Chronic lymphocytic leukemia (CLL) is indolent and is not curable by chemotherapy. Most patients with this disease do not require immediate treatment; treatment should be deferred until patients develop significant symptoms.

A. Chemotherapy is not curative in CLL.

B. Bone marrow transplantation is not curative and is very risky in older patients.

C. This describes infectious mononucleosis, a disease characterized by large, atypical lymphocytes on peripheral smear. CLL is not infectious and does not resolve spontaneously.

E. The life expectancy in newly diagnosed CLL is usually 2 to 10 years, depending on stage at diagnosis.

34. E

This patient has signs and symptoms that are highly suggestive of ruptured abdominal aortic aneurysm (AAA). In hemodynamically unstable patients with symptoms suggestive of ruptured AAA, immediate surgical intervention is essential and should not be delayed for radiologic evaluation.

A. This patient is clearly hypotensive at rest and orthostatic changes would certainly be present.

B, C, and D are incorrect because the correct management is immediate surgical intervention for likely ruptured AAA. Surgery should not be delayed for radiologic studies. In hemodynamically stable patients, immediate CT is occasionally obtained in consultation with the surgical service in order to plan emergent AAA repair. However, this patient is clearly hemodynamically unstable and surgery should not be delayed.

35. A

This woman has the psychiatric and neurologic manifestations of Wilson's disease. Her eye exam is notable for golden-brown rings known as Kayser-Fleischer rings.

B. This response describes chemosis, edema of the conjunctiva that is shown as a bulge when one uses the lower lid to press against it.

C. This answer describes a pterygium, an inflammatory structure forming secondary to chronic eye irritation, such as from wind and dust.

D. Visible dots in the cornea are found in Fanconi syndrome, which results in cystine deposits in the cornea without an inflammatory component.

E. This response describes arcus senilis, a normal finding in the elderly.

36. C

This is a case of human papillomavirus (HPV). Topical podophyllin or trichloroacetic acid is the initial treatment of choice. Refractory cases may require cryosurgery or excision. HPV 6 and 11 more commonly are associated with anorectal and genital warts; HPV 16 and 18 more commonly are associated with cervical cancer.

A. Benzathine penicillin G is for the treatment of syphilis, which can present with painless ulcers.

B. Health professionals always recommend condoms as a form of barrier protection, but they may not cover enough of the anatomy to prevent the transmission of HPV.

D. These growths may be mistaken for hemorrhoids, for which topical steroids can be prescribed.

E. Only refractory cases may require cryosurgery or excision.

37. B

The patient has bacterial endocarditis with a previous history of what sounds like rheumatic fever. Funduscopic findings that are present in a quarter of these patients are the classic Roth spots described in choice B.

A. Papilledema, which is associated with increased intracranial pressure, is described. There is no indication that this patient has high ICP.

C. The folded elevations describe a retinal detachment; the elevations being the detached portions of the retina.

D. This describes the hyperproliferative appearance of diabetic retinopathy. Given that the patient is on no diabetic medications and denies polydipsia, polyuria, fatigue, or weight loss, this is unlikely.

E. This choice describes cotton wool patches (soft exudates) seen in hypertension, which is not present in this patient.

38. C

Testicular torsion should be strongly considered in this patient and is therefore a surgical emergency. Doppler ultrasound will allow assessment of testicular artery flow, but surgical consultation and likely intervention should not be delayed. Delay of more than several hours in surgical decompression of testicular compression will result in infarction and require removal of the testicle.

A. This choice describes the treatment of epididymitis, which may mimic testicular torsion. However, epididymitis cannot be presumed without first ruling out testicular torsion.

B. This response describes the early treatment of nephrolithiasis, which is not appropriate in this patient.

D. Testicular torsion is a surgical emergency and definitive treatment should not be delayed by testing.

E. A CT will not provide additional information concerning testicular torsion.

39. D

Factors to balance here are (a) confidentiality to the daughter or (b) maintaining therapeutic trust between doctor and father. Choice D provides the best balance between these two conflicting needs.

A. This is not required by law (though some states require parental consent for a minor who wishes an abortion).

B. While technically true, this does not maintain the trust between the doctor and the father.

C. This response violates the confidentiality of the patient.

E. This does not uphold trust with the father and serves no purpose except to pressure the daughter to reveal her pregnancy.

40. E

Polycythemia vera is characterized by symptoms related to increased blood viscosity: headache, fatigue, and blurred vision. Pruritis classically occurs during showers and results from histamine release due to increased basophilia. Plethora, splenomegaly, and a high hematocrit with normal morphology are also present in polycythemia vera.

A. Hepatic failure may result in pruritis, but would not be expected to result in the other findings.

B. Chronic renal failure would result in a decreased hemoglobin and hematocrit.

C. Idiopathic myelofibrosis results in a decreased hemoglobin and abnormal morphology. Red cells are described as "teardrop cells."

D. An elevated platelet count is not present in this patient; therefore, this response is incorrect.

41. B

A unilateral, periorbital headache in a 20-year-old man is a classic presentation for a cluster headache.

A. Migraine typically involves a entire hemicranium and, in the classic form, involves visual field cuts (scotomas) accompanied by visual phenomenon such as scintillating lights.

C. Subarachnoid hemorrhage presents as the "worst headache of my life." Causative mechanisms include head trauma, ruptured aneurysm, and AVM. Subarachnoid hemorrhage would not be expected to occur every evening.

D. A simple partial seizure would be expected to have some motor activity, which is not present in this patient's presentation.

E. Hypoglycemia can produce headache; however, the lack of history, polydipsia, or polyuria rule this out.

42. A

This is a man with likely hepatic encephalopathy as indicated by the history and physical. The presence of asterixis helps to distinguish a metabolic disturbance versus a neurological disturbance. The main use for an ammonia level here is to follow its downward course with therapy rather than for diagnostic purposes.

B. A CT scan would be best for diagnosing a hemorrhagic stroke.

C. EEGs are better used for diagnosing seizures.

D. A portable chest x-ray might be able to diagnose pulmonary disease with secondary sequelae of mental status changes, but would not explain the tremors or asterixis.

E. An EMG would be indicated if the patient had noted muscular weakness.

43. D

Thiazide-type diuretics decrease renal excretion of calcium. The other choices are well-known risk factors for osteoporosis.

A. Caucasians and Asians are at increased risk for osteoporosis when compared to African Americans.

B. Postmenopausal status is a major risk factor for osteoporosis.

C. A thin build predisposes to osteoporosis, while obesity is protective against osteoporosis.

E. Smoking is strongly associated with osteoporosis.

44. D

Patients with chickenpox (Varicella-Zoster virus) are contagious until the lesions crust over. Parents may choose to expose their child to a contagious child, but the contagious child should not expose the other children in day care unless asked. Ideally, this parent would not bring this child into the office because your entire practice would be exposed.

A, B, C, and E are all incorrect because they all have the child returning to class before the lesions have crusted over.

45. A

Painless jaundice and depressed mood in the elderly is suggestive of pancreatic cancer. The CT shows a large, ill-defined mass in the body of the pancreas consistent with pancreatic adenocarcinoma. Jaundice is explained by blockage of biliary drainage.

B. The mass is poorly defined and of tissue density. Pancreatic pseudocyst results in a well-defined, low-density mass.

C. This mass is located in the pancreas and is not contiguous with the aorta.

D. This is clearly a mass composed of tissue rather than blood vessels.

E. The gall bladder is visualized in this view and appears normal.

46. A

You can advise your patient to first expect testicular enlargement (average age 11.5 years), then an increased penile length, then pubic hair, then his growth spurt (approximately 2 years after testicular enlargement).

B. This response is not the first sign of puberty.

C. When and how much a boy's voice will change is individualized.

D and E are both incorrect; they are not the first sign of puberty.

47. A

Total cholesterol and HDL are affected the least by recent consumption and can be used as screening tests in this setting.

B. Both LDL and triglyceride levels can be grossly affected by recent eating.

C. LDL tests require fasting.

D. Albumin levels are not part of the cholesterol screening panel.

E. Both components are best interpreted if the patient is fasting.

48. B

This patient has psoriasis, which commonly presents on extensor surfaces and fingernail pitting. It can cause arthritis and is distinguished by the Auspitz sign and the Koebner phenomenon. Patients with psoriasis are treated with P-UVA or immunosuppressants.

Do not confuse psoriasis with sarcoidosis, which is primarily a pulmonary disease, but can affect virtually any body system, and can have a variety of rashes, including erythema nodosum

A. Causes for a number of rashes present on palms and soles, include Rocky Mountain Spotted Fever, Kawasaki's, and other diseases.

C. In infants, "cradle cap" (seborrheic dermatitis) can spread to the face.

D. Intertriginal areas are affected by scabies, *Candida*, or tinea.

E. Eczema is linked to asthma (the atopic patient).

49. C

The suspicion for malignancy should be very high in this patient with extensive weight loss and smoking history. Chest CT is reasonable when the suspicion of lung cancer is very high.

A. Chest radiograph is not highly sensitive in the detection of lung cancer.

B. Routine screening of patients who smoke with chest radiography has not been shown to be effective in the early detection of lung cancer and does not improve outcomes or prognosis.

D. Full-body CT is unnecessary in this patient until lung cancer is ruled out with chest CT.

E. These antibody tests are expensive and not indicated at this time.

50. D

Criteria for receiving influenza vaccine include age greater than 50 years, presence of heart disease/lung disease, and those who work in high risk environments such as health care workers. This patient fulfills both the age cutoff as well as the pulmonary disease criteria.

A. This response fulfills none of the criteria.

B. This patient is considered too young, and her controlled hypertension would not put her at risk.

C. This patient would qualify *if not for her allergy*; the vaccine is made in eggs and is contraindicated in those with a chicken egg allergy.

E. Well-controlled minor asthma would not call for a vaccine.

51. C

Hand-Schuller-Christian, the more chronic-progressive of the histiocytosis X syndromes, has the classic triad of exophthalmos, skull findings, and diabetes insipidus.

A. One can see splenomegaly with a variety of conditions, including sickle-cell disease.

B. One can see hepatomegaly with Letterer-Siwe disease (usually fatal in infants).

D. One can see hilar prominence with a variety of diseases, including tuberculosis.

E. Sinus involvement is not associated with histiocytosis.

52. D

The patient's symptoms of nausea, vomiting, and tinnitus are consistent with salicylate overdose. The patient is clearly hyperventilating and is alkalemic due to respiratory alkalosis. In addition, an anion gap metabolic acidosis is present. The anion gap is calculated by the formula $[Na] - [Cl] - [HCO_3^-] = 30$ (8–12 is normal). A combined respiratory alkalosis and metabolic acidosis with increased anion gap are classic findings in salicylate overdose.

A and C. A metabolic acidosis (low bicarbonate level) and respiratory alkalosis (low CO_2) are clearly present.

B. Respiratory compensation for a primary metabolic acidosis would not "overcorrect" the pH to greater than 7.4.

E. A young, healthy person who is hyperventilating can have a PO_2 greater than 100 mm Hg.

53. B

This patient may have primary biliary cirrhosis (PBC), an autoimmune disease characterized by cholestasis due to destruction of the intrahepatic bile ducts. PBC is associated with Raynaud's syndrome, scleroderma, Sjögren's syndrome and autoimmune thyroiditis. It typically presents in middle-aged women with elevated alkaline phosphatase in its early stages and elevated bilirubin and jaundice in later stages. It is diagnosed by antimitochondrial antibodies and confirmed by liver biopsy.

A. Liver transaminases (AST, ALT) are normal in this patient and would be markedly elevated in acute viral hepatitis.

C. Significant hepatocellular damage due to acetaminophen would result in elevated liver transaminases, not present in this patient.

D. Hemolysis is not responsible for this hyperbilirubinemia, which is primarily direct (conjugated).

E. Any patient with jaundice needs a complete work-up to determine the etiology.

54. A

This patient has hemolytic anemia that appears to coincide with administration of medications with oxidative properties. Glucose-6-phosphate dehydrogenase (G6PD) deficiency is an X-linked, recessive enzyme deficiency often observed in African American men. It results in hemolytic anemia with administration of certain drugs, including antimalarials (primaquine, quinine), sulfonamides, and nitrofurantoin. In patients with G6PD deficiency, red blood cells are unable to generate reduced glutathione, which protects hemoglobin from oxidative denaturation.

B. Sickle-cell anemia would certainly be a previously discovered disease in a 65-year-old man and would not result in hemolysis only with medication administration.

C. Hereditary spherocytosis results in a chronic hemolytic anemia not associated with medications.

D. Paroxysmal nocturnal hemoglobinuria is an acquired stem cell disorder that predisposes red blood cells to lysis by complement. It is not associated with medications.

E. Folic acid deficiency results in macrocytic anemia rather than hemolysis.

55. A

This patient has right heart failure due to lung disease, a condition known as cor pulmonale. The physical examination and chest radiograph do not provide evidence of pulmonary edema due to left heart failure. Symptoms of right heart failure should respond to appropriate treatment of emphysema with supplemental oxygen, bronchodilators, and steroids. Supplemental oxygen will decrease pulmonary artery pressure, resulting in improved blood flow through the pulmonary circulation.

B. Although there may be a secondary role for diuretics in reducing fluid overload in right heart failure, this will not result in immediate improvement.

C. Digoxin is not indicated for right heart failure except in the presence of atrial fibrillation.

D. Beta blockers may exacerbate bronchoconstriction and pulmonary hypertension in this patient.

E. Aspirin will not benefit this patient with COPD and right heart failure.

56. A

Criteria for a positive tuberculin skin testing are as follows:

Low-risk patients (not normally tested):	>15 mm
High-risk patients (health care workers):	>10 mm
Very high-risk patients (HIV, close contact):	>5 mm

This patient/physician does not have HIV or a close contact with active TB; induration of 10 mm or greater is required for tuberculin skin test conversion.

B. Chest radiography is required for patients with skin test conversion to evaluate for active disease.

C. Isoniazid is only required for positive PPD.

D. Multidrug therapy is only required for active tuberculosis.

E. This patient's test is not positive. In any case, new skin test conversions are treated with isoniazid prophylaxis, not just if symptoms develop.

57. A
Diastolic murmurs are not normal findings in pregnancy.

B. Because of an increase in flow and the many changes associated with pregnancy, S_3 gallop can be a normal finding in a pregnant patient.

C. Because of an increase in flow and the many changes associated with pregnancy, systolic ejection murmur can be a normal finding in a pregnant patient.

D. Because of an increase in flow and the many changes associated with pregnancy, increased S_2 split can be a normal finding in a pregnant patient.

E. Because of an increase in flow and the many changes associated with pregnancy, distended neck veins can be a normal finding in a pregnant patient.

58. C
Causes for postoperative fever include atelectasis, urinary tract infection, wound infection, deep venous thrombosis, and drug fever. In this patient who takes oral contraceptive pills and has not been ambulating, deep venous thrombosis with pulmonary embolism should be strongly considered. Lower extremity ultrasound is the test of choice to confirm the diagnosis. V/Q scan or fine cut spiral CT can then be ordered if lower extremity doppler results are suspicious or positive.

A. In the presence of a normal chest x-ray, noncontrast chest CT will likely provide minimal additional information.

B. Blood cultures may be obtained, but initiation of broad-spectrum antibiotics is not indicated at this time because no source of infection has been identified.

D. D-dimer levels have very low specificity for deep venous thrombosis, especially in postoperative patients.

E. Repeating urinalysis is unlikely to provide additional information in this patient without urinary symptoms.

59. D
Sarcoidosis is a systemic disease characterized by granulomatous inflammation of multiple organs. The etiology is unknown. Radiographic findings often include bilateral hilar adenopathy and eggshell calcification of lymph nodes. Biopsy is required for definitive diagnosis. Elevated serum ACE levels are observed in a majority of patients with active sarcoidosis.

A. Small cell lung cancer typically presents with unilateral adenopathy and is very uncommon in nonsmokers.

B. Miliary tuberculosis results in multiple, small lung densities on chest radiograph rather than hilar adenopathy.

C. Radiograph shows no evidence of pulmonary edema.

E. Like miliary tuberculosis, extrinsic allergic alveolitis normally results in multiple, small lung densities on chest radiograph.

60. E

The explanation of why this answer is correct is stated in choice E: the child is not at risk.

A. Acetaminophen is a fine adjuvant and may make the child more comfortable, but it does not prevent febrile seizures.

B. Answer A is also true for ibuprofen.

C. Aspirin should only be given under doctor's orders (as in the case of Kawasaki's syndrome).

D. Many children are drowsy after a seizure; this has no known prognostic value.

61. D

This patient is having a myocardial infarction, as indicated by typical signs and symptoms and positive cardiac enzymes. EKG changes are not necessary for the diagnosis of myocardial infarction. In this case, anemia is resulting in decreased oxygen supply to the myocardium and must be immediately corrected. Blood transfusions should be given with a goal of maintaining hemoglobin greater than 10.0 g/dL in patients with coronary artery disease. If blood pressure permits, beta blockade will decrease oxygen demand, and should also be initiated.

A. Thrombolytics are strictly contraindicated in this patient with recent gastrointestinal bleeding.

B. Heparin is of no proven benefit unless TPA is used to lyse a clot and is *not* a good choice in a patient with recent bleeding.

C. Coronary artery bypass grafting is not indicated acutely and could not be performed until after coronary angiography.

E. Lidocaine drips are not beneficial in reducing the incidence of ventricular fibrillation in patients with ectopy.

62. A

This is likely a case of coarctation of the aorta, which has a continuous murmur that often does not present at birth. Key to the diagnosis is the murmur and 4-extremity blood pressure.

B. An egg-shaped heart is seen in patients with transposition of the great vessels (which would have presented earlier in life).

C. A boot-shaped heart is seen in patients with tetralogy of Fallot.

D. Hyperinflation is seen in patients with asthma or foreign body aspiration.

E. A chest x-ray may be normal in one of these patients, but one would more likely expect to see the classic picture of "rib-notching."

63. E

First, remember the key dermatology definitions: macule = flat, <1 cm; patch = flat, >1 cm; papule = raised, <1 cm; plaque = raised, >1 cm.

Although it is possible this mother has been tripping over toys, leading to bruises, or the sock lines are indicative of regular leg swelling seen in pregnancy, one cannot afford to overlook a complication of severe pregnancy-induced hypertension (PIH): the HELLP syndrome (hemolysis, elevated liver enzymes, and low platelets). PIH progresses to this syndrome in 5% to 10% of pregnancies (more commonly in older, multiparous patients). The only cure is delivery, with supportive care as needed.

A. While abuse certainly is something one does not want to miss, having the patient admitted can afford precious time to further investigate the social setting if the medical work-up is negative.

B. Bed rest will not alleviate the problems this patient presented with.

C. This condition has nothing to do with sunburn.

D. While it certainly would benefit this patient to have her children become helpful, this will not address her medical situation.

64. E

Children do vary in activity level and food consumption as they go through stages, but the combination of this with constipation is concerning.

This patient could well have infantile botulism. The parent probably followed folklore, giving the constipated child Karo syrup or honey. These food additives have been linked to infantile botulism in patients under age 1. Infantile botulism can lead to acute, flaccid paralysis; because the patient may need to be intubated for respiratory support, the baby should be monitored in a hospital.

A. Drooling is a developmental step, but there are more symptoms to note here that should cause a higher index of suspicion.

B. Although constipation causes discomfort, there are more symptoms to note here that should cause a higher index of suspicion.

C. He should return to the clinic if he were to develop these symptoms at home. He is already in your clinic so choice E is better. Always be extra cautious in such a young infant, especially given the change in mental status.

D. One would send for urine organic acids if one was concerned for a metabolic disorder; this is not the case in this patient.

65. E

Pregnancy is a hypercoagulable state, therefore this patient is at increased risk for a pulmonary embolism (PE). (The degree of your patient's agitation is also consistent with a PE.) Only after the spiral CT is cleared can you employ facets of the other answer choices. In pregnant women, 80% of DVTs occur postpartum.

A. While deep-breathing exercises can be helpful for general stress, one cannot afford to discount these severe symptoms.

B. Prolonged bedrest will only exacerbate hypercoagulable state.

C. While most people should increase their water consumption, that would neither cause edema nor "flush it out."

D. It is true that all pregnant women experience some shortness of breath related to the decrease in functional residual capacity by almost 20%. But these symptoms are much more severe.

66. A

This patient is suffering from polycystic ovarian syndrome (PCOS), the most common cause of androgen excess and hirsutism. For a patient who hopes to become pregnant, weight loss is the first step in improving the androgen excess and its associated effects. One expects the LH:FSH ratio to be about 3:1.

B. In patients who do not desire to become pregnant, hormonal contraceptives can help interrupt the feedback cycle, leading to decreased LH production.

C. Glucocorticoids are used for congenital adrenal hyperplasia, in which case the DHEA would have been elevated.

D. Mineralocorticoids have no role in this patient.

E. Surgery would be indicated if a tumor, such as a Sertoli-Leydig cell tumor (causing testosterone secretion but decreased LH/FSH) was present.

67. D

This patient has porphyria cutanea tarda, characterized by blistering, increased hair on temples and cheeks, and no abdominal pain. The disease is transmitted via an autosomal dominant pattern, thus the similarity in her siblings. The urine of these patients fluoresces an orange-pink color under the Wood's lamp due to increased uroporphyrins.

A. Often the gold standard for diagnosis in dermatology, a skin biopsy would not be helpful in this case.

B. Pemphigus vulgaris has immunofluorescence surrounding epidermal cells, showing a "tombstone" pattern; immunofluoresence in bullous pemphigoid shows a linear band around the basement membrane, with increased eosinophils in the dermis. Therefore, a skin biopsy with immunofluorescence would not be helpful.

C. While some dermatological conditions have known chromosomal abnormalities, diagnosis usually is obtained clinically or through biopsy and only confirmed by chromosomal analysis.

E. Urine porphyrobilinogen is the test for acute intermittent porphyria, which is associated with abdominal pain.

68. D

This is the classic presentation of Guillain-Barré syndrome. There is typically an antecedent gastrointestinal or upper respiratory illness, followed by steadily progressive ascending paralysis with loss of reflexes. The classic CSF finding is "cyto-albumino dissociation," which basically means high protein with few white blood cells.

A and B responses are both incorrect because meningitis typically presents with headache, photophobia, neck pain, and neck stiffness.

C. The ascending pattern of paresis and its rapid progression are not consistent with Tabes Dorsalis of neurosyphilis.

E. Amyotrophic lateral sclerosis is a chronic degenerative disease, and would not progress this quickly. It typically causes weakness with muscle fasciculations, and often hyperreflexia.

69. C

This is a very unusual patient, with a marked impairment of gas diffusion across his alveoli (in this case likely due to pulmonary alveolar proteinosis, a rare disease).

A. Hypoventilation is ruled out by normal PCO_2. PCO_2 changes inversely and linearly with ventilation, so hypoventilation *always* causes CO_2 retention and vice versa.

B. Patients inspiring low FIO_2 (when are you ever going to see this clinically?) do not have increased A-a differences.

D. V/Q mismatch and diffusion impairment can only be distinguished by pulmonary function testing, and specifically measuring DLCO. In your career, you will see many, many more patients with V/Q mismatch than diffusion impairment.

E. Hypoxia from shunts does not improve much with administration of exogenous oxygen.

70. B

According to published 2000 guidelines, all patients at increased risk for TB exposure should have PPDs read as positive at 10 mm. This includes health care workers, like medical students, regardless of other risk factors. Also, patients with immunocompromised states, such as cancer, diabetes, chronic renal failure, homeless patients, and patients from endemic areas are also positive at 10 mm. HIV patients, patients with evidence of old TB on chest x-ray, and known exposures of patients with active TB have positive PPDs at 5 mm.

A, C, and D are incorrect because they measure either under or over the guideline.

E. Medical students are at risk.

Index

Note: Page numbers followed by *f* indicate figures; those followed by *t* indicate tables.

Lymphogranuloma Venereum